Eicosanoids in the Cardiovascular and Renal Systems

ADVANCES IN EICOSANOID RESEARCH

Series Editor Keith Hillier

Eicosanoids and Reproduction
Edited by Keith Hillier

Eicosanoids in the Gastrointestinal Tract
Edited by Keith Hillier

Eicosanoids in Inflammatory Conditions of the Lung, Skin and Joints
Edited by Martin Church and Clive Robinson

Eicosanoids in the Cardiovascular and Renal Systems
Edited by Perry Halushka and Dale Mais

ADVANCES IN EICOSANOID RESEARCH

Series Editor Keith Hillier

Eicosanoids in the Cardiovascular and Renal Systems

Edited by

P. V. Halushka

Professor of Pharmacology and Medicine
Burroughs Wellcome Scholar in
Clinical Pharmacology

and

D. E. Mais

Assistant Professor of Pharmacology

Department of Pharmacology
Medical University of South Carolina
USA

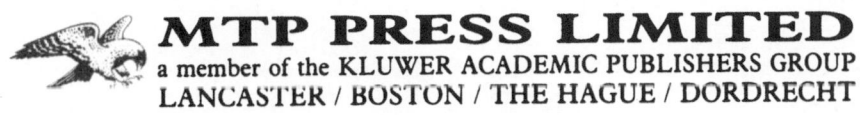

MTP PRESS LIMITED
a member of the KLUWER ACADEMIC PUBLISHERS GROUP
LANCASTER / BOSTON / THE HAGUE / DORDRECHT

Published in the UK and Europe by
MTP Press Limited
Falcon House
Lancaster, England

British Library Cataloguing in Publication Data

Eicosanoids in the cardiovascular and renal systems.
  1. Man.   Eicosanoids
  I. Halushka, P. V. (Perry Victor)
  II. Mais, D. E.
  612′.405

Published in the USA by
MTP Press
A division of Kluwer Academic Publishers
101 Philip Drive
Norwell, MA 02061, USA

Library of Congress Cataloging in Publication Data

Eicosanoids in the cardiovascular and renal systems/edited by P. V. Halushka
  and D. E. Mais.
        p.   cm. — (Advances in eicosanoid research series)
    Includes bibliographies and index.
    ISBN-13: 978-94-010-7071-3   e-ISBN-13: 978-94-009-1285-4
    DOI: 10.1007/978-94-009-1285-4
    1. Heart—Pathophysiology. 2. Kidneys—Pathophysiology.
  3. Arachidonic acid—Derivatives—Physiological effect.
  I. Halushka, Perry V. II. Mais, Dale E. (Dale Eugene) 1952–
  III. Series.
    [DNLM: 1. Arachidonic Acids—metabolism. 2. Cardiovascular System—metabolism.
  3. Eicosanoic Acids—metabolism. QU 90 E345]
  RC669.9.E38 1987
  616.1′207—dc19
  DNLM/DLC
  for Library of Congress   87-36644
                                                                              CIP

Typeset by Lasertext, Stretford, Manchester.

Contents

List of contributors

P.G. Baer
Dept of Molecular Pharmacology
Glaxo Incorporated
5 Moore Drive
Research Triangle Park, NC 27709
USA

H.A. Ball
Deutsches Krebsforschungszentrum
P 101949
6900 Heidelberg 1
W. Germany

S.W. Chang
Cardiovascular Pulmonary Research
  Laboratory and
Webb Waring Lung Institute
University of Colorado
Denver, Colorado 80262
USA

J.A. Cook
Department of Physiology
Medical University of South Carolina
171 Ashley Avenue
Charleston, SC 29425
USA

D.J. Fitzgerald
Department of Pharmacology
Vanderbilt University
School of Medicine
Nashville, TN 37232
USA

G.A. FitzGerald
Department of Pharmacology
Vanderbilt Univeristy
School of Medicine
Nashville, TN 37232
USA

P.V. Halushka
Dept of Cell/Molecular Pharmacology
and Experimental Therapeutics
Medical University of South Carolina
171 Ashley Avenue,
Charleston, SC 29425
USA

V.E. Kelley
Department of Medicine
Laboratory of
  Immunogenetics/Transplantation
Brigham and Women's Hospital
75 Francis Street
Boston, MA 02115, USA

S. Lear
Department of Medicine/Renal Division
Charles A. Dang Research Institute,
Harvard Thorndike Laboratory of the Beth
  Israel Hospital
Harvard Medical School
Boston, MA 02215
USA

J. MacDermot
Department of Pharmacology
University of Birmingham
The Medical School
Vincent Drive, Birmingham B15 2TJ
UK

D.E. Mais
Department of Cell/Molecular
  Pharmacology
and Experimental Therapeutics
Medical University of South Carolina
171 Ashley Avenue,
Charleston, SC 29425
USA

G. Matera
Department of Microbiology
University of Saskatchewan
Health Sciences Building
Saskatoon, Saskatchewan
Canada S7N OW0

J.C. McGiff
Department of Pharmacology
New York Medical College
Valhalla, NY 10595
USA

A. Nasjletti
Department of Pharmacology
New York Medical College
Valhalla, NY 10595
USA

J. Quilley
Department of Pharmacology
New York Medical College
Valhalla, NY 10595
USA

H.D. Reines
Department of Anesthesiology
Medical University of South Carolina
171 Ashley Avenue
Charleston, SC 29425
USA

D.L. Saussy, Jr
Department of Molecular Pharmacology
Smith Kline and French
PO Box 7929
Philadelphia, PA 19101
USA

J.B. Smith
Department of Pharmacology
Temple University School of Medicine
3420 N Broad Street
Philadelphia, PA 19140
USA

W.L. Smith
Department of Biochemistry
Michigan State University
East Lansing
MI 48824
USA

W.K. Sonnenburg
Department of Biochemistry
Michigan State University
East Lansing
MI 48824
USA

G.E. Tempel
Department of Physiology
Medical University of South Carolina
171 Ashley Avenue
Charleston, SC 29425
USA

K. Umegaki
Department of Biochemistry
Michigan State University
East Lansing
MI 48824
USA

N.F. Voelkel
Cardiovascular Pulmonary Research
    Laboratory and
Webb Waring Lung Institute
University of Colorado
Denver, Colorado 80262
USA

T. Watanabe
Department of Biochemistry
Michigan State University
East Lansing
MI 48824
USA

W.C. Wise
Department of Physiology
Medical University of South Carolina
171 Ashley Avenue
Charleston, SC 29425
USA

Series Editor's Foreword

The original series, *Advances in Prostaglandin Research*, edited by Sultan M. M. Karim, was published by MTP Press in three volumes in 1975 and 1976. A glance at those books illustrates the progress that has been made since then. The thromboxanes were mentioned twice (first publication 1975) and prostacyclin not once (first publication 1976); leukotrienes were only on the horizon.

The amazing generation of research data in the last 10–15 years has given new, broad insights into many areas, including asthma, inflammation, renal, cardiovascular and gastrointestinal diseases and in reproduction, and has led in some instances to real clinical benefit.

This series, *Advances in Eicosanoid Research*, reflects the current understanding of prostaglandins, thromboxanes and leukotrienes. The aim is to provide an introductory background to each topic and the most up-to-date information available.

Although each book stands alone, the eicosanoids cut across many boundaries in their basic actions; selected chapters from each book in the series will provide illuminating and productive information for all readers which will advance their education and research.

In the production of this series, I must acknowledge with pleasure my collaboration with editors and authors and the patient endeavours of Dr Michael Brewis and the staff at MTP Press.

KEITH HILLIER
University of Southampton
England

Preface

The prostaglandins, once called the glamour compounds of the 1970s, have not lost any of their lustre in the 1980s. Indeed, there appears to be a resurgence of interest in these natural products, in part because of their potential pathophysiological role in diseases. Following the isolation and identification of thromboxane A_2 and prostacyclin in the 1970, and the leukotrienes in the early 1980s, interest in these and related compounds increased dramatically and has resulted in a large body of information indicating that the compounds may be involved in physiological processes such as haemostasis, and pathophysiologically in vasospasm, circulatory shock, asthma, arterial thrombosis, coronary artery and renal diseases. In the last few years, interest has arisen in the use of thromboxane synthesis inhibitors and receptor antagonists and leukotriene synthesis inhibitors and antagonists as potential therapeutic agents in some cardiovascular and renal diseases. Indeed, early clinical trials of some of these compounds are underway and are providing some exciting data.

In addition to the initial physiological and pharmacological data, molecular and biochemical studies are now actively being pursued. The advent of tritiated and radioiodinated analogues have facilitated the extensive study of eicosanoid receptors. Concurrent with the study of these receptors, biochemical and cellular mechanisms of the action of the eicosanoids are being further elucidated.

This volume represents a timely and up-to-date review of the roles of arachidonic acid metabolites in the cardiovascular and renal systems. The intent of the editors was to bring together in one book a compilation of information which spans basic, clinical and molecular studies of the roles of the eicosanoids in these two systems. The book is divided into three parts. The first part reviews platelet and renal arachidonic acid metabolism while the second part addresses possible roles of these metabolites in various cardiovascular and renal diseases. The last part, of a more basic nature, discusses the current knowledge of various eicosanoid receptors and describes possible mechanisms of action.

PERRY V. HALUSHKA
DALE E. MAIS

1
Arachidonic acid metabolism and platelet function

J. B. Smith

INTRODUCTION

It is the intent of this chapter to summarize the role of arachidonic acid metabolism in platelet function from start to finish. The chapter starts by discussing the presence and distribution of arachidonic acid in platelets and then describes the studies done to determine the phospholipid sources of arachidonic acid involved in thromboxane synthesis. The second section of the chapter deals with the mechanism of biosynthesis of prostaglandin endoperoxides and thromboxane A_2 and then turns to a discussion of the development and effects of aspirin and other non-steroidal anti-inflammatory drugs, of thromboxane synthase inhibitors, and of thromboxane receptor agonists and antagonists. The effect of inhibitory prostaglandins on platelets, and the presence of platelet lipoxygenase are mentioned briefly. Certain areas are dealt with in greater depth than others, for example, one area which has not been dealt with, but which is covered in detail in another Chapter, is the work that has been done on the receptors for prostaglandins and thromboxane A_2 present on the surface of platelets. This reflects the biases of the author and the desire to make arachidonic acid, and not its transformation products, the central theme.

ARACHIDONIC ACID

Presence and distribution in platelets

Arachidonic acid is present in high concentrations in ester form in most animal fats and so can be assimilated by man directly in his diet. Alternatively, mammals may biosynthesize arachidonic acid from linoleic acid via desaturation to γ-linolenic acid, chain elongation to dihomo-γ-linolenic acid, and then further desaturation to arachidonic acid.

1

Approximately 30% of position sn-2 in human platelet phospholipids consists of arachidonate. Of course, the percentage of arachidonate varies within the different phospholipids species and the amounts of the different species of phospholipid vary in the platelet. This is illustrated in Table 1.1. which shows that sphingomyelin contains essentially ᵣo arachidonic acid while ethanolamine-phospholipids contain the most arachidonic acid. Although phosphatidylinositol is the phospholipid species that is most enriched in arachidonic acid, its contribution to the total content of arachidonate in blood platelets is small[1,2].

The choline- and ethanolamine-containing phospholipids of human platelets can be subdivided, based on the nature of the linkage to the fatty acid residue at the sn-1 position of the glycerol backbone, into 1,2-diacyl,1-O-alkyl-2-acyl and 1-O-alk-1'-enyl-2-acyl species (Table 1.2). The majority of arachidonic acid in the phosphatidylcholines is present in the diacyl species while 1-O-alk-1'enyl-2-acyl-PE (plasmalogen) contains most of the arachidonic acid in the phosphatidylethanolamines[2]. The amount of arachidonic acid present in the diacyl species of phosphatidylethanolamine is similar to that in diacyl phosphatidylcholine. Perret et al.[3] have shown that the distribution of arachidonate in the phospholipids of the platelet plasma membrane is asymmetric, the majority of it being present in the inner leaflet.

Table 1.1 Composition and arachidonate content of human platelet phospholipids

	Mass (nmol/10⁹ cells)	Mole %AA	Mass of AA (nmol/10⁹ cells)
Sphingomyelin	67.3	ND	ND
Choline-phospholipids	144.4	25.4	36.6
Phosphatidyl-inositol	16.7	93.8	15.7
Ethanolamine-phospholipids	96.1	63.6	61.1
Phosphatidylserine	41.1	46.0	18.9
Total	365.6	—	132.3

ND: not detectable

Table 1.2 Subspecies and arachidonate content of human platelet choline and ethanolamine phospholipids

	Mass (nmol/10⁹ cells)	Mole %AA	Mass of AA (nmol/10⁹ cells)
PC			
1,2-Diacyl-PC	118.0	23.2	27.4
1-O-alkyl-2-acyl-PC	14.0	43.7	6.1
1-O-alk-1'-enyl-2-acyl-PC	12.7	25.1	3.2
Total	144.7	—	36.7
PE			
1,2-Diacyl-PE	34.7	60.0	20.8
1-O-alkyl-2-acyl-PE	3.4	20.4	0.7
1-O-alk-1'-enyl-2-acyl-PE	58.0	68.4	39.7
Total	96.1	—	61.2

2

Sources of arachidonic acid involved in thromboxane synthesis

The fact that oxygenated products of arachidonic acid are produced when platelets are treated with thrombin suggested to early investigators that this fatty acid becomes available to prostaglandin and thromboxane synthases by being released from ester linkage in the platelet membrane phospholipids[4,5]. Support for this concept was forthcoming from numerous investigators[6-8] who demonstrated that unstimulated platelets suspended in plasma or albumin-containing media progressively incorporate radiolabelled arachidonic acid into their phospholipids during incubation at $37°C$ and subsequently release this radiolabel on stimulation with thrombin. In most of these studies, the losses in radiolabel occurred mainly in phosphatidylcholine and phosphatidylinositol with little change in phosphatidylethanolamine and no change in phosphatidyl-serine.

There has been disagreement in the literature about the amount and phospholipid source of arachidonic acid liberated in thrombin-stimulated platelets, and the issue of whether this release is selective or not. Bills et al.[7] used $30 \mu mol L^{-1}$ eicosatetraynoic acid to inhibit oxygenation of arachidonic acid and reported that 20 nmol of arachidonic acid per 10^9 cells was selectively released in thrombin-treated cells. They suggested that the majority of arachidonic acid was released from phosphatidylcholine by the selective action of phospholipase A_2. Bell et al.[9] reported that about 6 nmol of arachidonic acid per 10^9 platelets accumulated in platelets treated with thrombin in the presence of $5-15 \mu mol L^{-1}$ eicosatetraynoic acid. They were unable to detect sufficient phospholipase A_2 activity in disrupted platelets to release substantial amounts of arachidonic acid, and, furthermore, found that the activity that they studied did not possess the required 2-arachidonyl specificity as it acted equally well on 2-oleoyl phospholipids. They suggested that the selectivity of arachidonic acid release was explained by its release from phosphatidylinosi-tol, a phospholipid highly enriched in arachidonate (Table 1.1), by the actions of phospholipase C and diacylglycerol lipase. Broekman et al.[10] reported that similar, small amounts of several fatty acids, including arachidonic acid, were released in thrombin-stimulated cells and questioned whether the release of arachidonic acid was selective at all.

In showing that the release of arachidonic acid was selective, Bills et al.[7] had studied the incorporation of several radiolabelled fatty acids into the complex lipids of human platelets and the subsequent fate of the radiolabel after stimulation of the platelets with thrombin. They found a dramatically greater loss from phosphatidylcholine of radioactive arachidonic acid compared with the other radiolabelled fatty acids. By contrast, Mahadevappa and Holub[11] observed decreases in all the molecular species of phosphatidylcholine after thrombin treatment of platelets prelabelled with radioactive glycerol. They concluded that arachidonate is not selectively released from this phospholipid because the results obtained with radioactive fatty acids were due to unique patterns of incorporation, while those obtained with radioactive glycerol represented the endogenous phospholipid pool.

The above studies suffered from one or other of two weaknesses. Either, one, they relied on the results obtained with radiolabel to draw conclusions

3

about mass changes or, two, they did not totally prevent arachidonic acid from being oxygenated to thromboxanes and other oxygenated products before measuring free fatty acid release. When mass changes are measured in the presence of agents, such as BW755C and propylgallate, at concentrations that totally inhibit both the cyclo-oxygenase and lipoxygenase pathways in platelets, the increases in arachidonic acid induced by thrombin are much greater than the increases in the other free fatty acids. The average increases in free fatty acids (in nmol 10^{-9} platelets) are 1 for linoleic acid, 3.6 for oleic acid, 4.5 for palmitic acid, 7.6 for stearic acid and 32.0 for arachidonic acid[12] (Figure 1.1).

The release of 32 nmol of arachidonic acid per 10^9 platelets obtained using 5U/ml thrombin represents the hydrolysis of approximately 25% of the total arachidonate present in platelet phospholipids (Table 1.1) and is approximately twice the mass of phosphatidylinositol. Thus, the total hydrolysis of phosphatidylinositol by either a phospholipase A_2 pathway acting on this phospholipid[13] or a phospholipase C-diglyceride lipase pathway could at the

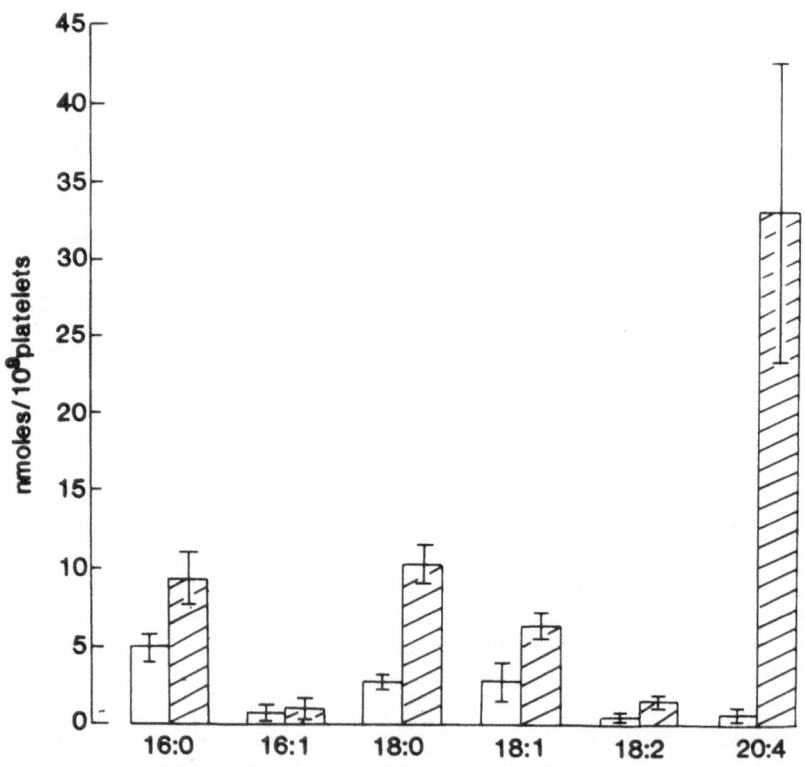

Figure 1.1 Average increase in free fatty acids induced by thrombin using the platelets from eight donors. Gel-filtered platelet suspensions were preincubated with 100 μM BW 755 C for 1 min at 37°C and then incubated with 5 u/ml thrombin for a further 5 min at 37°C. Free fatty acids were extracted and analysed as methyl esters by GLC Reproduced from Smith *et al.*, *Biochim. Biophys. Acta*, **835**, 344, 1985 with permission

most account for 15.7 nmol of arachidonic acid per 10^9 platelets (Table 1.1). However, only 50% of phosphatidylinositol is hydrolysed in response to thrombin stimulation. Moreover, 40% of the decrease in the mass of phosphatidylinositol that occurs can be accounted for by the synthesis of 1-stearoyl-2-arachidonoylphosphatic acid due to phosphorylation of the 1-stearoyl-2 arachidonoylglycerol formed by the action of phospholipase C on phosphatidylinositol[2]. These studies indicate that phosphatidylinositol could contribute a maximum of 4–5 nmol of arachidonic acid per 10^9 platelets to the total arachidonic acid liberated by thrombin (i.e. less than 15%).

The other sources of the arachidonic acid released by platelets in response to thrombin are phosphatidylcholine and phosphatidylethanolamine (Table 1.1). However, each of these phospholipids exists as three species in platelets, namely as the diacyl-, 1-O-alkyl-, or 1-O-alk-1′enyl- forms (Table 1.2). Table 1.2 also shows that 1-O-alkyl-2-acyl-PC and 1-O-alk-1′enyl-2-acyl-PE are enriched in arachidonic acid relative to the other classes of PC or PE, giving rise to the idea that they could serve as important sources of arachidonic acid in stimulated platelets. Purdon and Smith[14] prelabelled platelets with [^{3}H]-arachidonic acid and followed the changes in the different species of PC and PE following thrombin stimulation. It was found that while there was a decrease in radiolabel of both 1,2-diacyl-PC and 1,2-diacyl-PE at all times studied, there was no decrease in the other species of PC or PE, and, indeed, radiolabel in 1-O-alkyl-2-acyl-PC and 1-O-alk-1′-enyl-2-acyl-PE increased at later time points (3–5 min) after thrombin. The thrombin-induced incorporation of arachidonic acid in plasmalogen PE was observed previously by others[15]. Purdon and Smith[14] concluded that, upon stimulation of human platelets, arachidonic acid is released from both 1,2-diacyl-PC and 1,2-diacyl-PE for metabolism by cyclo-oxygenase and lipoxygenase, while certain other pools of phosphatidylcholine and phosphatidylethanolamine act to collect arachidonic acid.

While arachidonic acid is selectively released in thrombin-stimulated platelets, small amounts of palmitic, stearic and oleic acids are also released (Figure 1.1). The most likely explanation of this is that they are released by the action of lysophospholipase on the 1-acyl-2-lyso-PC or 1-acyl-2-lyso-PE formed after selective phospholipase A_2 hydrolysis of 1-acyl-2-arachidonyl-PC or 1-acyl-2-arachidonyl-PE. It has been reported that palmitate, stearate and oleate occupy more than 90% of the 1-position of platelet PC[16]. Furthermore, it has been shown that thrombin treatment of platelets prelabelled with [^{14}C]stearic or [^{14}C]palmitic acids induces the formation of both radioactive lysophosphatidylcholine and free fatty acids[17]. This subsequent hydrolysis by lysophospholipase also explains why the amounts of lysophosphatidylcholine that accumulate in thrombin-treated platelets[18] are considerably lower than the amounts of arachidonic acid which are released.

Figure 1.2 suggests a mechanism for arachidonic acid release in thrombin-stimulated human blood platelets. Phospholipase A_2 acts selectively on 1-acyl-2-arachidonoyl-phospholipids, of which the most important quantitatively is phosphatidylcholine, to liberate arachidonic acid and produce lysophospholipids. These lysophospholipids are subsequently hydrolysed in part by lysophospholipase to produce mainly glycerophosphocholine and smaller

5

$$\begin{array}{c} \text{diacyl-PC} \\ \text{diacyl-PE} \end{array} \xrightarrow{\text{PLA}_2} \begin{array}{c} 20{:}4 + \text{LPC} \\ \text{LPE} \end{array}$$

$$\downarrow$$

$$\text{Lysophospholipase}$$

$$\downarrow$$

$$\text{GPC} + \text{GPE} + 16{:}0 + 18{:}0 + 18{:}1$$

Figure 1.2 Hypothetical scheme which explains the release of large amounts of arachidonic acid (20:4) and smaller amounts of other fatty acids. It is proposed that phospholipase A$_2$ (PLA$_2$) acts on an arachidonate-enriched domain of membrane to selectively release arachidonic acid and form lysophospholipids. The 1-acyl-lysophospholipids are subsequently partially hydrolysed to glycerophosphocholine, glycerophosphoethanolamine and free fatty acids

amounts of glycerophosphoethanolamine[19] as well as palmitic, stearic and oleic acids. In keeping with this mechanism, we have recently demonstrated significant decreases in the amounts of diacyl-PC and diacyl-PE following thrombin stimulation of platelets[20].

No absolute fatty acid specificity has yet been demonstrated[21] for platelet phospholipase A$_2$. Thus, it is possible that the specificity of arachidonic acid release does not depend on the enzyme itself but rather the fact that the platelet contains specific arachidonate-enriched membrane domains, such as the inner plasma membrane[3], in which the 1-acyl-2-arachidonoyl-phospholipids are located.

The mechanism by which thrombin activates phospholipase A$_2$ is presently unknown. Touqui *et al.*[22] have provided evidence for the presence of the phospholipase A$_2$ inhibitor, lipocortin, in blood platelets and have suggested that its phosphorylation during the platelets' response to thrombin relieves inhibition and allows arachidonic acid release. On the other hand, Apitz-Castro *et al.*[21] have suggested that phosphatidic acid (made available subsequent to phospholipase C acting on phosphoinositides) changes the state of organization of the phospholipids in the platelet membrane making them more susceptible to attack by phospholipase A$_2$.

Thrombin is by far the most efficient stimulus in releasing arachidonic acid from platelets and consequently has been the most studied. Collagen is also able to release substantial amounts of arachidonic acid by a mechanism that seems to depend on positive feedback by formed prostaglandin endoperoxides[23] but most other platelet agonists, such as ADP, serotonin and platelet activating factor, are weak inducers of arachidonic acid release.

PROSTAGLANDIN ENDOPEROXIDES AND THROMBOXANE A$_2$

Mechanism of biosynthesis

The biosynthetic conversion of arachidonic acid into PGE$_2$ was simultaneously demonstrated in 1964 by two groups[24,25]. Subsequently, the precursors of PGE$_1$ and PGE$_3$ were shown to be the dihomo-γ-linolenic acid and eicosapentaenoic acid, respectively[26,27]. Dihomo-γ-linolenic acid is present in appreciable amounts in seminal vesicles[28], explaining the presence of PGE_1 in human semen. However, both it and eicosapentaenoic acid are normally present only in trace amounts in most human tissues. Arachidonic acid is by far the most prevalent prostaglandin precursor.

The formation of PGE_2 is known to involve the actions of two enzymes, prostaglandin endoperoxide synthase and PGH-PGE isomerase. Prostaglandin endoperoxide synthase is a membrane-bound enzyme with a molecular weight of about 124 000 daltons. On sodium dodecyl sulphate polyacrylamide gel electrophoresis, a single polypeptide of 72 000 daltons is observed, indicating that the enzyme has two subunits[29]. PGH-PGE isomerase has been solubilized and isolated from the microsomes of bovine seminal vesicles, and was shown to require glutathione as a cofactor to catalyse the formation of E-type prostaglandins[30].

The mechanism of prostaglandin endoperoxide formation from arachidonic acid initially involves the stereospecific abstraction of a proton from carbon-13, followed by a lipoxygenase-like reaction with the introduction of a molecule of oxygen at carbon-11. This peroxy fatty acid is subsequently transformed by intramolecular rearrangement (with the introduction of a second molecule of oxygen) into PGG_2. The cyclic endoperoxide PGG_2 contains a 15S-hydroperoxy group and is converted enzymatically into PGH_2 with a 15S-hydroxy group. These unstable endoperoxides, PGG_2 and PGH_2, were first isolated in 1973 by Nugteren and Hazelhof[31] and Hamberg et al.[32].

The prostaglandin endoperoxides are unstable under aqueous conditions and decompose with a half-life of 5 min in buffer at pH7.4 and 37°C. However, they can be stored in dry organic solvents at reduced temperatures for several months. PGG_2 and PGH_2 induce the aggregation of platelets[32] and constrict porcine, cat and canine coronary arteries. The paradoxical relaxation of bovine coronary arteries by PGH_2 and PGG_2 was shown to be due to their conversion into a potent but unstable vasodilator[33], later identified as prostacyclin[34].

The discovery that PGG_2 and PGH_2 induce the aggregation of platelets provided explanations for the earlier observations that platelet aggregation ensues when arachidonic acid is incubated with platelet-rich plasma[35] and for the labile aggregation stimulating substance (LASS) produced when arachidonic acid is incubated with an endoperoxide synthase preparation from seminal vesicles[36]. PGG_2 is about 3 times more potent than PGH_2 as an aggregating agent and its threshold concentration[32] for inducing aggregation in human citrated platelet-rich plasma is about 0.3 μmol L^{-1}.

When human platelets are incubated with arachidonic acid[37,38] or thrombin[39], they produce a potent constrictor of vascular smooth muscle and platelet-aggregating factor. This factor was shown not to be prostaglandin endoperoxides because it was more potent and more unstable[5]. In studying the biochemical transformation of arachidonic acid or PGG_2 by platelets, it was observed that an intermediate was formed whose time-course correlated with that of the constrictor and aggregating factor (i.e. it had a half-life of about 30 s at 37°C). The structure of this intermediate was proposed to be a novel bicyclic oxetane and it was given the name[5] thromboxane A_2. The stable hydration product of thromboxane A_2 was named thromboxane B_2. It is known that micromolar amounts of thromboxane B_2 are produced when human platelets are treated with thrombin[40].

Recently, synthetic material having the structure proposed for thromboxane A_2 was shown to be indistinguishable from platelet-derived thromboxane A_2 in various biological assays, strongly suggesting that the structure of thromboxane A_2 is correct. The synthetic thromboxane A_2 caused aggregation in human citrated platelet-rich medium at a threshold concentration of 0.05 μmol L^{-1}, indicating[41] that it is about 6 times more potent that PGG_2.

Aspirin and other non-steroidal anti-inflammatory drugs

Aspirin and other non-steroidal anti-inflammatory drugs, such as indomethacin, inhibit prostaglandin endoperoxide synthase[4] and therefore prevent platelets from converting arachidonic acid into prostaglandin endoperoxides and thromboxane A_2. Aspirin is known to act by acetylating a hydroxy serine group in the catalytic site of prostaglandin endoperoxide synthase[42]. Aspirin inhibits the second wave of platelet aggregation induced by ADP or epinephrine as well as the single wave of aggregation induced by arachidonic acid or collagen in citrated platelet-rich plasma. These events are normally associated with prostaglandin endoperoxide and thromboxane A_2 formation. Aspirin does not inhibit the first wave of aggregation induced by epinephrine, ADP, serotonin or platelet activating factor and it is known that these events are not associated with prostaglandin formation[43]. Paradoxically, aspirin does not inhibit platelet aggregation or secretion induced by thrombin even though this agonist is the most effective inducer of arachidonic acid release and thromboxane synthesis.

Inhibitors of thromboxane synthase

Thromboxane synthase, the enzyme responsible for the conversion of PGH_2 into TxA_2, is present in the membrane fraction of platelets and has been solubilized and separated from prostaglandin synthase[44]. Besides converting PGH_2 into TxA_2, thromboxane synthase simultaneously converts PGH_2 into 12-hydroxy-5-cis,8-trans-,10-trans-heptadecatrienoic acid (HHT) and the 3-carbon containing compound, malondialdehyde. Mechanistic studies indicate that two molecules of PGH_2 interact with thromboxane synthase to produce approximately equimolar amounts of TxA_2, HHT, and malondialdehyde by a dismutase reaction[45]. These studies also indicate that HHT and malondialdehyde are not normally produced by breakdown of TxA_2, although, at strong acid pH, either PGH_2 or TxA_2 will be cleaved into these products[31]. Thromboxane synthase has a molecular weight of 58 800 daltons and is present in platelet microsomes[46].

The first truly selective inhibitor of thromboxane synthase described, which was not also a receptor antagonist (see below), was imidazole[47,48,49]. Subsequently, 1-carboxyalkyl derivatives of imidazole were found to be more potent inhibitors of thromboxane synthase than imidazole and to act in a non-competitive fashion[50]. Recently, even more specific inhibitors, such as

OKY-046, CV-4151 and CGS-12970, have been described in the literature[51,52,53]. These compounds resemble imidazole in having an aromatic, heteroatom nucleus linked to a carboxyalkyl side chain.

Needleman et al.[48] studied the effects of imidazole on arachidonic acid-induced aggregation of human blood platelets in vitro and found that it had very little inhibitory activity even though it inhibited TxA_2 formation, as shown by reduced contraction of rabbit aortic strips. They concluded that TxA_2 was no more effective than prostaglandin endoperoxides in inducing platelet aggregation but was considerably more potent that PGH_2 as a contractor of aortic smooth muscle. On the other hand, Gorman et al.[54] found that 15-deoxy-9,11-azo-PGH_2, another potent inhibitor of thromboxane synthase, abolished platelet aggregation induced by arachidonic acid or PGH_2. They concluded that the formation of TxA_2 is obligatory for endoperoxide-induced platelet aggregation. The solution to these contradictory conclusions came with the finding that 15-deoxy-9,11-azo-PGH_2 not only inhibits thromboxane synthase but also is a potent endoperoxide receptor antagonist[55]. For example, it inhibits platelet aggregation induced by 9,11-epoxymethano-PGH_2, a stable PGH_2 mimetic which cannot be converted into TxA_2. The concept that prostaglandin endoperoxides alone are able to cause platelet aggregation is now fairly well accepted[56].

Moncada and Vane[57] found that microsomes prepared from blood vessels convert PGH_2 into prostacyclin, the very potent inhibitor of platelet aggregation. They proposed that the blood vessels 'steal' the endoperoxides from aggregating platelets. It follows that if this hypothesis is correct, thromboxane synthase inhibitors should be much more active in vivo than in vitro because, by allowing PGH_2 to be released from aggregating platelets, they would cause increased prostacyclin formation. However, Carey and Haworth[58] have been unable to confirm this assumption in an acute challenge model which involved the intravenous injection of collagen, thrombin or arachidonic acid into rats.

All thromboxane synthase inhibitors investigated prolong the rat tail bleeding time in a dose-related fashion[59]. As the compounds have little effect on collagen-induced rat platelet aggregation in vitro, Butler et al.[59] have postulated that the inhibitors produce their effect, not by inhibiting platelet aggregation or blood coagulation, but rather by preventing the vasoconstriction which would normally be caused by thromboxane A_2.

Stable thromboxane receptor agonists and antagonists

Because of the inherent lability of the prostaglandin endoperoxides and thromboxane A_2, it is important and desirable to have chemically- and metabolically-stable thromboxane receptor agonists so that one can determine the biochemical, physiological and pharmacological profile of this important compound. Several laboratories have reported the synthesis and biological actions of a number of prostaglandin endoperoxide analogs which are thromboxane receptor agonists or are both thromboxane agonists and thromboxane synthetase inhibitors. These include[60,61] 9,11-epoxymethano-PGH_2, 9,11-methanoepoxy-PGH_2 and 9,11-azo-PGH_2. A series of 7-oxabicycloheptane derivatives of prostaglandins, including SQ 24,775, SQ 24,810 and SQ 26,538, have also been shown to be stable thromboxane receptor agonists[62]. These compounds mimic the prostaglandin endoperoxides and thromboxane A_2 in that they induce platelet aggregation and cause contraction of isolated rabbit aorta and coronary arteries.

A number of stable thromboxane receptor antagonists have been reported. These include 13-aza-prostanoic acid[63], pinane thromboxane A_2[64] and the 7-oxabicycloheptane compounds, SQ 26,536[62] and SQ 29,548[65].

INHIBITORY PROSTAGLANDINS

Like aspirin, prostaglandin endoperoxide and thromboxane A_2 receptor antagonists inhibit platelet aggregation induced by arachidonic acid, prostaglandin endoperoxides, thromboxane A_2, or collagen in platelet-rich plasma but do not inhibit primary platelet aggregation induced by other agonists, such as ADP, platelet-activating factor or thrombin. Two derivatives of arachidonic acid, prostacyclin and PGD_2, as well as PGE_1, a derivative of dihomo-γ-linolenic acid, by contrast inhibit platelet aggregation induced by all of these agents. Prostacyclin produces its effects at nanomolar concentrations and is the most potent known inhibitor of platelet aggregation. These prostaglandins act by elevating cyclic AMP in platelets, a subject which has been reviewed elsewhere[66].

PLATELET LIPOXYGENASE

Arachidonic acid is rapidly oxygenated when it is incubated with human platelets in the absence of albumin[67]. Of course, three of the major oxygenated derivatives produced are thromboxane B_2, HHT and malondialdehyde which are formed as a result of the action of thromboxane synthase on prostaglandin endoperoxides. A fourth derivative, which is produced somewhat more slowly as a result of the action of platelet lipoxygenase on arachidonic acid, is 12-hydroxy-8,10,14-eicosatetraenoic acid (12-HETE). It has been shown that micromolar amounts of all four of these derivatives are synthesized when washed human platelets are treated with thrombin[38]. As aspirin inhibits prostaglandin endoperoxide synthase but not platelet lipoxygenase, thrombin treatment of platelets from donors who have taken aspirin results in markedly diminished formation of the derivatives of the prostaglandin endoperoxide—thromboxane synthases and increased formation of 12-HETE. Although the platelet lipoxygenase pathway has been the subject of several studies, its relevance to platelet physiology has not been established[68].

CONCLUDING REMARKS

Remarkable progress has been made in understanding the biochemical and pharmacological aspects of arachidonic acid metabolism and platelet function since the initial discovery[4] that platelets make prostaglandins in 1971. It is now apparent that platelets are poised to selectively release large amounts of arachidonic acid when they come into contact with collagen or thrombin. This arachidonic acid is rapidly converted by membrane-bound enzymes into thromboxane A_2, a potent but labile inducer of platelet aggregation and constrictor of blood vessels. The role of this thromboxane A_2 appears to be to recruit other platelets to platelets that are already adhering to collagen. This explains why inhibitors of cyclo-oxygenase, such as aspirin and other non-steroidal anti-inflammatory drugs, as well as thromboxane A_2 receptor antagonists, inhibit collagen-induced platelet aggregation. The fact that thromboxane synthetase inhibitors are less active inhibitors of aggregation is explained by the realization that prostaglandin endoperoxides have aggregating activity in their own right. The effect of aspirin on platelets may explain why aspirin is effective in reducing myocardial infarction and death in patients with unstable angina, a syndrome thought to involve platelet thrombus formation in atherosclerotic blood vessels[69]. Additionally, the vasoconstrictive effect of thromboxane A_2 may play a role in unstable angina.

The facile pathway by which human platelets make thromboxane A_2 should not cause the physiological role of thromboxane A_2 to be overestimated. It is clear that other agonists, such as ADP, platelet activating factor and serotonin, can induce platelet aggregation without stimulating thromboxane synthesis. Thrombin, the most active inducer of thromboxane synthesis, still causes platelet aggregation and nucleotide secretion when thromboxane synthesis is abolished using non-steroidal anti-inflammatory drugs[4]. Thus, platelets are still able to perform their haemostatic function in the absence of thromboxane synthesis. Indeed, platelets obtained from ruminants, such as cow and sheep, have very little capacity for thromboxane synthesis in response to thrombin, even under normal conditions[70]. The role of thromboxane A_2 seems to be that of a back up system for platelet aggregation in the event that thrombin formation is in some way compromised. It is well known that haemophiliacs who have a deficiency of one of the coagulation proteins required for thrombin formation bleed profusely if they damage a blood vessel after aspirin ingestion.

As well as the apparent pathological role that thromboxane A_2 plays in unstable angina, it also seems to be involved in the transient ischaemic attacks that occur in stroke patients. Aspirin is recommended by the FDA for treating these patients. The evaluation of thromboxane synthase inhibitors and prostaglandin endoperoxide–thromboxane A_2 receptor antagonists in the clinical setting will doubtless reveal pathological roles for thromboxane A_2 in other human diseases.

REFERENCES

1. Mueller, H.W., Purdon, A.D., Smith, J.B. and Wykle, R.L. (1983). 1-O-Alkyl-linked phosphoglycerides of human platelets: Distribution of arachidonate and other acyl residues in the ether-linked and diacyl species. *Lipids*, **18**, 814–881
2. Mauco, G., Dangelmaier, C.A. and Smith, J.B. (1984). Inositol lipids, phosphatidate and diacylglycerol share stearoylarachidonoylglycerol as a common backbone in thrombin-stimulated human platelets. *Biochem. J*, **224**, 933–940

11

3 Perret, B., Chap, H.J. and Douste-Blazy, L. (1979). Asymmetric distribution of arachidonic acid in the plasma membrane of human platelets. A determination using purified phospholipases and a rapid method for membrane isolation. Biochim. Biophys. Acta, 556, 434–446

4. Smith, J.B. and Willis, A.L. (1971). Aspirin selectively inhibits prostaglandin production in human platelets. Nature New Biol., 231, 235–237

5. Hamberg, M., Svensson, J. and Samuelsson, B. (1975). Thromboxanes—A new group of biologically active compounds derived from prostaglandin endoperoxides. Proc. Natl. Acad. Sci. USA, 72, 2994–2998

6. Bills, T.K., Smith J.B. and Silver, M.J. (1976). Metabolism of [14C] arachidonic acid by human platelets. Biochim. Biophys. Acta, 424, 303–314

7. Bills, T.K., Smith, J.B. and Silver, M.J. (1977). Selective release of arachidonic acid from the phospholipids of human platelets in response to thrombin. J. Clin. Invest., 60, 1–6

8. Flower, R.J. and Blackwell, G.J. (1976). The importance of phospholipase A₂ in prostaglandin biosynthesis. Biochem. Pharmacol., 25, 285–291

9. Bell, R.L., Kennerly, D.A., Stanford, N. and Majerus, P.W. (1979). Diglyceride lipase: a pathway for arachidonate release from human platelets. Proc. Natl. Acad. Sci. USA, 76, 3238–3241

10. Broekman, M.J., Ward, J.W. and Marcus, A.J. (1981). Fatty acid composition of phosphatidylinositol and phosphatidic acid in stimulated platelets. J. Biol. Chem., 256, 8271–8274

11. Mahadevappa, V.G. and Holub, B.J. (1984). Relative degradation of different molecular species of phosphatidylcholine in thrombin-stimulated human platelets. J. Biol. Chem., 259, 9369–9373

12. Smith, J.B., Dangelmaier, C. and Mauco, G. (1985). Measurement of arachidonic acid liberation in thrombin-stimulated human platelets. Use of agents that inhibit both the lipoxygenase and cyclooxygenase enzymes. Biochim. Biophys. Acta, 835, 344–351

13. Billah, M.M. and Lapetina, E.G. (1982). Formation of lysophosphatidylinositol in platelets stimulated with thrombin or ionophore. J. Biol. Chem., 257, 5196–5200

14. Purdon, A.D. and Smith, J.B. (1985). Turnover of arachidonic acid in the major diacyl and ether phospholipids of human platelets. J. Biol. Chem., 260, 12700–12704

15. Rittenhouse-Simmons, S., Russel, F.A. and Deykin, D. (1976). Transfer of arachidonic acid to human platelet plasmalogen in response to thrombin. Biochem. Biophys. Res. Commun., 70, 295–302

16. Mahadevappa, V.G. and Holub, B.J. (1982). The molecular species composition of individual diacyl phospholipids in human platelets. Biochim. Biophys. Acta, 713, 73–79

17. Bills, T.K., Smith, J.B. and Silver, M.J. (1977). Platelet uptake, release and oxidation of [14C]arachidonic acid. In Silver, M.J., Smith, J.B. and Kocsis, J.J. (eds.) Prostaglandins in Hematology, pp. 17–55. (New York: Spectrum Publications Inc.)

18. McKean, M.L., Smith, J.B. and Silver, M.J. (1982). Phospholipid biosynthesis in human platelets. Formation of phosphatidylcholine from 1-acyl--lysophosphatidylcholine by acyl-CoA: 1-acyl-sn-glycero-3-phosphocholine acyl transferase. J. Biol. Chem., 257, 11278–11283

19. Koslowski, A. and Smith, J.B. Unpublished observations.

20. Purdon, A.D., Patelunas, D. and Smith, J.B. (1987). Resolution of radiolabelled molecular species of phospholipid in the human platelets. Lipids 22, 116–120

21. Apitz-Castro, R., Cruz, R., Mas, M. and Jain, M.K. (1981). Further studies on a phospholipase A₂ isolated from human platelet plasma membranes. Thrombosis. Res., 23, 347–354

22. Touqui, L., Rothhut, B., Shaw, A.M., Fradin, A., Vargaftig, B.B. and Russo-Maria, F. (1986). Platelet activation – a role for a 40 K anti-phospholipase A₂ protein indistinguishable from lipocortin. Nature (London), 321, 177–180

23. Rittenhouse, S.E. and Allen, C.L. (1982). Synergistic activation by collagen and 15-hydroxy-9α, 11α-peroxidoprosta-5,13-dienoic acid (PGH₂) of phosphatidylinositol metabolism and arachidonic acid release in human platelets. J. Clin. Invest., 70, 1216

24. Bergström, S., Danielsson, H. and Samuelsson, B. (1964). The enzymatic formation of prostaglandin E₂ from arachidonic acid. Prostaglandins and related factors 32. Biochim. Biophys. Acta, 90, 207–210

25. Van Dorp, D.A., Beerthuis, R.K., Nugteren, D.M. and Vonkeman, H. (1964). The biosynthesis of prostaglandins. Biochim. Biophys. Acta, 90, 204–207

26. Nugteren, D.H., Beerthuis, R.K. and Van Dorp, D.A. (1966). The enzymatic conversion of all-*cis* 8,11,14-eicosatrienoic acid into prostaglandin E_1. *Rec. Trav. Chim. Pays-Bas*, **85**, 405–419
27. Struijk, C.B., Beerthuis, R.K., Pabon, H.J.J. and Van Dorp, D.A. (1966). Specificity in the enzymatic conversion of polyunsaturated fatty acids into prostaglandins. *Rev. Trav. Chim. Pays-Bas*, **85**, 1233–1253
28. Lands, W.E.M. and Samuelsson, B. (1968). Phospholipid precursors of prostaglandins. *Biochim. Biophys. Acta*, **164**, 426–429
29. Van der Ouderaa, F.J. Buytenhek, M., Nugteren, D.H. and Van Dorp, D.A. (1977). Purification and characterization of prostaglandin endoperoxide synthetase from sheep vesicular glands. *Biochim. Biophys. Acta*, **487**, 315–331
30. Ogino, N., Miyamoto, T., Yamamoto, S. and Hayaishi, O. (1977). Prostaglandin endoperoxide E isomerase from bovine vesicular gland microsomes, a glutathione-requiring enzyme. *J. Biol. Chem.*, **252**, 890–895
31. Nugteren, D.H. and Hazelhof, E. (1973) Isolation and properties of intermediates in prostaglandin biosynthesis. *Biochim. Biophys. Acta*, **326**, 448–461
32. Hamberg, M., Svensson, J., Wakabayashi, T and Samuelsson, B. (1974). Isolation and structure of two prostaglandin endoperoxides that cause platelet aggregation. *Proc. Natl. Acad. Sci. USA*, **71**, 345–349
33. Kulkarni, P.S., Roberts, R. and Needleman, P. (1976). Paradoxical endogenous synthesis of a coronary dilating substance from arachidonate. *Prostaglandins*, **12**, 337–353
34. Needleman, P., Kulkarni, P.S. and Raz, A. (1977). Coronary tone modulation: Formation and actions of prostaglandins, endoperoxides and thromboxanes. *Science*, **195**, 409–412
35. Silver, M.J., Smith, J.B., Ingerman, C. and Kocsis, J.J. (1973). Arachidonic acid-induced human platelet aggregation and prostaglandin formation. *Prostaglandins*, **4**, 863–875
36. Willis, A.L., Vane, F.M., Kuhn, D.C., Scott, C.G. and Petrin, M. (1974). An endoperoxide aggregator (LASS), formed in platelets in response to thrombotic stimuli – Purification, identification and unique biological significance. *Prostaglandins*, **8**, 453–507
37. Vargaftig, B.B. and Zirinis, P. (1973). Platelet aggregation induced by arachidonic acid is accompanied by release of potential inflammatory mediators distinct from PGE_2 and $PGF_{2\alpha}$. *Nature (London)*, **244**, 114–116
38. Hamberg, M., Svensson, J. and Samuelsson, B. (1974). Prostaglandin endoperoxides: A new concept concerning the mode of action and release of prostaglandins. *Proc. Natl. Acad. Sci. USA*, **71**, 3824–3828
39. Ellis, E. F., Oelz, O., Roberts, L.J. II, Payne, N.A. Sweetman, B.J., Nies, A.S. and Oates, J.A. (1976). Coronary arterial smooth muscle contraction by a substance released from platelets: Evidence that it is thromboxane A_2. *Science*, **193**, 1135–1137
40. Smith, J.B. (1978). Prostaglandins and platelet function. In Mielke, C.H. Jr. and Rodvien, R. (eds.) *Mechanisms of Hemostasis and Thrombosis*, pp.59–71. (Miami, FL: Symposia Specialists, Inc.)
41. Bhagwat, S.S., Hamann, P.R., Still, W.C., Bunting, S. and Fitzpatrick, F.A. (1985). Synthesis and structure of the platelet aggregation factor thromboxane A_2. *Nature (London)*, **315**, 511–512
42. Nugteren, D.H., Buytenhek, M., Christ-Hazelhof, E., Moonen, P. and van der Ouderaa, F.J. (1981). Enzymes involved in the conversion of endoperoxides. *Prog. Lipid Res.*, **20**, 169–172
43. Smith, J.B., Ingerman, C.M., Kocsis, J.J. and Silver, M.J. (1973). Formation of prostaglandins during the aggregation of human blood platelets. *J. Clin. Invest.*, **52**, 965–969
44. Hammarström, S. and Falardeau, P. (1977). Resolution of prostaglandin endoperoxide synthase and thromboxane synthase of human platelets. *Proc. Natl. Acad. Sci. USA*, **64**, 3691–3695
45. Anderson, M.W., Crutchly, D.J., Tainer, B.E. and Eling, T.E. (1978). Kinetic studies on the conversion of prostaglandin endoperoxide PGH_2 by thromboxane synthase. *Prostaglandins*, **16**, 563–570
46. Haurand, M. and Ullrich, V. (1985). Characterization of thromboxane synthase from human platelets as a cytochrome P-450 enzyme. *J. Biol. Chem.*, **260**, 15057–15059
47. Needleman, P., Bryan, B., Wyche, A., Bronson, S.D., Eakin, E., Ferrendelli, J.A. and Minkes, M. (1977). Thromboxane synthetase inhibitors as pharmacological tools: Differential biochemical and biological effects on platelet suspension. *Prostaglandins*, **14**, 897–907

13

48. Needleman, P., Raz, A., Ferrendelli, J.A. and Minkes, M. (1977). Application of imidazole as a selective inhibitor of thromboxane synthetase in human platelets. *Proc. Natl. Acad. Sci. USA*, **74**, 1716–1720

49. Moncada, S., Bunting, S., Mullane, K., Thorogood, P., Vane, J.R., Raz, A. and Needleman, P. (1977). A selective inhibitor of thromboxane synthetase. *Prostaglandins*, **13**, 611–618

50. Yoshimoto, T., Yamamoto, S. and Hayaishi, O. (1978). Selective inhibition of prostaglandin endoperoxide thromboxane isomerase by 1-carboxyalkylimidazoles. *Prostaglandins*, **16**, 529–540

51. Terashita, Z., Imura, Y., Tanabe, M., Kawazoe, K., Nishikawa, K., Kato, K. and Terao, S. (1986). CV-4151–A potent, selective thromboxane A$_2$ synthetase inhibitor. *Thrombosis Res.*, **41**, 223–237

52. Garcia-Szabo, R., Kern, D.F. and Malik, A. B. (1984). Pulmonary vascular response to thrombin: Effects of thromboxane synthetase inhibition with OKY-046 and OKY-1581. *Prostaglandins*, **28**, 851–866

53. Ambler, J., Butler, K.D., Ku, E.C., Maguire, E.D., Smith, J.R. and Wallis, R.B. (1985). CGS 12970: A novel, long acting thromboxane synthetase inhibitor. *Br. J. Pharmac.*, **86**, 497–504

54. Gorman, R.R., Bundy, G.L., Peterson, D.C., Sun, F.F. and Miller, O.V. (1977). Inhibition of human platelet thromboxane synthetase by 9,11-azoprosta-5,13-dienoic acid. *Proc. Natl. Acad. Sci. USA*, **74**, 4007–4011

55. MacIntyre, D.E. (1981). Platelet prostaglandin receptors in platelets in biology and pathology. In Dingle, J.L. and Gordon, J.L. (eds.) *Research Monographs in Cell and Tissue Physiology*, Vol. 5, pp. 211–244. (Amsterdam: Elsevier)

56. Grimm, L.J., Knapp, D.R., Senator, D. and Halushka, P. (1981). Inhibition of platelet thromboxane synthesis by 7-(1-imidazolyl) heptanoic acid: dissociation from inhibition of aggregation. *Thrombosis Res.*, **24**, 307–317

57. Moncada, S. and Vane, J.R. (1982). The role of prostaglandins in platelet-vessel wall interactions. In Nossel, H.L. and Vogel, H.J. (eds.) *Pathobiology of the Endothelial Cell*, pp. 252–275. (New York: Academic Press)

58. Carey, F. and Haworth, D. (1986) Thromboxane synthase inhibition: implications of prostaglandin endoperoxide metabolism. *Prostaglandins*, **31**, 47–59

59. Butler, K.D., Maguire, E.D., Smith, J.R., Turnbull, A.A., Wallis, R.B. and White, A.M. (1982). Prolongation of rat tail bleeding time caused by oral doses of a thromboxane synthetase inhibitor which have little effect on platelet aggregation. *Thromb. Haem. (Stutgt)*, **47**, 46–49

60. Malmsten, C. (1976). Some biological effects of prostaglandin endoperoxide analogs. *Life Sci.*, **18**, 169–176

61. Corey, E. J., Nicolaou, K.C., Yoshimasa, M., Malmsten, C.L. and Samuelsson, B. (1975). Synthesis and biological properties of a 9,11-azo-prostanoid. Highly active biochemical mimic of prostaglandin endoperoxides. *Proc. Natl. Acad. Sci. USA*, **72**, 3355–3358

62. Harris, D.N., Phillips, M.B., Michel, I.M., Goldenberg, H.J., Heikers, J.E., Sprague, P.W. and Antonaccio, M.J. (1981). 9α-Homo-9,11-epoxy-5,13-prostadienoic acid analogs: Specific stable agonist (SQ 26,538) and antagonist (SQ 26,536) of the human platelet thromboxane receptor. *Prostaglandins*, **22**, 295–307

63. Venton, D.L., Enke, S.E. and LeBreton, G.C. (1979). Azaprostanoic acid derivatives. Inhibitors of arachidonic acid induced platelet aggregation. *J. Med. Chem.*, **22**, 824–830

64. Nicolaou, K.C., Magolda, R.L., Smith, J.B., Aharony, D., Smith, E.F. and Lefer, A.M. (1979). Synthesis and biological properties of pinane-thromboxane A$_2$, a selective inhibitor of coronary artery constriction, platelet aggregation, and thromboxane formation. *Proc. Natl. Acad. Sci. USA*, **76**, 2566–2570

65. Darius, H., Smith, J.B. and Lefer, A.M. (1985). Beneficial effects of a new potent and specific thromboxane receptor antagonist (SQ 29,548) *in vitro* and *in vivo*. *J. Pharm. Exp. Ther.*, **235**, 274–280

66. Haslam, R.J., Davidson, M.M., Davies, T., Lynham, J.A. and McClenaghan, M.D. (1978). Regulation of blood platelet function by cyclic nucleotides In George, W.J. and Ignarro, L.J. (eds.) *Advances in Cyclic Nucleotide Research*. Vol. 9, p. 533. (New York: Raven Press)

67. Hamberg, M. and Samuelsson, B. (1974). Prostaglandin endoperoxides – Novel transformations of arachidonic acid in human platelets. *Proc. Natl. Acad. Sci. USA*, **71**, 3400–3404

68. Aharony, D., Smith, J.B and Silver, M.J. (1984). Platelet arachidonate lipoxygenase. In Chalkin, E. (ed.) *The Leukotrienes*, pp. 104–122. (New York: Academic Press)
69. Lewis, M.D. Jr., Davis, J.W., Archibald, D.G. *et al.* (1983): Protective effects of aspirin against acute myocardial infarction and death in men with unstable angina: results of a Veteran Administration cooperative study. *N. Engl. J. Med.*, **309**, 396–403
70. Meyers, K.M., Katz, J.B., Clemmons, R.M., Smith, J.B. and Holmsen, H. (1980). An evaluation of the arachidonate pathway of platelets from companion and food-producing animals, mink and man. *Thrombosis Res.*, **20**, 13–15

2
Renal arachidonic acid metabolism

J. Quilley and J. C. McGiff

The 'ubiquity' of prostaglandin-generating capacity of cells is usually cited as a general principle within the first paragraph of reviews of prostaglandins. This principle and others need amending in view of recent studies. As for ubiquity, within the past several years, the ability of some cell types to synthesize prostaglandins has been challenged following the application of immunodissection and cytochemical methods and cell separation techniques to the study of renal arachidonic acid (AA) metabolism[1,2]. There are cells which either do not generate prostaglandins or have a greatly reduced capacity to synthesize them. For example, within the nephron, there are segments which lack cyclo-oxygenase[3] or show negligible capacity to transform added AA to prostanoids[4]. In contrast, within the vasculature, cyclo-oxygenase is found in abundance although the principal products vary both longitudinally along the vasculature and cross-sectionally within the blood vessel wall; e.g. endothelium versus vascular smooth muscle[5,6]. The construct that the profile of vascular prostanoids differs between the microcirculation and large blood vessels can also be cast in terms of renal and other visceral blood vessels compared with those supplying the limbs, as well as the coronary vasculature compared with the cerebral vasculature[5,7,8]. Further, within an organ, regional variations of AA metabolism occur[9]. Zonal variations in renal prostaglandin synthesis are apparent when comparing the capacity of renal cortical and renal medullary slices to generate prostanoids from exogenous arachidonic acid[10]. Moreover, renal vascular elements differ both quantitatively and qualitatively in their capacity to generate eicosanoids. This capacity is subject to modification by disease and experimental conditions[11,12]. It appears that the profile of eicosanoids produced is similar for all preglomerular arterial elements[13]: differences in the prostanoid profile of arteries compared with that of the microcirculation are predictable as they have been described in all regional vascular beds studied thus far[7,8].

16

PROSTAGLANDIN-DEPENDENT VASCULAR MECHANISMS

The adaptation of the renal circulation to stress and disease has been defined in terms of prostaglandin dependency[14]. Prostaglandin-related vascular mechanisms, subserving the renal circulation, demonstrate minimal activity in the resting state as evidenced by low levels of prostaglandins in renal venous blood and negligible effects of inhibitors of cyclo-oxygenase on renal blood flow[15]. Vascular mechanisms mediated by prostaglandins can be evoked rapidly in response to stimulation, chiefly by vasoactive peptides and neurotransmitters. For example, injection of norepinephrine into the rat kidney caused a surge of prostaglandins into renal venous and urinary effluents[16]. Renal efflux of PGE_2 increased by as much as two hundred-fold within 90 s in response to norepinephrine and then declined over a period of several minutes. Prostaglandin-dependent mechanisms operating within the renal vasculature regulate renal blood flow and its regional distribution, particularly when the renin-angiotensin and adrenergic nervous systems are stimulated by, for example, contraction of extracellular fluid volume. Under these conditions, the renal circulation is maintained within normal levels because of activation of prostaglandin mechanisms intrarenally despite increased activity of pressor systems[17]. Although total renal blood flow is usually unaffected, there are major alterations in zonal perfusion of the kidney; viz, blood flow redistributes from the outer cortex to the inner cortex and medulla as a consequence of stimulation of renal prostaglandin synthesis[18]. The degree of stimulation of prostaglandin synthesis, as measured by efflux of PGE_2 into the renal venous effluent, is closely related to the level of activity of the renin–angiotensin system[15]. The importance of this prostaglandin-dependent mechanism to the renal circulation is readily demonstrated by inhibition of prostaglandin synthesis with indomethacin, resulting in acute decline of renal blood flow. This decline[19] predominates in the medulla and parallels reduced renal efflux of PGE_2.

Changes in renal prostaglandin synthesis should affect renal blood flow primarily to the medulla because of the high activity of cyclo-oxygenase in the renal medulla and the relative absence of prostaglandin catabolizing enzymes in this region when compared with the cortex[20]. Moreover, the anatomical arrangements indicate that the inner cortical and medullary circulations are continuous because the vasa recta originate from the efferent arterioles of the inner cortex. Thus, inhibition of prostaglandin synthesis should affect inner cortical and medullary blood flow to the greatest degree. The canine blood-perfused, isolated kidney, perfused at constant pressure, has been used in order to study the effect of changes in prostaglandin synthesis on the renal circulation independently of extrarenal haemodynamic and hormonal influences[18,19]. Blood flow increased with time, particularly that fraction to the inner cortex[18]. The greatest rate of increase of renal blood flow and its inner cortical component occurred when the rate of increase of PGE_2 levels in the perfusate was most rapid. Inhibition of renal prostaglandin synthesis with either indomethacin or meclofenamate resulted in reduced renal blood flow, particularly to the inner cortex and presumably by anatomical extension to the renal medulla for reasons cited above. Moreover, the relatively selective reduction by indomethacin of inner cortical blood flow could not be reversed by exogenous PGE_2, suggesting that PGE_2 acts as a local hormone to effect increases in inner cortical and medullary blood flow[18]. The inner cortical and medullary circulations are, then, subject to regulation by vasodilator prostaglandins, such as PGE_2, acting as local hormones within the kidney. More direct measurements of renal blood flow[21] have confirmed the changes in renal medullary blood flow deduced in the earlier study.

Kinins dilate the renal vasculature through a direct action[22] as well as a secondary effect mediated by vasodilator prostaglandins[23]. Therefore, stimulation or inhibiton of the renal kallikrein–kinin system should result in corresponding changes in renal prostaglandin levels as reflected by altered concentrations in renal venous and urinary effluents[24] as well as by alterations in renal blood flow. Inhibition of kininase II, the principal renal kinin catabolizing enzyme, with an angiotensin converting enzyme inhibitor will increase the activity of the renal kallikrein–kinin system as reflected in renal vasodilatation, natriuresis and diuresis[25]. Aprotinin, an inhibitor of serine proteases, including renal kallikrein, prevented the accompanying renal vasodilatation, diuresis, natriuresis and elevated plasma renin activity caused by inhibition of kininase II[25]. Inhibition of cyclo-oxygenase with indomethacin had effects similar to those produced by aprotinin on the actions of the angiotensin converting enzyme inhibitor with the exception that the natriuresis, which is prevented by aprotinin, was unaffected by indomethacin. These results provide evidence for prostaglandin-related mechanisms mediating the effects of kinins on renal blood flow, renin release and water excretion. However, the natriuresis was assumed to be a direct action of kinins as it was not prevented by indomethacin. In addition, administration of either aprotinin or indomethacin prevented the redistribution of cortical blood flow from the superficial to the deep cortex and medulla, consequent to administration of the angiotensin converting enzyme inhibitor. Kramer et al. have also observed that aprotinin decreased blood flow to the inner cortex[26]. Thus, inhibition of either kallikrein or cyclo-oxygenase caused similar effects on the distribution of renal blood flow. Together, these studies strongly support the view that the renal kallikrein–kinin and prostaglandin systems act in concert to regulate renal blood flow and its zonal distribution.

The above studies were acute and, therefore, limited by the period of observation and precluded general conclusions on the long-term consequences of kinin–prostaglandin interactions. Nasjletti et al. have conducted a study[27] in rats extending over a period of three weeks and have measured simultaneous changes in the renal kallikrein–kinin and prostaglandin systems as reflected in excretion of kallikrein and prostaglandins in response to stimulation and inhibition of the former (Figure 2.1). Either augmentation or depression of urinary kallikrein excretion resulted in corresponding changes in excretion of PGE_2. Mineralocorticoids were administered to increase the activity of the renal kallikrein–kinin system, and aprotinin was given to reverse the stimulatory effects of mineralocorticoids. Aldosterone administered over a period of up to two weeks in the conscious rat produced an initial transient antinatriuresis. A diuresis appeared on the second day of steroid treatment and persisted for the remainder of the study, associated with a three-fold

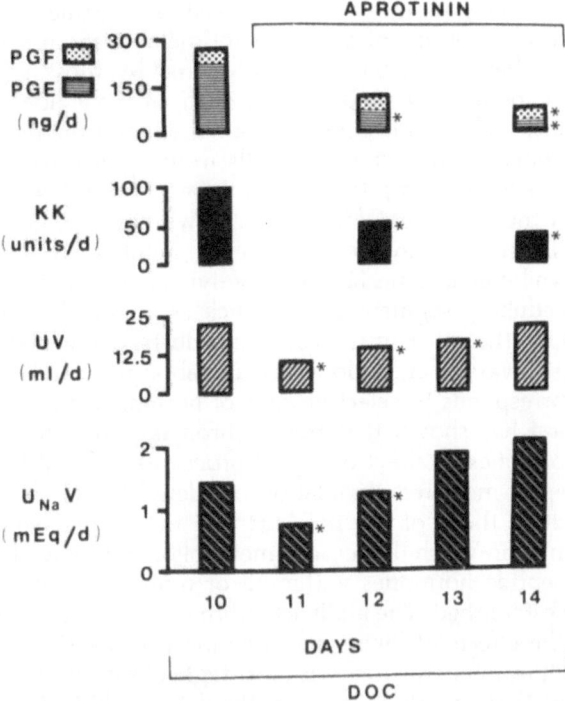

Figure 2.1 Excretion of urinary prostaglandins E (PGE)- and F (PGF)-like substances, kallikrein (KK), urine volume (UV), and sodium excretion ($U_{Na}V$) in rats injected with deoxycorticosterone (DOC), 5 mg day^{-1} for 14 days. From day 11, aprotinin, 50 000 kiu was injected subcutaneously twice daily for 4 days. Values are means; *indicates significant differences ($p < 0.05$) compared with control values

increase in excretion of kallikrein and PGE_2. Injection of aprotinin in the face of continued administration of the mineralocorticoids resulted in a rapid decline in urinary kallikrein activity and a secondary reduction in excretion of PGE_2. The importance of renal prostaglandins to the excretion of water was suggested by the increased urinary efflux of prostaglandins during the diuresis induced by the mineralocorticoid. Further, reduced PGE_2 excretion in response to aprotinin in rats receiving mineralocorticoids was associated with decreased water excretion lasting several days. This study, then, strongly endorses previous proposals that the kallikrein–kinin and prostaglandin systems are closely linked within the kidney[28]. The concerted actions of these systems is important to the regulation of renal haemodynamics, particularly the allocation of blood flow to the inner cortex and medulla, and to attendant effects on the regulation of extracellular fluid volume.

ARACHIDONIC ACID METABOLISM IN THE NEPHRON

In contrast to the widespread mobilization of prostaglandin mechanisms within the renal vasculature, stimulation of renal arachidonic acid metabolism can be more discrete – localized to specific cells and segments of the nephron. The functional implications of arachidonate metabolism in specific segments of the nephron have been blurred or obscured by those studies based on conventional experimental preparations, such as renal homogenates, slices and microsomes. The application of immunodissection methods and cell separation techniques to isolation of cells from a particular segment of the nephron has resulted in important discoveries concerning arachidonic acid metabolism in these segments[1,2]. There are two sites within the nephron of commanding interest as they are critical to the regulation of extracellular fluid volume and exhibit unique mechanisms involving arachidonic acid metabolites, one in the medullary segment of the thick ascending limb of the loop of Henle (mTALH), the other in the collecting ducts. Segmental distribution of the different pathways of arachidonic acid metabolism, including prostaglandin generation, corresponds to selective sites of hormonal stimulation within the nephron. Morel has shown that the nephron is segmented relative to the capacity of hormones to affect transport processes and that this selectivity is linked to receptor-mediated stimulation of adenylate cyclase for a particular cell type, such as those of the mTALH and the cortical collecting ducts[29]. Whether or not an arachidonic acid metabolite is involved in the cellular response to peptide hormones within all or most segments of the nephron remains to be established. The evidence is firmest for the cells of the collecting ducts where the effects of kinins and arginine vasopressin (AVP) have been shown to result from interactions with prostaglandins[30]. In the mTALH, recent studies suggest that peptide hormones stimulate arachidonic acid metabolism via a cytochrome P450-dependent mechanism[1]. Several metabolites of arachidonic acid have been identified in mTALH which can affect transport in this segment of the nephron as well as dilate blood vessels and can be stimulated by AVP[31].

The initial studies of Grantham and Orloff on modulation of the hydro-osmotic action of AVP by prostaglandins of the E series[32] have been extended by Smith and his associates to include AVP-prostanoids and prostanoid–prostanoid interactions which differ depending on the side of the cell; viz, urinary compartment or vascular-interstitial compartment[30]. In addition, the presence of kinins generated by kininogenases released from the distal convoluted tubules can affect the response to AVP in the collecting ducts probably through a prostaglandin-related effect[33]. Further, arachidonic acid metabolites arising from non-cyclo-oxygenase pathways in response to stimulation by AVP in the mTALH, probably determine the tonicity of the medulla and thereby the hydro-osmotic effect of AVP in the collecting tubules[31]. As the mTALH establishes the solute gradient on which the hydro-osmotic action of AVP depends, regulation of transport function in mTALH by arachidonate metabolites presumably determines the effect of AVP on water absorption in the collecting ducts. Further, there is evidence that AVP can affect mTALH transport function and, thereby, influence its final effect on water movement in the distal tubules. The interactions of arachidonate metabolites with AVP at several levels in the nephron are complemented by those existing extrarenally, and together constitute a hormonal system

20

demonstrating a multiplicity of check points which co-operate to achieve a final effect – viz, the regulation of extracellular fluid volume.

Before examining peptide–eicosanoid interactions in mTALH, a general statement regarding the effects of eicosanoids on the activity of peptide hormones is in order. The concept that prostaglandins and other arachidonate metabolites act locally as either modulators or mediators of peptide hormones and neurotransmitters aids in understanding the multiple and overlapping spheres of biological activity and diverse effects of products of arachidonic acid metabolism[34]. For example, peptide-induced formation of prostaglandins by blood vessels[35] results in changes in the intensity and range of the vascular effects of the peptide. This is accomplished in several ways: by modulating or mediating some of the peptide's effects and by regulating release/activation of proteases – kallikrein and renin – responsible for liberating vasoactive peptides, angiotensin and kinins from inactive substrate. Thus, a prostaglandin-dependent mechanism is intimately related to regulating renin release[36], and, perhaps, kallikrein release[37]. The synchronization and integration of hormonal systems in various target organs and tissues are related to prostaglandin-dependent mechanisms, particularly under conditions of stress and disease. The network of ADH-prostaglandin interrelationships reflects the importance of eicosanoids to the integrated actions of peptide hormones. A system of great complexity and multiple control points is disclosed, one that facilitates expression of the action of the peptide hormone in terms of homoeostasis. At each control point, ADH can interact with either prostaglandins or other arachidonic acid metabolites which affect the activity of the peptide. Products of the arachidonic acid cascade arising from cyclo-oxygenase may either augment (TxA_2)[38] or attenuate (PGE_2)[32] ADH-dependent water flow. A prostaglandin-related mechanism participates in the regulation of ADH release from the posterior pituitary[39]. Additional interactions involving ADH and arachidonic acid metabolites are those on the systemic vasculature[40], on redistribution of renal blood flow to juxtamedullary nephrons[41] and on sodium excretion[42], in addition to negative feedback control of ADH-mediated permeability changes in the collecting ducts[32].

CYTOCHROME P450-RELATED METABOLISM OF ARACHIDONIC ACID

The above digression on the far-reaching implications of peptide hormone–eicosanoid interactions is a prelude to examination of an AVP–eicosanoid interaction, localized to a segment of the nephron, the mTALH, of overriding importance to the regulation of extracellular fluid volume[43] and the activity of AVP. The mTALH has been shown to possess negligible cyclo-oxygenase activity in agreement with other studies[4,30], although this segment avidly metabolizes arachidonic acid to novel products. The biochemical pathway in mTALH which oxygenates arachidonic acid has been identified as a cyto-chrome P450 species and is stimulated by AVP. Although the hepatic cytochrome P450 system is well characterized, less is known concerning the renal cytochrome P450 system. The renal content of the components of

21

the cytochrome P450-dependent, mixed-function oxidase system has been measured, and, in most species studied, it was found to be small compared with this system in the liver[44]. The highest levels of cytochrome P450 and the components of this system were present in the renal cortex[45]. Since cytochrome P450 exists in multiple forms[46], the predominance of one of these reactions over the other may be controlled by the isoenzyme composition of each tissue or cell type. Furthermore, a particular form may be detected only after its induction with a specific drug.

Two arachidonate metabolites generated by a cytochrome P450-dependent mono-oxygenase and released from isolated mTALH cells (Figure 2.2) possess important biological effects. One of these novel products inhibits Na^+-K^+-ATPase activity, and the other relaxes blood vessels, each in $nmol\,L^{-1}$ concentrations. As the mTALH has one of the highest concentrations in mammalian tissues of the enzyme, Na^+-K^+-ATPase, which drives active sodium transport, natural substances which have the capacity to influence segmental renal tubular transport function and the contiguous medullary microcirculation, are of the greatest importance to understanding renal regulatory mechanisms.

If, as appears to be the case for most arachidonate metabolites, the microenvironment of the cell of origin is the principal site of their activity and their degradation occurs rapidly within this restricted area, then establishing the

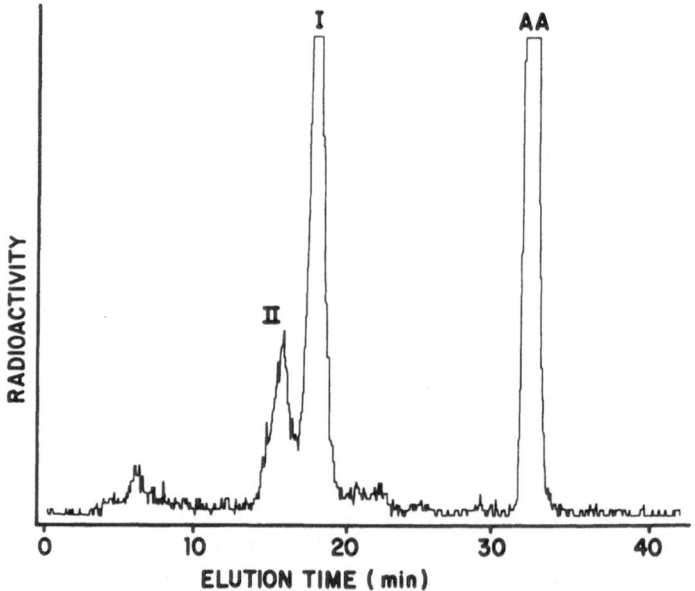

Figure 2.2 Separation by reverse-phase high-performance liquid chromatography of ^{14}C-labelled oxygenated metabolites of arachidonic acid (AA). Medullary thick ascending loop of Henle cells ($3 \times 10^6\,cell\,ml^{-1}$) were incubated with $[^{14}C]AA$ for 45 min. Cells were removed by centrifugation and the media extracted. Arachidonic acid metabolites were separated on a Bondapak C_{18} microcolumn, using a linear solvent gradient ranging from water:acetonitrile (1:1, containing 0.1% acetic acid); the rate of change was 1.25% per min at a flow rate of 1 ml min^{-1}. Radioactivity was monitored continuously using a radioactive flow detector

structural identity and precise physiological role of these products will be a difficult task. Ferreri *et al.* first reported on the presence of a cytochrome P450-dependent mono-oxygenase in mTALH cells having a preference for arachidonic acid as substrate[1]. Isolated cells were selected for study as they allow characterization of transport processes and biochemical pathways in the absence of complicating factors. Moreover, a relatively homogeneous population of intact cells was required as hormonal responsiveness of a specific nephron segment was deemed essential to this study, and biochemical pathways and products that require intact cells for their demonstration might have been overlooked if homogenates or subcellular fractions had been used. A suspension of outer medullary cells obtained from the rabbit kidney was separated into several fractions by centrifugal elutriation. Two cell fractions were prepared, one enriched with mTALH cells and the residue, outer medullary cells depleted of TALH cells. In the enriched fraction, 80% of the cells were mTALH based on histochemical, morphological and biochemical criteria:

(1) A two- to three-fold increase in Na^+-K^+-ATPase activity, a non-specific marker; a three-fold reduction in a negative marker, alkaline phosphatase identified with proximal tubular cells; and immuno-fluorescent localization of Tamm–Horsfall protein, a specific marker for mTALH cells.

(2) Electron microscopic criteria established that approximately 80% of these cells were mTALH in origin.

(3) These cells responded only to those hormones, AVP and salmon calcitonin (SCT), which have been reported to increase adenylate cyclase activity in this segment of the nephron[29].

Incubation of mTALH cells with ^{14}C-labelled arachidonic acid resulted in formation of oxygenated metabolites separated into peaks I and II by reverse-phase chromatography (Figure 2.2). The metabolites accounted for 30 to 40% of the recovered radioactivity and their formation was not affected by indomethacin. These products of arachidonate metabolism were considered to arise from a cytochrome P450-related mono-oxygenase based on the following findings:

(1) They did not demonstrate UV absorbance at 234 nm and 276 nm, indicating the absence of a conjugated diene or triene structure, respectively.

(2) Generation of the metabolites by cell-free homogenates of mTALH was dependent on the presence of NADPH.

(3) SKF-525A and carbon monoxide inhibited their formation.

(4) The metabolites recovered from peaks I and II had different retention times on reverse-phase HPLC from arachidonic acid products formed by lipoxygenases.

(5) Induction of cytochrome P450 with 3-methylcholanthrene and β-naphthoflavone increased formation of the products.

23

AVP and SCT stimulated arachidonic acid metabolism in mTALH cells prelabelled with [^{14}C]arachidonic acid (Figure 2.3). The concentrations of AVP and SCT that stimulated arachidonic acid metabolism via cytochrome P450-dependent mono-oxygenase in mTALH corresponded to those concentrations that stimulated adenylate cyclase activity in this nephron segment[29]. Moreover, the phosphodiesterase inhibitor 1-isobutyl 3-methylxanthine (IBMX) (10 μmol L^{-1}), increased formation of peaks I and II two-fold as did dibutyryl cyclic AMP (1 nmol L^{-1}). Bradykinin and angiotensin II, only at concentrations two to three orders of magnitude greater than AVP and SCT, increased formation of the arachidonic acid metabolites and then only minimally. Further, parathormone and isoproterenol, which do not affect adenylate cyclase in this nephron segment[29], did not increase arachidonic acid metabolism by mTALH. This study, when considered in the light of those of Morel and associates[29], indicates that adenylate cyclase in mTALH transduces the hormonal signal elicited by either AVP or SCT after formation of a hormone-receptor complex. Then cyclic AMP acts as a second messenger to initiate the events leading to arachidonic acid product formation.

ARACHIDONATE METABOLITES: MODULATORS OF Na$^+$-K$^+$-ATPase?

The major arachidonate metabolites generated by mTALH have been designated as peaks I and II based on reverse phase HPLC separation (Figure 2.2). Fractions containing peaks I and II were collected separately and tested

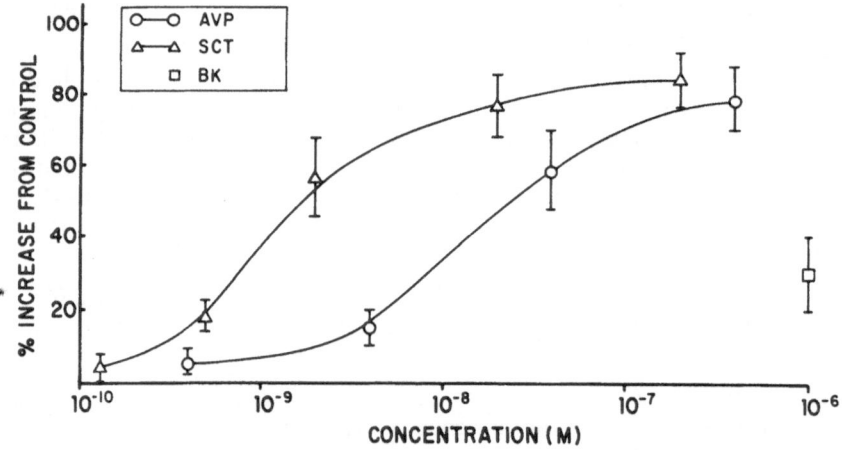

Figure 2.3 Hormonal stimulation of arachidonic acid (AA) metabolism by medullary thick ascending loop of Henle cells prelabelled with [^{14}C]AA (0.4 μCi per 3 × 10^6 cells for 90 min at 37°C). Following incubation with AVP (O, 4 × 10^{-10} to 4 × 10^{-7} mol L^{-1}), SCT ($\triangle$, 10^{-10} to 2 × 10^{-7} mol/L) and bradykinin ($\square$, 10^{-6} mol L^{-1}), the AA metabolites were separated by thin-layer chromatography. Radioactive zones corresponding to P$_1$ and P$_2$ were cut and counted using a liquid scintillation counter. The percentage increase in the formation of P$_1$ and P$_2$ above the unstimulated control value was plotted. The means ± SEM for four experiments are shown

for their ability to inhibit Na^+-K^+-ATPase, using a purified microsomal preparation from the canine heart[31]. Arachidonic acid metabolites recovered from the more polar peak, peak II, inhibited Na^+-K^+-ATPase activity in a dose-dependent fashion, whereas peak I contained far less inhibitory activity. In contrast, arachidonic acid metabolites associated with peak I relaxed precontracted rabbit pulmonary arteries in low, $nmol\,L^{-1}$, concentrations, whereas peak II, containing high Na^+-K^+-ATPase inhibitory activity, was devoid of vasoactivity.

Based on these findings, one can conclude that arachidonic acid metabolism in mTALH via the cytochrome P450-dependent pathway is stimulated by either AVP or SCT via an adenylate cyclase-coupled receptor. Moreover, one or more of the arachidonic acid metabolites formed modulate Na^+-K^+-ATPase activity and thereby contribute to the regulation of extracellular fluid volume. A factor which diminishes the activity of Na^+-K^+-ATPase in the mTALH has been postulated to account for exaggerated natriuresis in response to volume expansion in hypertension[47].

An endogenous modulator of Na^+-K^+-ATPase activity has long been sought[48]. Previous studies based on this hypothesis have focused on a **circulating factor** of low molecular weight having the capacity to displace digitalis-like compounds from binding sites on cell membranes[49]. The factor is thought to be synthesized within the central nervous system from which it is released in response to expansion of extracellular fluid volume. An important feature of the putative circulating Na^+-K^+-ATPase inhibitor is its capacity to elevate blood pressure consequent to increasing intracellular sodium which affects calcium binding and results in elevated intracellular free calcium concentration[50]. The latter is the final common pathway mediating enhanced reactivity of vascular smooth muscle as well as promoting increased secretory activity of many tissues, including autonomic nerves. On the other hand, the studies on mTALH have addressed potential regulators of Na^+-K^+-ATPase and local blood flow **generated within the target tissue**. Transporting epithelia, those of the mTALH[1] and cornea[51], have been studied thus far. These novel arachidonate metabolites, formed by a cytochrome P450 mono-oxygenase pathway, may link epithelial Na^+-K^+-ATPase activity to changes in local blood flow, and, thereby, couple a metabolic event to regulation of regional blood flow.

Cytochrome P450 dependent arachidonate metabolism has been designated the third pathway[52], assuming that the several lipoxygenases represent the second pathway and cyclo-oxygenase the first. The cytochrome P450-dependent metabolic pathway in the mTALH which is highly selective in responding to circulating hormones also demonstrates large changes in product formation when challenged by either elevated blood pressure or increased salt intake[53]. These findings may provide answers and future directions to major questions that have been raised by physiologists regarding regulation of the activity of Na^+-K^+-ATPase in the short term, i.e. Na^+-K^+-ATPase can participate in rapid adjustments of transport processes[48]. In addition, abnormalities of Na^+-K^+-ATPase activity have been described in essential hypertension[49] as well as in experimental hypertension[47], i.e. a reduction in the reabsorptive capacity of the TALH has been found and has been proposed to be an early lesion in hypertension[54]. An endogenous inhibitor of sodium transport operating in this segment of the nephron and affected by AVP has been postulated by Fejes-Toth and Szenasi[55]. Moreover, AVP stimulates adenylate cyclase activity in the mTALH and the dibutyryl analogue of cyclic AMP also stimulates arachidonic acid metabolism in this segment[31], suggesting that the effects of AVP on cytochrome P450-dependent arachidonic acid metabolism in mTALH requires a receptor linked to an adenylate cyclase step.

The flux of arachidonic acid through the mTALH can be manipulated by induction or depletion of cytochrome P450 in this zone of the kidney, the outer medulla. Zonal stratification of arachidonic acid metabolism within the kidney by the cytochrome P450-dependent mono-oxygenase has received support from a recent study[44]. In this study, because of quantitative limitations of cell separation techniques, microsomes were used rather than separated cells in order to answer questions concerning regional and zonal differences in cytochrome P450-dependent oxygenation of arachidonic acid. Microsomes were obtained from the three major renal zones: cortex, outer medulla and inner medulla, and the following questions were posed:

(1) As the content of cytochrome P450 can be altered in either direction intrarenally, is this associated with corresponding changes in mono-oxygenase activity?
(2) If so, are there associated changes in arachidonic acid metabolism?
(3) Are the changes in arachidonic acid metabolism reflected to a greater degree in a particular region within the kidney?
(4) Do changes in arachidonic acid metabolism within the outer medulla correspond to those in the mTALH?

The renal content of cytochrome P450 was increased by treatment with 3-methylcholanthrene and β-napthoflavone and decreased by treatment with cobalt. Cobalt stimulates haeme oxygenase resulting in accelerated degradation of haeme and reduction of cytochrome P450, a haemoprotein. The outer medulla displayed an exceedingly high rate of haeme oxygenase activity. The kidney, therefore, must be considered another site for haeme degradation in addition to the liver which is well known for prominent haeme degradative activity. Microsomes, obtained from the three major zones, were incubated with arachidonic acid, indomethacin and an NADPH-generating system. Arachidonic acid product formation was inhibited by SKF-525A. Determination of changes in cytochrome P450 function was assessed by measuring aryl hydrocarbon hydroxylase activity (expressed in terms of hydroxylation of benzo-(a)-pyrene). Under control conditions, aryl hydroxylase activity was detectable in all zones of the kidney, activity ranging from 3 to 10% of that of the liver. This activity was increased and decreased proportionately to those directional changes in cytochrome P450 content produced by 3-methylcholanthrene together with β-napthoflavone and by cobalt. For example, the decrease in hepatic and renal cytochrome P450 produced by cobalt treatment was accompanied by a substantial decrease in aryl hydrocarbon hydroxylase activity in the liver and kidney. Thus, mixed-function oxidase activity can be manipulated by changing the tissue content of cytochrome P450 intrarenally. This observation substantiates the finding on the presence and induction of cytochrome P450 in the inner stripe of the outer medulla. Perturbations in cytochrome P450 systems were also reflected in arachidonic acid metabolism by mTALH cells. Arachidonic acid conversion by mTALH cells via cytochrome P450 systems was increased by 3-methylcholanthrene and β-napthoflavone treatment and decreased by cobalt treatment.

Thus, changing the cytochrome P450 content results in corresponding alterations in cytochrome P450-dependent mono-oxygenase activity and associated changes in arachidonic acid metabolism expressed either in renal microsomes or in the cells separated from the medullary portion of the thick ascending limb of the loop of Henle (mTALH). The finding that outer medullary cytochrome P450 isoenzyme(s)-specific activity directed towards arachidonic acid metabolism is much higher than that observed in the liver is important in terms of the potential contribution of these arachidonic acid metabolites to renal function. The cytochrome P450 species that is specific for arachidonic acid metabolism appears to predominate in the kidney, an interpretation based on the comparison of the capacities of liver and kidney for the metabolism of arachidonic acid by cytochrome P450-dependent enzymes. Moreover, the highest concentration of this cytochrome P450 species is present in the inner stripe of the outer medulla, the zone from which TALH cells are isolated. The outer medullary microsomes converted arachidonic acid in the presence of NADPH mainly via ω and ω-1 hydroxylation pathways to form the 20- and 19-hydroxyeicosatetraenoic acids. This is in agreement with the results reported by other investigators[56,57]. In addition, renal microsomes possess epoxygenase activity as well as epoxide hydrolase activity, and, thereby, can convert arachidonic acid into epoxides and diols. The epoxides of arachidonic acid have been shown to stimulate secretion of hormones and to inhibit chloride transport[58,59].

The following conclusions regarding metabolism of arachidonic acid by renal cytochrome P450-linked oxygenase can be made:

(1)   The highest concentration of the cytochrome P450 species which metabolizes arachidonic acid is present in the outer medulla, i.e. the zone from which mTALH cells are obtained.
(2)   The flux of arachidonic acid can be controlled by changing the levels of cytochrome P450.
(3)   Arachidonate metabolites of this pathway probably contribute to the regulation of renal transport function and to local renal circulatory changes.

PROSTAGLANDIN-RELATED RELEASE OF KALLIKREIN AND RENIN

The initial description of biological activities of arachidonic acid metabolites arising from cytochrome P450 mono-oxygenases reveals similarities to prostanoids, i.e. they can act as secretagogues[58] and local modulators of circulating hormones[31] and their principal activity is circumscribed to the microenvironment of the cell of origin. The physiological role of renal prostaglandins, the products of the first pathway, seems established, at least in terms of their acting as local modulators and sometimes as mediators of the activity of the renin–angiotensin and kallikrein–kinin systems, as well as modulators of autonomic nervous activity and circulating hormones, particularly AVP[34]. Generalizations like these, however, ignore the equally important function of prostanoids acting as secretagogues, whereby the initial step in the activation of the systemic or local hormone is regulated by a prostaglandin-dependent mechanism. For example, release of renin[36] and glandular kallikrein[37] from the kidney is under the partial control of prostanoids acting as secretagogues.

Studies on the participation of prostaglandin-dependent mechanisms in regulating kallikrein release are few and only touch upon this event tangentially[60,61]. For example, furosemide causes immediate release of renal kallikrein, as well as renin, and, as the drug-induced effect on renin is related to a prostaglandin-dependent mechanism, it may be inferred that kallikrein release is too[60]. In support of this interpretation is the finding that, in Bartter's syndrome, which is characterized by salt wasting, activation of the renin–angiotensin system and increased excretion of prostaglandins, kallikrein excretion is also elevated and, like the other abnormalities, is corrected by indomethacin treatment[61]. More to the point is the study of Vio et al. which directly addressed the question of whether a prostaglandin-dependent mechanism participates in the regulation of kallikrein release[37]. They showed that arachidonic acid caused a dose-related increase of kallikrein release into the venous effluent of the rat isolated kidney, an effect dependent upon transformation of arachidonic acid to a prostaglandin as it was prevented by indomethacin.

Products of arachidonic acid metabolism particularly via the cyclo-oxygenase pathway, have also been implicated in renin release through their direct effects on juxtaglomerular cells as well as indirectly through macula densa, baroreceptor and β-adrenoreceptor mechanisms of renin release. Studies of arachidonic acid metabolism have shown that the glomerulus possesses both cyclo-oxygenase and lipoxygenase enzymes and may synthesize PGE_2, $PGF_{2\alpha}$ and PGI_2 as well as 5- and 12-HETEs, depending upon the species[62]. Immunocytochemical procedures have localized the cyclo-oxygenase complex in the kidney to vascular endothelial cells, glomerular mesangial cells and epithelial cells of Bowmans capsule[3]. Products of arachidonic acid metabolism via the cyclo-oxygenase pathway were shown to stimulate renin release in vivo and in vitro using renal cortical slices and isolated glomeruli[63,64]. Arachidonic acid, PGE_2 and PGI_2 stimulated renin secretion. The effect of arachidonic acid was blocked by inhibitors of cyclo-oxygenase. Further evidence for a role of prostaglandins in renin release arose from studies with cyclo-oxygenase inhibitors which suppressed stimulated (but not basal) release of renin associated with inhibition of angiotensin converting enzyme[65], furosemide administration[66], salt depletion[67] and Bartter's syndrome[68]. More recently, in vitro studies have indicated that products via the lipoxygenase pathway of arachidonate metabolism inhibit renin release[69] and thereby may provide a tonic control mechanism.

28

A prime candidate for mediating prostaglandin-stimulated renin release is PGI_2^{70}, a major prostanoid in blood vessels of the renal cortex[13]. PGI_2 is degraded intrarenally to a number of metabolites via 15-hydroxyprostaglandin dehydrogenase followed by $\Delta 13,14$-reductase, as well as by β-oxidation[71]. Prostacyclin can also be transformed to a stable metabolite, 6-keto-PGE_1 by the enzyme 9-hydroxyprostaglandin dehydrogenase[72]. This prostanoid is a more potent renin secretagogue than PGI_2, with a greater duration of action which could explain the prolonged renin secretory response to PGI_2 in renal cortical slices[70] (Figure 2.4). Studies have shown that the kidney possesses the enzymic machinery necessary to convert PGI_2 to 6-keto-PGE_1 and, recently, 6-keto-PGE_1 release from the isolated rabbit kidney has been documented[73]. However, a coincident rise in 6-keto-PGE_1 and renin secretion has not been shown.

The role of prostaglandins in renin release mediated by β-adrenergic stimulation, the macula densa or vascular baroreceptors has received considerable attention but results have been conflicting. Available evidence indicates that a prostaglandin mechanism forms an integral part of renin release in response to changes in renal blood flow or perfusion pressure, particularly

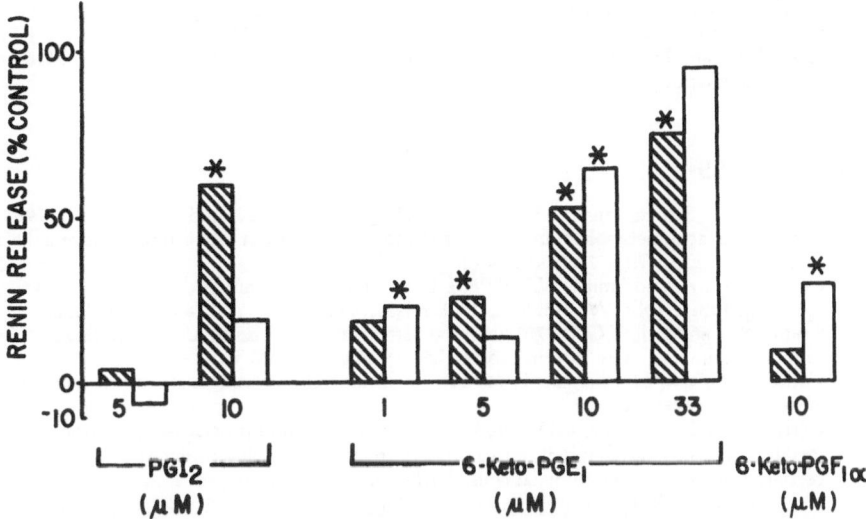

Figure 2.4 Effects of prostacyclin (PGI_2), 6-keto-prostaglandin E_1 (6-keto-PGE_1), and 6-keto-$PGF_{1\alpha}$ on renin release from rabbit renal cortical slices. Renal slices were incubated in Krebs–Ringer solution for four successive 20 min periods (I–IV) and medium was collected for renin assay after each period. Renin release did not increase during periods I–IV in vehicle-treated slices. Prostaglandins were added, only once, at the beginning of period III; the final concentrations achieved are indicated. Between periods III and IV, the incubate was aspirated and replaced with fresh medium after rinsing. Thus, periods I and II indicated basal release, period III agonist-evoked release, and period IV was intended as a recovery period. Renin release during periods III (diagonally hatched columns) and IV (open columns) is expressed as a percentage of the control period II value. Statistical significance was determined by Student's paired t test; $^*p < 0.05$, compared with renin release during the control period; $n = 4$–6 tissue incubations for each test agent

within the autoregulatory range[74]. Moreover, evidence is available to suggest a role for arachidonic acid metabolites in the tubular signal arising from the macula densa to influence renin release[75]. In contrast, a prostaglandin component to adrenergically-stimulated renin release appears to have a permissive role. Thus, PGI_2 has been shown to act synergistically with isoproterenol[76] in stimulating renin release. In this respect, it is of great interest that acetylcholine, in the presence of vascular endothelium, enhances renin release in response to PGE_2, i.e. acetylcholine, which of itself was without effect on renin release, sensitizes the kidney to PGE_2 (personal communication from Dr Beierwaltes). As PGE_2 has been shown to release renin only in the presence of the macula densa, it is of interest that PGE_2 affects sodium chloride reabsorption in the thick ascending limb[77]. Thus, isolated glomeruli show no increase in renin release in response to PGE_2. These results suggest that the inhibitory action of the macula densa on juxtaglomerular cells may be suppressed by PGE_2 resulting in release of renin through removal of an endogenous inhibitor of the renin-releasing mechanism.

ACKNOWLEDGEMENTS

We thank P. Blank, S. Klein and S. McGiff for their help in preparing the manuscript. This work was supported by NYS Health Research Council #HRC D3-035, NIH Grant # R01-HL25394, Program Project Grant # P01-HL34300, and G. Harold and Leila Y. Mathers Charitable Foundation.

REFERENCES

1. Ferreri, N.R., Schwartzman, M., Ibraham, N.G., Chander, P.N. and McGiff, J.C. (1984). Arachidonic acid metabolism in a cell suspension isolated from rabbit renal outer medulla. *J. Pharmacol. Exp. Ther.*, **231**, 441–448
2. Garcia-Perez, A. and Smith, W.L. (1983). Use of monoclonal antibodies to isolate cortical collecting tubule cells: AVP induces PGE release. *Am. J. Physiol.*, **244**, C211–C220
3. Smith, W.L. and Bell, T.G. (1978). Immunohistochemical localization of the prostaglandin-forming cyclooxygenase in renal cortex. *Am. J. Physiol.*, **235**, F451–F457
4. Currie, M.G. and Needleman, P. (1984). Renal arachidonic acid metabolism. *Ann. Rev. Physiol.*, **46**, 327–341
5. Gerritsen, M.E. and Cheli, C.D. (1983). Arachidonic acid and prostaglandin endoperoxide metabolism in isolated rabbit and coronary microvessels and isolated and cultivated coronary microvessel endothelial cells. *J. Clin. Invest.*, **72**, 1658–1671
6. Moncada, S. and Vane, J.R. (1979). Pharmacology and endogenous roles of prostaglandin endoperoxides, thromboxane A_2 and prostacyclin. *Pharmacol. Rev.*, **30**, 293–331
7. Myers, T.O., Messina, E.J., Rodrigues, A.M. and Gerritsen, M.E. (1985). Altered aortic and cremaster muscle prostaglandin synthesis in diabetic rats. *Am. J. Physiol.*, **249**, E374–E379
8. Gerritsen, M.E. and Printz, M.P. (1981). Prostaglandin D synthase in microvessels from the rat cerebral cortex. *Prostaglandins*, **22**, 553–556
9. Tomasi, V., Meringolo, C., Bartolini, G. and Orlandi, M. (1978). Biosynthesis of prostacyclin in rat liver endothelial cells and its control by prostaglandin E_2. *Nature (London)*, **273**, 670–671
10. Larsson, C. and Anggard, E. (1973). Regional differences in the formation and metabolism of prostaglandins in the rabbit kidney. *Eur. J. Pharmacol.*, **21**, 30–36
11. Lonigro, A.J., Itskovitz, H.D., Crowshaw, K. and McGiff, J.C. (1973). Dependency of renal blood flow on prostaglandin synthesis in the dog. *Circ. Res.*, **32**, 712–717

12. Dunn, M.J. and Zambraski, E.J. (1980). Renal effects of drugs that inhibit prostaglandin synthesis. *Kidney Int.*, **18**, 609–622
13. Terragno, N.A., McGiff, J.C. and Terragno, D.A. (1979). Synthesis of prostaglandins by vascular and nonvascular renal tissues and the presence of an endogenous prostaglandin synthesis inhibitor in the cortex. In Vargaftig, B.B. (ed.) *Advances in Pharmacology and Therapeutics.* Vol. 4, pp. 39–46. (Oxford and New York: Pergamon Press)
14. Blasingham, M.C., Shade, R.E., Share, L. and Nasjletti, A. (1980). The effect of meclofenamate on renal blood flow in the unanesthetized dog: relation to renal prostaglandins and sodium balance. *J. Pharmacol. Exp. Ther.*, **214**, 1–4
15. Terragno, N.A., Terragno, D.A. and McGiff, J.C. (1977). Contribution of prostaglandins to the renal circulation in conscious, anesthetized, and laparotomized dogs. *Circ. Res.*, **40**, 590–595
16. Ferreri, N.R., McGiff, J.C., Miller, M.J.S., Schwartzman, M., Spokas, E.G. and Wong, P.Y-K (1983). The kidney and arachidonic acid metabolism. In Samuelsson, B., Paoletti, R. and Ramwell, P. (eds.) *Advances in Prostaglandin, Thromboxane, and Leukotriene Research.* Vol. 11, pp. 481–485. (New York: Raven Press)
17. McGiff, J.C., Crowshaw, K., Terragno, N.A. and Lonigro, A.J. (1970). Renal prostaglandins: possible regulators of the renal actions of pressor hormones. *Nature (London)*, **227**, 1255–1257
18. Itskovitz, H.D., Terragno, N.A. and McGiff, J.C. (1974). Effect of a renal prostaglandin on distribution of blood flow in isolated canine kidney. *Circ. Res.*, **34**, 770–776
19. Itskovitz, H.D. and McGiff, J.C. (1974). Hormonal regulation of the circulation. *Circ. Res.*, **34** and **35** (Suppl. 1) 65–73
20. Anggard, E. and Oliw, E. (1981). Formation and metabolism of prostaglandins in the kidney. *Kidney Int.*, **19**, 771–780
21. Lemley, K.V., Schmitt, S.L., Holliger, C., Dunn, M.J., Robertson, C.R. and Jamison, R.L. (1984). Prostaglandin synthesis inhibitors and vasa recta erythrocyte velocities in the rat. *Am. J. Physiol.*, **247**, F562–F567
22. McGiff, J.C., Itskovitz, H.D. and Terragno, N.A. (1975). The actions of bradykinin and eledoisin in the canine isolated kidney: relationships to prostaglandins. *Clin. Sci. Mol. Med.*, **49**, 125–131
23. McGiff, J.C., Terragno, N.A., Malik, K.U. and Longiro, A.J. (1972). Release of a prostaglandin E-like substance from canine kidney by bradykinin. *Circ. Res.*, **31**, 36–43
24. Colina-Chourio, J., McGiff, J.C., Miller, M.P. and Nasjletti, A. (1976). Possible influence of intrarenal generation of kinins on prostaglandin release from rabbit perfused kidney. *Br. J. Pharmacol.*, **58**, 165–172
25. Abe, Y., Miura, K., Imanishi, M., Yukimura, T., Komori, T., Okahara, T. and Yamamoto, K. (1980). Effects of an orally active converting enzyme inhibitor (YS-980) on renal function in dogs. *J. Pharmacol. Exp. Ther.*, **214**, 166–170
26. Kramer, H.J., Glanzer, K. and Dusing, R. (1981). Role of prostaglandins in the regulation of renal water excretion. *Kidney Int.*, **19**, 851–859
27. Nasjletti, A., McGiff, J.C. and Colina-Chourio, J. (1978). Interrelationships of the renal kallikrein–kinin system and renal prostaglandins in the conscious rat: influence of mineralocorticoids. *Circ. Res.*, **43**, 799–807
28. McGiff, J.C., Itskovitz, H.D., Terragno, A. and Wong, P.Y-K (1976). Modulation and mediation of the action of the renal kallikrein–kinin system by prostaglandins. *Fed. Proc.*, **35**, 175–180
29. Morel, F. (1981). Sites of hormone action in the mammalian nephron. *Am. J. Physiol.*, **240**, F159–F164
30. Smith, W.L. and Garcia-Perez, A. (1980). A two-receptor model for the mechanism of action of prostaglandins in the renal collecting tubule. In Bailey, J.M. (ed.) *Prostaglandins, Leukotrienes, and Lipoxins*, pp. 35–45. (New York and London: Plenum Press)
31. Schwartzman, M., Ferreri, N.R., Carroll, M.A., Songu-Mize, E. and McGiff, J.C. (1985). Renal cytochrome P450-related arachidonate metabolite inhibits (Na^+-K^+)ATPase. *Nature (London)*, **314**, 620–622
32. Grantham, J.J. and Orloff, J. (1968). Effect of prostaglandin E_1 on the permeability response of the isolated collecting tubule to vasopressin, adenosine 3′, 5′-monophosphate, and theophylline. *J. Clin. Invest.*, **47**, 1154–1161

33. Grenier, F.C., Rollins, T.E. and Smith W.L. (1981). Kinin-induced prostaglandin synthesis by renal papillary collecting tubule cells in culture. *Am. J. Physiol.*, **241**, F94–F104
34. McGiff, J.C. (1980). Interactions of prostaglandins with the kallikrein–kinin and renin–angiotensin systems. *Clin. Sci.*, **59**, 105s–116s
35. Terragno, D.A., Crowshaw, K., Terragno, N.A. and McGiff, J.C. (1975). Prostaglandin synthesis by bovine mesenteric arteries and veins. *Circ. Res.*, **36**, 1–76; **37**, 1–80
36. Larsson, C., Weber, P. and Anggard, E. (1974). Arachidonic acid increases and indomethacin decreases plasma renin activity in the rabbit. *Eur. J. Pharmacol.*, **28**, 391–394
37. Vio, C.P., Churchill, L., Terragno, A., McGiff, J.C and Terragno, N.A. (1982). Arachidonic acid stimulates renal kallikrein release in isolated rat kidney. *Clin. Sci.*, **63**, 235s–237s
38. Burch, R.M., Knapp, D.R. and Halushka, P.V. (1980). Vasopressin-stimulated water flow is decreased by thromboxane synthesis inhibition or antagonism. *Am. J. Physiol.*, **239**, F160–F166
39. Yamamoto, M., Share, L. and Shade, R.E. (1976). Vasopressin release during ventriculo-cisternal perfusion with prostaglandin E_2 in the dog. *J. Endocrinol.*, **71**, 325–331
40. Glanzer, K., Prussing, B., Dusing, R. and Kramer, H.J. (1982). Hemodynamic and hormonal responses to 8-arginine-vasopressin in healthy man: effects of indomethacin. *Klin. Wochenschr.*, **60**, 1234–1239
41. Davis, J.M. and Schnermann, J. (1971). The effect of antidiuretic hormone on the distribution of nephron filtration rates in rats with hereditary diabetes insipidus. *Pflugers Arch.*, **330**, 323–334
42. Fejes-Toth, G., Zahajszky, T. and Filep, J. (1980). Effect of vasopressin on renal kallikrein excretion. *Am. J. Physiol.* **239**, F388–F392
43. Jorgensen, P.L. (1980). Sodium and potassium ion pump in kidney tubules. *Physiol. Rev.*, **60**, 864–917
44. Schwartzman, M.L., Abraham, N.G., Carroll, M.A., Levere, R.D. and McGiff, J.C. (1986). Regulation of arachidonic acid metabolism by cytochrome P-450 in rabbit kidney. *Biochem. J.*, **238**, 283–290
45. Zenser, T.V., Mattamal, M.B. and Davis, B.B. (1978). Differential distribution of the mixed-function oxidase activities in rabbit kidney. *J. Pharmacol. Exp. Ther.*, **207**, 719–725
46. Lu, A.Y.H. and West, S.B. (1979). Multiplicity of mammalian microsomal cytochromes P-450. *Pharmacol. Rev.*, **31**, 277–295
47. Postnov, Y.U., Reznikova, M. and Boriskina, G. (1976). Na-K-adenosine triphosphatase in the kidney of rats with renal hypertension and spontaneously hypertensive rats. *Pflugers Arch.*, **362**, 95–99
48. Katz, A.I. (1985). Renal Na-K-ATPase: its role in tubular sodium and potassium transport. *Am. J. Physiol.*, **242**, F207–F219
49. de Wardener, H.E. and Clarkson, E.M. (1985). Concept of natriuretic hormone. *Physiol. Rev.*, **65**, 658–759
50. Blaustein, M.P. (1977). Sodium ions, calcium ions, blood pressure regulation, and hypertension: a reassessment and a hypothesis. *Am. J. Physiol.*, **232**, C165–C173
51. Schwartzman, M.L., Abraham, N.G., Masferrer, J., Dunn, M.W. and McGiff, J.C. (1985). Cytochrome P450-dependent metabolism of arachidonic acid in bovine corneal epithelium. *Biochem. Biophys. Res. Commun.*, **132**, 343–351
52. Schwartzman, M., Carroll, M.A., Ibraham, N.G., Ferreri, N.R., Songu-Mize, E. and McGiff, J.C. (1985). Renal arachidonic acid metabolism; the third pathway. *Hypertension*, **7** (Suppl. 1), 1–136, 1–144
53. Carroll, M.A., Schwartzman, M.A., Abraham, N.G., Pinto, A. and McGiff, J.C. (1986). Cytochrome P450-dependent arachidonate metabolism in renomedullary cells: formation of Na^+-K^+-ATPase inhibitor. *J. Hypertension*, **4** (Suppl. 4), S33–S42
54. Baldwin, D.S., Biggs, A.W., Goldring, W., Hulet, W.H. and Chasis, H. (1985). Exaggerated natriuresis in essential hypertension. *Am. J. Med.*, **24**, 893–902
55. Fejes-Toth, G. and Szenasi, G. (1981). The effect of vasopressin on renal tubular ^{22}Na efflux in the rat. *J. Physiol. (London)*, **318**, 1–7
56. Oliw, E.H. and Oates, J.A. (1981). Rabbit renal cortical microsomes metabolize arachidonic acid to trihydroxyeicosatrienoic acids. *Prostaglandins*, **22**, 863–871
57. Morrison, A. and Pascoe, N. (1981). Metabolism of arachidonate through NADPH-dependent oxygenase of renal cortex. *Proc. Natl. Acad. Sci. USA*, **78**, 7375–7378

58. Capdevila, J., Chacos, N., Falck, J.R., Manna, S., Negro-Vilar, A. and Ojeda, S.R. (1983). Novel hypothalamic arachidonate products stimulate somatostatin release from the median eminence. *Endocrinology*, **113**, 421–423
59. Jacobson, H.R., Corona, S., Capdevila, J., Chacos, N., Manna, S., Womack, A. and Falck, J.R. (1984). Effects of epoxyicosatrienoic acids on ion transport in rabbit cortical collecting tubules. In Braquet, P., Garay, R.P., Frolich, J.C. and Nicosia, S. (eds.) *Prostaglandins and Membrane Ion Transport*, pp. 311–318. (New York: Raven Press)
60. Abe, K., Irokawa, N., Yasujima, M., Seino, M., Chiba, S., Sakurai, Y., Yoshinaga, K. and Saito, T. (1978). The kallikrein–kinin system and prostaglandins in the kidney. *Circ. Res.*, **43**, 254–260
61. Vinci, J.M., Gill, J.R., Bowden, R.E., Pisano, J.J., Izzo, J.L., Radfar, N., Taylor, A.A., Zusman, R.M. and Bartter, F.C. (1978). The kallikrein–kinin system in Bartter's syndrome and its response to prostaglandin synthetase inhibition. *J. Clin. Invest.*, **61**, 1671–1682
62. Morrison, A.R. (1986). Biochemistry and pharmacology of renal arachidonic acid metabolism. *Am. J. Med.*, **80**, 3–11
63. Weber, P.C., Larsson, C., Anggard, E., Hamberg, M., Corey, E.J., Nicolaou, K.C. and Samuelsson, B. (1976). Stimulation of renin release from rabbit renal cortex by arachidonic acid and prostaglandin endoperoxides. *Circ. Res.*, **39**, 868–874
64. Beierwaltes, W.H., Schryver, S., Sanders, E., Strand, J. and Romero, J.C. (1982). Renin release selectively stimulated by prostaglandin I_2 in isolated rat glomeruli. *Am. J. Physiol.*, **243**, F276–F283
65. DeForrest, J.M., Davis, J.O., Freeman, R.H., Seymour, A.A., Rowe, B.P., Williams, G.M. and Davis, T.P. (1980). Effects of indomethacin and meclofenamate on renin release and renal hemodynamic function during chronic sodium depletion in conscious dogs. *Circ. Res.*, **47**, 99–107
66. Frolich, J.C., Hollifield, J.W., Dormois, J.C., Frolich, B.L., Seyberth, H., Michelakis, A.M. and Oates, J.A. (1976). Suppression of plasma renin activity by indomethacin in man. *Circ. Res.*, **39**, 447–452
67. Oates, J.A., Whorton, A.R., Gerkens, J.F., Branch, R.A., Hollifield, J.W. and Frolich, J.C. (1979). The participation of prostaglandins in the control of renin release. *Fed. Proc.*, **38**, 72–74
68. Gill, J.R., Frolich, J.C., Bowden, R.E., Taylor, A.A., Keiser, H.R., Seyberth, H.W., Oates, J.A. and Bartter, F.C. (1976). Bartter's syndrome: a disorder characterized by high urinary prostaglandins and a dependence of hyperreninemia on prostaglandin synthesis. *Am. J. Med.*, **61**, 43–51
69. Antonipillai, I., Robin, E.C., Nadler, J.L. and Horton, R. (1986). Evidence for the inhibitory role of lipoxygenase products in renin release. Presented at the *6th International Conference on Prostaglandins and Related Compounds*, June 3–6, Florence, Italy
70. Whorton, A.R., Misono, K., Hollifield, J., Frolich, J.C., Inagami, T. and Oates, J.A. (1977). Prostaglandins and renin release from rabbit renal cortical slices by PGI_2. *Prostaglandins*, **14**, 1095–1104
71. Wong, P.Y-K, McGiff, J.C., Cagen, L.M., Malik, K.U. and Sun, F.F. (1979). Metabolism of prostacyclin in the rabbit kidney. *J. Biol. Chem.*, **254**, 12–14
72. McGiff, J.C., Spokas, E.C. and Wong, P.Y-K (1982). Stimulation of renin release by 6-oxo-prostaglandin E_1 and prostacyclin. *Br. J. Pharmacol.*, **75**, 137–144
73. Pieroni, J.P., Dray, F. and McGiff, J.C. (1985). Renal production of 6-keto-prostaglandin E_1. *Clin. Res.*, **33**, 496A
74. Blackshear, J.L., Spielman, W.S., Knox, F.G. and Romero, J.C. (1979). Dissociation of renin release and renal vasodilation by prostaglandin synthesis inhibitors. *Am. J. Physiol.*, **237**, F20–F24
75. Schnermann, J. and Weber, P.C. (1982). Reversal of indomethacin-induced inhibition of tubuloglomerular feedback by prostaglandin infusion. *Prostaglandins*, **24**, 341–361
76. Henrich, W.L. and Campbell, W.B. (1984). Relationship between PG and β-adrenergic pathways to renin release in rat renal cortical slices. *Am. J. Physiol.*, **247**, E343–E348
77. Stokes, J.B. (1979). Effect of prostaglandin E_2 on chloride transport across the rabbit thick ascending limb of Henle. *J. Clin. Invest.*, **64**, 495–502

3
Arachidonic acid metabolism in renal disease

S. Lear and V. E. Kelley

INTRODUCTION

Arachidonic acid (AA) metabolites are produced by a variety of renal cells, although the eicosanoid profile varies among different cell types and regions of the kidney. The details of eicosanoid biosynthesis and metabolism are discussed in a preceding chapter. The importance of arachidonic acid metabolites in renal disease has emerged from experimental studies and clinical evaluation of immunologically mediated, as well as non-immune, forms of renal injury. Since arachidonic acid metabolites (eicosanoids), in particular thromboxane (TxA_2), prostacyclin (PGI_2), prostaglandin E_2 (PGE_2) and leukotrienes (LT), can regulate haemodynamic and immunological/inflammatory events, an alteration in the metabolism of any of these molecules can promote or protect the formation of renal injury.

This review will be concerned with two families of AA products called eicosanoids, which are processed by the cyclo-oxygenase and the lipoxygenase enzymes (Figure 3.1), and their role in the pathogenesis of renal disease. Prostaglandins (PG) of the E and F series are especially abundant in the renal medulla and collecting tubules, where they act as autacoids, i.e. local hormones. PG exert diverse actions in the kidney. These metabolites promote water excretion, are natriuretic, stimulate renin release, and modulate renal haemodynamics, both by increasing overall renal blood flow (RBF) and by preferentially increasing blood flow to the inner cortical and medullary regions. In addition, the action of PG is inextricably intertwined with the actions of other hormones and factors on the kidney. Although it is well established that cyclo-oxygenase derivatives of AA are involved in renal pathophysiological states, products of non-cyclo-oxygenase pathways may play a pathogenetic role in human renal disease which is as yet to be elucidated. The first section of this chapter will focus on the effect of endogenous renomedullary PG in the physiology and pathophysiology of salt and water excretion, the role of renal PG in specific kidney disease and pharmacological inhibition of PG.

34

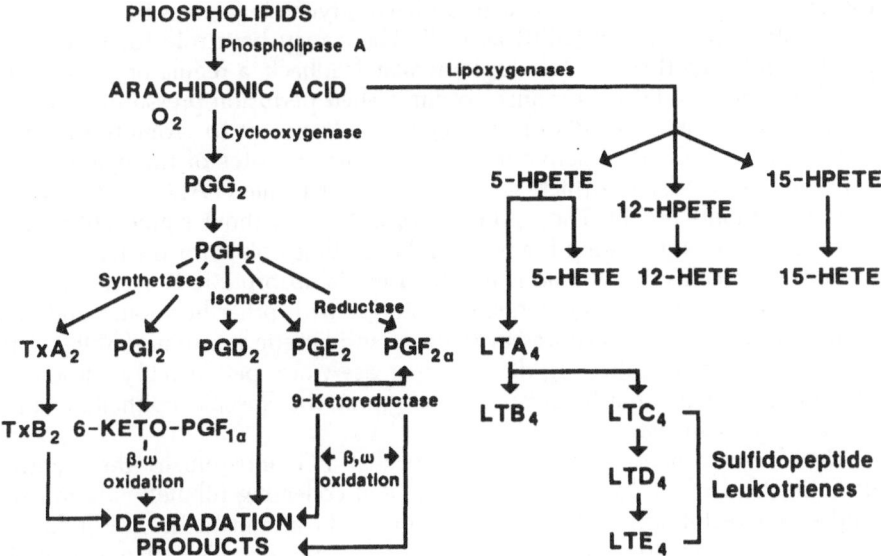

Figure 3.1 Metabolism of arachidonic acid

Increased renal TxA_2 levels have recently been implicated in the inexorable progression of induced and spontaneous experimental models of renal injury and has been documented in several clinical studies of patients with loss of renal function. In the second section of this chapter, we will discuss the role of thromboxane in renal injury, the source of enhanced generation of this metabolite, the rationale and data for using omega-3 fatty acids, found in fish oil, to regulate eicosanoids and protect from autoimmune and cyclosporine-induced renal damage.

THE ROLE OF PG IN THE PATHOPHYSIOLOGY OF RENAL DISEASE

In order to understand the potential for PG involvement in the pathogenesis of renal disease, we will first review the role of PG in renal physiology. The effect of PG on salt homeostasis is the subject of a vast literature. Although the role of PG in the promotion of salt and water excretion has been well established in the mammalian kidney, whole animal and human studies have not produced a clear picture of the effect of PG in renal regulation of total body salt and water homeostasis. Acute and chronic salt loading in mammals, including man, has been associated with[1] decreased, increased or unchanged urinary excretion of PGE_2 (an index of renal PG metabolism)[2]. However, studies on isolated renal tubular epithelia have provided a means of understanding the significance of PG in renal pathophysiology.

Vasodilatory prostanoids tend to promote renal salt and water excretion. The natriuretic effect of PG is in part related to their positive influence on

35

RBF, but is not solely dependent upon haemodynamic factors. PG modulate glomerular filtration rate (GFR) as well. There may be a role for enhanced prostaglandin synthesis in tubuloglomerular feedback, a regulatory response which preserves GFR in response to diminished perfusion pressures. Finally, there is a direct effect of PG on transepithelial transport to promote salt and water diuresis. PG affect active ion transport in two sites of the mammalian nephron, specifically the thick ascending limb of Henle (TALH) and cortical collecting tubule (CCT). The TALH absorbs NaCl without significant water absorption, thereby diluting the urine and providing solute for the hypertonic medulla. The collecting tubule is involved in Na absorption, K secretion and water handling. In both segments, PG interact with other hormones and are known to antagonize vasopressin (VP) or antidiuretic hormone (ADH). VP acts on mammalian collecting ducts to increase water permeability, although the precise cellular mechanisms depend upon the specific epithelium and require further investigation.

Orloff and others first demonstrated that PG antagonizes the hydro-osmotic effect of VP in the toad bladder[3] and collecting tubule[4]. Subsequent studies suggest that, while prostanoid products attenuate the VP-induced decrease in water flow in amphibian tissues[5-7] and a variety of mammalian collecting tubule preparations[8,9], TxA_2 and similar compounds act as positive mediators of VP-stimulated water flow in the toad bladder[10,11]. In addition, the vasopressin effect is enhanced by inhibitors of prostaglandin synthesis (although there is debate as to the exact mechanism of this effect). Micropuncture studies[12] show that PG inhibition of electrogenic Na reabsorption in cortical collecting tubule is mediated by VP. In the outer medullary and papillary collecting duct, Na transport is also inhibited by PG[13,14].

The interaction of PG and VP may ultimately affect water excretion in several ways: regulation of hydraulic conductivity of the cortical collecting tubule, maintenance of the hypertonic milieu of the renal medulla, regulation of medullary blood flow, and modulation of biosynthesis of arachidonic acid metabolites. It has been suggested that the enhanced effect of VP seen with PG inhibition is a result of an increase in medullary tonicity, which contributes to a decrease in free water clearance. Inhibitors of PG synthesis enhance medullary tonicity by increasing interstitial Na or urea content[15-18]. Enhanced water reabsorption, caused by inhibitors of PG synthesis, occurs even in the absence of VP. Cyclo-oxygenase inhibitors increase urine osmolality and papillary solute concentration in the Brattleboro rat, a strain in which antidiuretic hormone is genetically absent[19]. PG, alone and with VP, regulate medullary blood flow, which in turn determines medullary solute content[20,21].

VP has a stimulatory effect on prostaglandin production in toad bladder[22,23], cultured renomedullary interstitial cells[24], isolated CCT[25], and the Brattleboro rat[26-28]. A negative feedback loop between VP and PG has been hypothesized[29], but is not well established in all species studied. In toad bladder epithelium, for example, VP stimulates PG production by activation of phospholipase in a cAMP-independent manner; the resultant increase in PG leads to inhibition of the hydro-osmotic effect of VP. A second negative feedback loop of cAMP-induced inhibition of prostaglandin synthesis may be present.

There is evidence that prostaglandins serve as endogenous modulators of active Cl reabsorption in the medullary TALH (mTALH). The data concerning the effect of PGE_2 in isolated perfused tubules of rabbit medullary TALH have been conflicting. Whereas Stokes demonstrated a reduction in transepithelial voltage (Vt), an index of net NaCl absorption, and net Cl efflux in the mTALH of rabbits[30], Fine and Trizna[31] showed no change in transepithelial PD and Na flux in the presence of high and low concentrations of several PG, including PGE_2. However, the latter experiments used plasma as the bathing solution. In cells isolated from rabbit mTALH, PGE_2 caused a dose-dependent inhibition of ouabain-sensitive (transport-dependent) oxygen consumption[32].

In contrast to rabbit mTALH, there is no effect of PGE_2 on spontaneous Vt or net Cl absorption in mouse mTALH[33]. NaCl absorption in mouse and rat mTALH is mediated by vasopressin as well as other hormones, such as glucagon. Unlike the rabbit mTALH, NaCl transport in mouse mTALH can be stimulated by VP, which acts through the second messenger, cAMP. In isolated perfused mouse mTALH, there is a dose-dependent inhibitory effect of PGE_2 on VP stimulation of Cl transport and Vt, although PGE_2 had no effect on the vasopressin-independent moiety of Vt. Further investigation revealed that PGE_2 exerts its inhibitory effect on or near the guanine nucleotide regulatory subunit of adenylate cyclase[34].

Renal prostanoids act via different cellular mechanisms depending upon the target cell. Prostaglandins interact with cyclic nucleotides in their modulation of renin release and hormone-sensitive water and electrolyte excretion. Glomerular adenylate cyclase is stimulated by PG to release renin[35,36]. The interaction between PG and VP is also mediated by cAMP in two nephron segments involved in salt and water excretion, the collecting duct and the TALH, where there is VP-sensitive adenylate cyclase. PG prevent VP-mediated stimulation of adenylate cyclase in rat mTALH[37] and toad bladder[4,38]. However, the precise nature of the interaction of PG, VP and cAMP in the collecting duct is somewhat confounded by methodological differences, including the use of preparations which contain more than one cell type. The use of isolated tubule segments and cultured cells has obviated one problem, but there is still no consensus on the interaction of PG, VP and cAMP in collecting duct. The original hypothesis[3] that PGE_2 antagonizes the VP-stimulated increase in cAMP production in isolated collecting duct has met with opposition. In primary culture of rat papillary collecting duct, AA and PGE_2 did not decrease VP-sensitive cAMP production[39]; the lack of PGE_2 effect was substantiated by other investigators[40,41]. On the other hand, PGE_2 inhibited vasopressin-dependent cAMP accumulation, but only at high concentrations (10 micromolar)[42]. Enhancement of VP-stimulated adenyl cyclase in collecting duct exposed to cyclo-oxygenase inhibitors was found[43,44]. PGE_2 suppressed VP-stimulated increases in cAMP in cortical collecting duct, but only in the absence of phosphodiesterase inhibition[37]. In addition, intracellular calcium may play a role in the interaction between VP and PG, independent of cAMP. VP and PG affect calcium fluxes in toad bladder, such that PGE increases certain pools of intracellular calcium[45]. The influence of prostaglandins on cellular levels of calcium requires further investigation.

37

A variety of endogenous factors influence PG metabolism through regulation of phospholipase A_2 (PLA_2) activity, which in turn governs AA release. Humoral stimulators of PLA_2 include angiotensin II[28,46], bradykinin[46,47], VP[48] and norepinephrine[49-51]; calcium[52], hypertonicity[52] and trauma[53] can enhance PLA_2 activity. Urea[52,54], cAMP[55], hyperkalemia[56] and glucocorticoids[57] can inhibit PLA_2 activity. In addition, ureteral and renal venous obstruction have been shown to stimulate cyclo-oxygenase[58-60].

Recent studies from several laboratories show that metabolites of the lipoxygenase pathway inhibit active sodium transport in renal epithelia[61], including inhibition of Na–K-ATPase in mTALH[62,63]. The pathophysiological significance of these inhibitors is the subject of intensified investigation.

RENAL EICOSANOIDS IN DISEASE

Hypertension

Prostaglandins have been studied extensively with respect to their role in the pathophysiology of systemic hypertension, as have other, non-prostanoid metabolites of AA. The role of PG in essential hypertension is the subject of several reviews[64,65]. The precise pathophysiological mechanisms which lead to the development of essential hypertension are still unknown. Renal PG, in multiple and complex interactions with renal kallikreins and kinins, contribute to the regulation of renal blood flow, renin release and salt handling, all factors which influence blood pressure. PG regulate the release of several circulating vasoconstrictors. PG stimulates kallikrein and renin, and products of these two systems in turn stimulate PG production in a positive feedback fashion. Kallikrein metabolites, like prostaglandins, increase RBF and are natriuretic. Most studies suggest that basal urinary kallikrein and possibly kinin excretion are reduced in essential hypertension, although there is not universal agreement on this point. It is generally accepted that urinary kallikrein excretion is increased in most patients with secondary hypertension due to primary hyperaldosteronism[66-68]. Through their influence on renin release, and possibly an independent effect on angiotensin, PG affect aldosterone secretion.

It is hypothesized that vasodilatory PG exert an action on systemic and renal vascular tone, so that a deficiency of PG would contribute to high blood pressure and may even be the fundamental abnormality. Reduction of urinary PGE_2 excretion has been noted in human essential hypertension[69-74]. Studies of experimental hypertension in rats suggest that renal prostaglandin synthesis is increased[64]. The use of PG as antihypertensive therapy in man has not proved tenable, although the intravenous administration of PGA_2 and PGI_2 effectively lowered blood pressure in limited, experimental settings[75-79]. Inhibition of PG synthesis with non-steroidal anti-inflammatory drugs (NSAID) has little or no effect on normal blood pressure (reviewed in ref. 64). However, NSAID cause elevations in blood pressure in the setting of pre-existing hypertension or after administration of vasoconstrictor agents (reviewed in ref. 64).

Acute renal failure

There are several potential mechanisms of PG involvement in the pathogenesis of acute renal failure (ARF). Vascular factors are pre-eminent in the initiation and maintenance of acute renal failure. These include control of RBF, autoregulation, tubuloglomerular feedback, the glomerular capillary ultrafiltration coefficient (Kf), the 'no-reflow' phenomenon (which is secondary to capillary endothelial injury and swelling), the renin–angiotensin system and endogenous vasoconstrictors (e.g. catecholamines).

A decrease in prostaglandin synthesis during ARF was shown in early studies[80–83]. In both haemodynamic (glycerol)[80,83] and nephrotoxic (mercuric chloride)[82] rabbit models of ARF, whole kidney PGE_2 levels were increased. There is also evidence for a protective effect of PGE_2 in haemodynamically mediated (norepinephrine-induced) ARF[84]. Furosemide, which stimulates prostaglandin production[70,85,86], has a protective effect on renal function in some models of ARF if administered prophylactically[87,88], whereas it is of no benefit in nephrotoxic models[89,90]. The beneficial effect may depend upon a combination of factors, including increased solute excretion and vasodilation; however, furosemide action at other nephron and vascular sites may explain this salutary effect.

Enhanced thromboxane synthesis, which would have a vasoconstrictor effect, has been demonstrated in some models of ARF[70], although its potential in human disease has not been fully explored.

ARF associated with the use of non-steroidal anti-inflammatory drugs will be discussed below under pharmacologic inhibition of prostaglandin synthesis.

Chronic renal failure

Urinary PGE_2 levels have been reported to be high, normal and low in patients with chronic renal failure (CRF)[83,91,92]. However, inhibition of prostaglandin with non-steroidal anti-inflammatory drugs in humans with chronic renal insufficiency of various aetiologies results in a significant decline in RBF and GFR[93–98], suggesting that endogenous prostanoids may be important in sustaining renal function. More dramatic effects of NSAID on GFR are noted in cases of primary glomerular[96–100], rather than tubulointerstitial[98,101], disease. Thus AA metabolites may be beneficial in the maintenance of renal function where there is pre-existing renal compromise.

Obstructive uropathy

Changes in the pattern of prostanoid production during obstructive uropathy affect renal function primarily through alterations in renal haemodynamics. In general, enhanced biosynthesis of vasodilatory prostanoids occurs with acute obstruction, while increases in thromboxane synthesis prevail in the later stages. The role of eicosanoids in obstruction will be discussed in detail below.

Bartter's syndrome

Bartter and associates[102] described a rare and often familial syndrome characterized by hypokalaemia, renal potassium wasting, chloride-resistant metabolic alkalosis, increase in plasma angiotensin II and urinary aldosterone, and hyperreninaemia, in the absence of oedema and hypertension. The associated histopathological lesion, hyperplasia of the JGA, is not pathognomonic. Increased urinary excretion of PG occurs frequently[100,103–107], but not invariably[108]. Urinary kallikrein excretion is highly correlated with the increase in PGE_2 excretion[51,109].

The primary pathogenetic mechanism of Bartter's syndrome is still unresolved. There is considerable evidence in support of the hypothesis that an overproduction of renal prostaglandins is the underlying abnormality[106,107,110–113]. Treatment with inhibitors of prostaglandin synthesis has proven beneficial in many[100,105–107,110,114], but not all, cases. PG synthesis inhibitors generally fail to reverse the potassium wasting[100,112]. Other states of potassium depletion have also been associated with increased PGE_2[115,116]. In addition, renomedullary interstitial cells, cultured from rabbit, show enhanced PGE_2 production when potassium is removed from the medium. In sum, the evidence points to prostaglandin excess as a secondary phenomenon.

An alternative theory which has received recent support proposes that impaired NaCl reabsorption, probably in the distal nephron, is the primary abnormality[117,118]. A defect in active chloride reabsorption in the TALH has been postulated[119,120], with a resultant increase in distal solute delivery which would promote potassium secretion. The resultant potassium depletion and hypokalaemia would enhance renal PG production, thereby stimulating renin and aldosterone secretion (which would further augment potassium losses) as well as bradykinin and kallikreins (which together with PG tend to reduce the vascular sensitivity to angiotensin and permit a normal systemic blood pressure). Volume depletion due to urinary salt loss would also activate the renin–angiotensin–aldosterone system. However, there are case reports of normal TALH function with a water load challenge[121–123]. A newer hypothesis proposes a more generalized transport defect: that an increase in cell Na permeability is the primary defect, which, in the distal nephron, would secondarily stimulate Na–K-ATPase and result in increased potassium loss into the urine[123–127].

Miscellaneous clinical disorders

Elevated urinary PG have been measured in a variety of tubulointerstitial disorders of polyuria and impaired renal concentrating ability, including hypokalaemia[128], lithium nephropathy[129], hypercalcaemia[130] and pyelonephritis[131]. Since PG antagonize the hydro-osmotic action of VP, PG have been implicated in the aetiology of these clinical syndromes. In fact, NSAID reverse the concentrating defect in some cases[129–131]. However, an increase in urine flow rate can *per se* enhance urinary PG excretion[129,132], as can hypokalaemia[133] and hypercalcaemia[52] (depending upon the experimental setting). There may also be a role for increased thromboxane synthesis in the

40

polyuria associated with potassium depletion[134,135]. However, it is difficult to prove experimentally that the primary disturbance is the proximate result of an imbalance in PG synthesis.

Hyporeninaemic hypoaldosteronism, a syndrome characterized by hyperkalaemia, low renin levels and inappropriately low aldosterone secretion in spite of normal glucocorticoid function, is seen in the elderly, diabetics and patients with varying degrees of renal insufficiency. Since vasodilatory renal prostaglandins are direct stimulators of renin release, impaired prostaglandin production has been implicated in the aetiology of hyporeninaemic hypoaldosteronism. Although earlier measurements of PGE_2 levels in hyporeninaemic hypoaldosteronism were conflicting (low or normal excretion), recent examination of prostacyclin (PGI_2) production, as determined by its stable urinary metabolite 6-keto-$PGF_{1\alpha}$, has revealed reduced basal and stimulated (by calcium and norepinephrine) excretion[136]. However, in the feedback scheme involving renal PG and the renin–angiotensin system, it is difficult to discern whether PGI_2 deficiency is cause or effect. An attractive alternative hypothesis proposes that increased production of atrial natriuretic peptide, a potent inhibitor of both aldosterone and renin, is the proximate cause of hyporeninaemic hypoaldosteronism. In patients with hyperkalaemia secondary to hyporeninaemic hypoaldosteronism, drugs that suppress renin and aldosterone, such as β-blockers, calcium-channel blockers and non-steroidal anti-inflammatory drugs (see below), should be avoided.

A subset of patients with hypercalcaemia related to a malignancy show no evidence of excess parathyroid hormone production or osseous metastases. PG have been implicated in the pathogenesis of malignancy-related hypercalcaemia, since PG enhance bone resorption, and are necessary for the synthesis of osteoclastic activating factor. Some patients with renal cell carcinoma and concomitant hypercalcaemia have been shown to have elevated renal PG levels which can be suppressed with indomethacin.

Pharmacological inhibition of PG synthesis

The use of compounds which affect enzymes in the metabolism of AA has contributed important insights into the role of eicosanoids in renal disease. Glucocorticoids[57], calcium channel blockers[137] and mepacrine[28] inhibit PLA_2. The largest number of compounds, and the most clinically relevant, are the inhibitors of cyclo-oxygenase. We will focus upon the effects of pharmacological inhibition of PG synthesis, with particular attention to non-steroidal anti-inflammatory drugs (NSAID). NSAID act as inhibitors of cyclo-oxygenase, thereby decreasing the synthesis of renal PG. However, NSAID may also affect the production of other eicosanoid compounds which possess either synergistic or antagonistic biological activity. Furthermore, these agents vary in their ability to block cyclo-oxygenase.

During the past fifteen years, there has been a proliferation of NSAID on the market. NSAID are in broad clinical use as therapy for arthritis and other inflammatory and painful conditions, as well as for less common disorders, such as patent ductus arteriosus. As the use of these drugs expands in the clinical sphere, the literature concerning the renal complications associated with their use grows. There are structurally distinct pharmacological classes of NSAID (Table 1). The effects of NSAID on renal function are described in several reviews[138-142]. Renal actions of NSAID in humans include decreased RBF, decreased GFR, sodium retention, hyperkalaemia, impaired water clearance, decreased plasma renin activity, hypertension and acute renal failure.

The effect of NSAID on GFR was studied in normal man and the results were conflicting, showing either no effect or a small decrease[93-98,143-150]. NSAID may interfere with salt and water excretion. In conditions of normal sodium intake and intact circulation, NSAID induce only transient Na retention and a mild decrease in GFR[28]. However, in conditions of volume depletion or impaired renal perfusion[101,150-154] where there is a compensatory increase in renal prostaglandin production, inhibition of PG causes marked functional changes. In patients with diminished effective intravascular volume and salt retention (e.g. congestive heart failure, nephrotic syndrome and cirrhosis), oedema worsens with the administration of NSAID[103]. In such patients, NSAID have been shown to antagonize the effect of diuretics when given concomitantly[148,155-159]. NSAID interfere with the therapeutic efficacy of various antihypertensive agents, including diuretics of different types (thiazides, furosemide and spironolactone) and β-adrenergic blockers. Concurrent use of triamterene and indomethacin has lead to renal insufficiency, even in healthy subjects[145,160], perhaps unmasking a nephrotoxic effect of triamterene. Indeed, several NSAID (particularly indomethacin and meclofenamate) have been used therapeutically in an effort to diminish the massive proteinuria seen in certain cases of nephrosis (particularly focal and segmental glomerulosclerosis and membranous nephropathy) because of their ability to reduce filtration[161-164].

PG promote free water excretion, probably by acting at several different sites. Cyclo-oxygenase inhibition with NSAID should, therefore, diminish

Table 3.1 Non-steroidal anti-inflammatory drugs

Chemical family	Generic name
Salicylic acid derivatives	Acetylsalicylic acid
	Sodium salicylate
	Choline salicylate
	Choline magnesium trisalicylate
Pyrazolone derivative	Phenylbutazone
Propionic acid derivatives	Ibuprofen
	Naproxen
	Fenoprofen calcium
	Benoxaprofen
Indoleacetic acid derivatives	Indomethacin
	Sulindac
	Tolmetin
Anthranilic acid derivatives	Meclofenamate sodium
	Mefenamate
Oxicam derivative	Piroxicam

water excretion. Consistent with this rationale, NSAID have been employed in nephrogenic diabetes insipidus (DI), a polyuric state in which the collecting duct is unresponsive to VP[165,166]. In a strain of rat with hereditary nephrogenic DI, low urinary PGE_2 excretion has been measured[44]. By enhancing water retention, NSAID could theoretically result in hyponatraemia. There are case reports of hyponatraemia in patients on NSAID; however, there is at least one other drug that could contribute to impaired water excretion in these cases[153,167,168].

Potassium secretion in the distal nephron is influenced by a variety of factors which are modulated by PG, including urinary flow rate, distal delivery of filtrate and aldosterone. Since PG tend to enhance distal delivery of filtrate and stimulate renin release, treatment with NSAID can cause hyperkalaemia. Administration of NSAID to people with normal[169] and impaired[170,171] renal function results in positive potassium balance. In the setting of renal failure, NSAID cause a syndrome virtually indistinguishable from hyporeninaemic hypoaldosteronism (also known as Type IV renal tubular acidosis)[97,172]. NSAID, therefore, should not be used concurrently with other pharmacological agents that lead to positive potassium balance.

The use of NSAID in patients with essential and renovascular hypertension is complicated largely because of negative interaction with other drug therapy. An important exception to this observation may be sulindac, a NSAID with the putative unique property of inhibiting only extrarenal PG synthesis[173,174]. However, the selective nature of sulindac's inhibition of PG synthesis has been disputed[175]. Sulindac potentiates, rather than antagonizes, the antihypertensive effect of thiazides in patients with essential hypertension[176]. However, there are case reports of nephrotic syndrome, sometimes associated with acute interstitial nephritis, related to sulindac therapy[177].

Syndromes of renal failure associated with NSAID

Inhibition of PG synthesis causes the most marked depression of GFR when there is pre-existing renal compromise, in the setting of both high and normal plasma renin activity (PRA).

Hypovolaemia and inadequate effective circulating arterial volume induce an increase in vasopressor substances, including PRA. In high renin states, renal PG may function as local vasolidators in order to maintain RBF and GFR. Hypovolaemia, salt depletion and disorders of diminished effective circulating blood volume, with the attendant inhibition of prostaglandin synthesis by high renin, result in a decrease in GFR. The use of NSAID in such clinical settings is associated with acute renal failure. RBF and GFR fell in cirrhotics given indomethacin[154,178], and there was a corresponding fall in urinary PGE_2. A decrement in renal function was observed in nephrotics on indomethacin[101], which was irreversible in one study of childhood nephrosis[179].

The hepatorenal syndrome is characterized by acute renal failure in the setting of advanced cirrhosis, sometimes with ascites. The diminution in renal function is felt to be due to marked vasoconstriction without any structural abnormality. A variety of vasoconstrictor substances have been implicated, but none definitively. Since enhanced production of vasodilatory PG is seen in cirrhosis[178,180], most likely in a compensatory attempt to maintain GFR[154,178,181], it is not unreasonable to suspect that the decrease in PG synthesis contributes to impaired RBF. An imbalance of eicosanoids has been found, with an increase in TxA_2 and a decrease in PGE_2 levels[180].

The decrease in RBF and GFR produced by cyclo-oxygenase inhibition is more pronounced in the anaesthetized than the conscious animal[182-185]. During anaesthesia, there are increased levels of circulating vasoconstrictor hormones, such as angiotensin II and catecholamines, which would require an increase in vasodilatory PG in order to counteract the expected renal vasoconstriction[186]. There are no comparable studies in anaesthetized humans.

Patients with chronic parenchymal renal disease show a fall in RBF and GFR during treatment with NSAID, including aspirin[93,96,97,187]. In chronic glomerulonephritis, afferent arteriolar dilatation may be a compensatory mechanism in the maintenance of filtration. A study of patients with systemic lupus erythematosus revealed an abnormal increase in basal PGE_2 excretion consistent with the postulated means of compensation[94]. In other aetiologies of renal insufficiency, including diabetes, hypertension and interstitial nephritis, there is acute worsening of renal function with NSAID[188-191].

Acute renal failure associated with NSAID falls into several categories: (1) acute interstitial nephritis with glomerular abnormalities, (2) functional acute renal failure, probably haemodynamic in nature, (3) papillary necrosis, and (4) phenylbutazone anuria.

Acute interstitial nephritis with nephrotic syndrome
Acute renal failure associated with acute interstitial nephritis has reportedly developed as an idiosyncratic reaction in patients within weeks to months of receiving NSAID; specifically fenoprofen, indomethacin, naproxen and tolmetin[192-201]. Interestingly, these drugs represent different pharmacological sub-types of NSAID. Interstitial nephritis is often associated with nephrotic-range proteinuria. The pathological glomerular abnormalities resemble the changes seen with lipoid nephrosis. Renal failure may be so severe as to necessitate dialysis. The syndrome resolves upon withdrawal of the offending NSAID after a variable period of time. Steroids have proven beneficial in some instances.

Functional acute renal failure
The functional variety of acute renal failure tends to appear in patients with pre-existing renal disease and factors predisposing to impaired renal perfusion, such as diminished effective intravascular volume from diuretic use or congestive heart failure (reviewed in ref. 138). In the few cases where renal biopsy was performed, histology was compatible with acute tubular necrosis[202,203]. The hypothesis proposed is that the nature of the primary insult is haemodynamic, and that inhibition of PG synthesis would worsen pre-existing circulatory compromise. In summary, this category would encompass cases of NSAID use resulting in acute tubular necrosis or poor renal perfusion with ARF.

Papillary necrosis

Necrosis of the renal papillae is a classic pathological finding of analgesic nephropathy, which presumes the ingestion of large amounts of compounds containing phenacetin, aspirin and acetaminophen. Salicylates are concentrated in the renal papilla which would tend to enhance toxicity. Inhibitors of PG synthesis reduce medullary blood flow and could thus contribute to papillary ischaemia. Although the pathogenesis of analgesic nephropathy is unclear, there is theoretical substantiation and experimental evidence for a role of PG inhibition in the development of papillary necrosis. Although suprapharmacological doses of phenacetin, aspirin or acetaminophen alone can cause papillary necrosis in experimental animals, the combination of at least two of these drugs seems to be synergistic in producing nephrotoxicity[204–206]. Papillary necrosis occurs in animals given meclofenamate, fenoprofen and phenylbutazone[207–209]. Papillary necrosis has been reported with NSAID therapy in man[210–212].

Phenylbutazone anuria

Oligoanuric acute renal failure has been described in patients on phenylbutazone[213–215]. A pathogenetic mechanism reponsible is the inhibition of the tubular reabsorption of uric acid, which results in hyperuricosuria, uric acid crystallization and, eventually, urethral obstruction. Another form of this syndrome, in which there is no evidence of hyperuricaemia, is felt to be an idiosyncratic reaction. The biopsy picture is consistent with acute tubular necrosis[216].

A ROLE FOR TxA$_2$ IN RENAL INJURY

The following section of this chapter presents the evidence implicating TxA$_2$ as an important mediator of renal injury.

Enhanced TxA$_2$ generation in experimental models

Increased levels of renal TxA$_2$ is a common feature of immune-mediated and physiologically induced loss of renal function. Numerous and diverse experimental and clinical studies have implicated TxA$_2$ in the progression of renal injury[217–234] (Table 3.2). Measurements of renal arachidonic acid metabolite levels in most experimental and clinical studies involve detection of the actual metabolites or stable breakdown products (i.e. TxB$_2$ the breakdown product of TxA$_2$ and 6-keto-PGF$_{1\alpha}$ the breakdown product of prostacyclin) by radioimmunoassays. The amount of generated renal eicosanoid is usually measured from samples of either supernatants containing the synthesized molecules from incubated kidney slices or amounts excreted in urine.

Exaggerated production of renal arachidonic acid metabolites (PGE$_2$ and TxA$_2$) was first noted in two non-immunologically mediated forms of renal injury, the obstructed rabbit kidney and spontaneous hypertensive rat[229–231]. In the unilateral obstructed rabbit kidney, enhanced PGE$_2$ and TxA$_2$ production

Table 3.2   Experimental forms of renal disease with increased renal TxA$_2$

Type of study	References
Experimental Animal Studies	
Lupus nephritis	Kelley et al. 1986 (264)
Anti-glomerular basement membrane	Lianos et al. 1983 (218)
Allograft rejection	Khirabadi et al. 1985 (233),
	Coffman et al. 1985 (220),
	Mangino et al. 1986 (221)
Endotoxaemia	Badr et al. 1986 (282)
Cyclosporine nephrotoxicity	Kawaguchi et al. 1985 (223),
	Elzinga et al. 1986 (224)
Subtotal renal ablation	Purkerson et al. 1985 (225)
Adriamycin nephrosis	Remuzzi et al. 1985 (226)
Glycerol-induced acute renal failure	Benabe et al. 1980 (227),
	Sraer et al. 1981 (228)
Hydronephrosis	Morrison et al. 1978 (229),
	Okegawa et al. 1983 (230)
Spontaneous hypertensive rat	Konieczkowski et al. 1983 (231)
Clinical Human Studies	
Lupus nephritis	Patrono et al. 1985 (232)
Allograft rejection	Foegh et al. 1981 (219),
	Steinhauer et al. 1984 (234)

was reported in renal cortical slices but was only increased after stimulation with vasoactive peptide molecules (bradykinin or angiotensin II). The physiological vasoconstriction caused by excess TxA$_2$ in these rabbits was reversible[235] with the TxA$_2$ synthetase inhibitor OKY-1581. Similarly, there is an increase in PGE$_2$ and TxA$_2$ in glomeruli from spontaneous hypertensive rats[231]. It was hypothesized that enhanced levels of glomerular TxA$_2$ could account for the increased renal resistance through direct vasoconstrictor action or alternatively that PGE$_2$ might cause vasoconstriction indirectly through stimulation of renin release and the formation of angiotensin.

The concept of TxA$_2$ as an important mediator of renal injury was strengthened when elevations in this metabolite were noted in glomeruli from rats with antiglomerular basement membrane (GBM) antibody-induced glomerulonephritis[218]. This form of glomerular immune injury is produced by the administration of rabbit antirat antibody to GBM (nephrotoxic serum). The early pathological phase of this renal disease is a heterologous reaction caused by antibody binding to GBM, an increase in mesangial and glomerular endothelial cells and an influx of polymorphonuclear and mononuclear cells and the detachment of endothelium from the capillary wall. The later phase of the disease (14 days) is caused by an autologous reaction including the binding of rat IgG and C3 to the GBM, mesangial proliferation, focal mononuclear cell infiltration and areas of glomerular sclerosis and more complete detachment of endothelium from the capillary wall. In the heterologous phase there is an elevation in glomerular TxA$_2$, PGE$_2$ and PGF$_{2\alpha}$ release, while in the autologous phase, enhanced eicosanoid metabolism was restricted to TxA$_2$ alone.

Enhanced renal TxA$_2$ generation occurs in two experimental immune-mediated forms of renal injury which are excellent models of human conditions:

mice with spontaneous systemic lupus erythematosus and rat cardiac allograft transplantation[218,220,221,233]. Studies indicate an overproduction of renal synthesis of TxA$_2$ in mouse strains with lupus nephritis including the MRL-*lpr* mice and the female NZB × NZW F1 hybrid (NZB × NZW). Although these autoimmune animal models share common denominators instrumental in the pathogenesis of lupus, they are each governed by distinct immunological and genetic factors which influence the tempo of disease expression.

The common features in the murine strains and human lupus include lymphoid abnormalities, lymphokine deficiencies, autoantibodies and immune complex-mediated renal disease. The tempo of expression of immunological changes and renal disease is slower in NZB × NZW F1 female hybrid (NZB × NZW) than in the MRL-*lpr* mice. The 50% mortality in this hybrid is at 10 months of age. Pathological proteinuria begins at 6 months of age and eventually 90% of the mice have extensive increases in urinary protein, are oedematous and die in renal failure[236]. Lymphoid abnormalities include a modest increase in T and B lymphocytes[237], deficiency in interleukin-2 (IL-2) production and responsiveness[238,239], loss of antigen-specific T cell suppression[240], and B cell hyperresponsiveness[241]. T helper lymphocytes and enhanced class II major histocompatibility complex molecules are important ingredients in the pathogenesis, as indicated by the ability of monoclonal antibodies to cell surface antigens such as anti-L3T4[242] and anti-Ia[232] given prophylactically to prolong survival and inhibit renal injury.

MRL-*lpr* strain is a particularly appealing strain for studies of lupus nephritis. Disease in these mice is rapidly progressive and regulated by a single autosomal recessive gene (*lpr*). This gene is responsible for a massive increase in a unique subset of lymphocytes capable of expressing both T (Thy1.2 + , Ly1 + 23 − ,L3T4 −) and B (2C2 +, 6B2 +, Ig −) lymphocyte markers *in vivo*, which do not express class II MHC (major histocompatibility complex) determinants[244-246]. These cells are divergent since, although they are rapidly dividing, they neither secrete nor respond to T cell growth factor, IL-2[238,239]. In addition, these unusual cells can elaborate a B cell differentiation factor which enhances B cell activation, promotes the switch from IgM to IgG and may account for heightened B cell function characteristic of autoimmune mice[247]. Expansion of this unique population of T cells regulates the expression of disease since suppressing their proliferation by a variety of treatments, including lymphoid irradiation[240] or pharmacological doses of PGE[248] and monoclonal anti-T cell antibody[249], arrests the course of renal disease.

Studies in our laboratory[250,251] demonstrated that when the *lpr* gene is transferred by a series of cross–intercross matings into mice not predisposed to autoimmunity, it induces autoantibodies and lymphoproliferation, shortens survival, but does not cause renal disease. Expression of this gene in several strains of mice is influenced by the background genome. This gene is an accelerating factor for the MRL − + + strain which has a late onset mild form of autoimmunity. Transferring the *lpr* gene onto this background converts a mild illness into an aggressive, fulminant renal disease. In MRL-*lpr* mice, lymphoid hyperplasia is prominent by 3 months of age and precedes enhanced expression of Ia antigens on the surface of resident peritoneal macrophages and the onset of renal disease[251]. The quantitative increase in

Ia is not limited to the peritoneal macrophages but is also prominent in renal tissue of proteinuric MRL-*lpr* mice. The cells within the kidney responsible for enhanced Ia determinants include the macrophage, endothelial cells, tubular cells and cells in the interstitium[252]. It has been hypothesized that interferon is the lymphokine released from the proliferating unique T cells responsible for inducing Ia synthesis in the MRL-*lpr*. However, the inability of these same T cells to induce Ia on other strains, coupled with a recent careful study showing that these cells are incapable of synthesizing this lymphokine, indicates that another factor must be responsible for the induction of these cell surface antigens which may promote immune-induced renal injury[251,253,254].

Experiments in MRL-*lpr* and NZB × NZW mice showed that renal biosynthesis of TxA$_2$ increased in lupus nephritis[217]. This increase in renal TxA$_2$ was progressive and proportional to the deterioration of renal function and increase in the degree of kidney pathological change. Renal TxA$_2$ increase was measured in the cortex, medulla and glomeruli. Treatment schemes capable of preventing renal disease in these autoimmune mice, including pharmacological doses of PGE$_1$ and fish oil diets rich in ω-3 fatty acids, prevented the enhanced renal TxA$_2$ production[255].

Enhanced TxA$_2$ generation in humans

In the search for alterations in arachidonate derivatives abnormally synthesized in human renal disease, evidence for a role for TxA$_2$ comes from two source – lupus nephritis and allograft rejection[219,232,234]. Patrono *et al.*[232] report that patients with systemic lupus erythematosus have excess urinary TxB$_2$ and reduced excretion of 6-keto-PGF$_{1\alpha}$ levels. In contrast to the urinary TxB$_2$, no increase was seen in TxB$_2$ in whole blood or in urinary 2,3-dinor-TxB$_2$, a major metabolite that primarily reflects extrarenal TxB$_2$ formation. Thus, the increased urinary TxB$_2$ indicates renal production of this metabolite. In addition, there was an inverse correlation between TxB$_2$ levels and creatinine clearances. These studies could not confirm earlier observations of Kimberly *et al.*[94] reporting enhanced renal synthesis of the vasodilator PGE$_2$. In another group of studies, human kidney allograft rejection was associated with an early increase in urinary TxB$_2$. Foegh *et al.* reported an increase in urinary immunoreactive TxB$_2$ one to three days before clinical apparent allograft rejection[219]. In another report, the clinical diagnosis of rejection was confirmed by an increase in TxB$_2$ in the urine[234]. Thus, urinary TxB$_2$ measurements appear to be an early, specific and sensitive marker of renal allograft rejection.

Although there is documentation of elevated renal TxA$_2$ in human kidney disease, it will be important to explore abnormal arachidonic acid metabolism in other forms of glomerulonephritis and non-immunological forms of injury to determine how generalized the concept of enhanced TxA$_2$ synthesis is in influencing the loss of renal function in humans.

Role of TxA$_2$ in renal disease

Experiments defining the role of TxA$_2$ in renal disease are based primarily on studies using thromboxane synthetase inhibitors. However, adequate inhibition of renal TxA$_2$ synthesis is difficult. While platelet TxA$_2$ inhibition occurs at relatively low doses, blocking renal TxA_2 production requires considerably higher levels of the synthetase inhibitor. In addition, some of these inhibitors which are imidazole derivatives have a short half-life and must be injected several times a day. Studies are further complicated since use of urinary TxB_2 measurements as indicators of renal thromboxane production may be complicated by the presence of TxB_2 and other metabolites from the systemic circulation and renal tubular processing of TxB_2. Intravenously injected $[^3H]TxB_2$ is excreted in the urine as 20 different TxB_2 metabolites of which 2,3-dinor-TxB_2 is the most abundant. Circulating TxA_2 may also be metabolized to 2,3-dinor-TxB_2 since it is transported by the organic acid secretory pathway. Since most of the TxB_2 antibodies used in radioimmunoassays cross-react with this metabolite, these urinary measurements may also include circulating thromboxane. Similarly, studies determining the degree of blocking of TxA_2 in which TxA_2 synthesis is measured *ex vivo* from incubating renal slices may not accurately represent the degree of effective inhibition since blockage may be altered when tissue is removed from the animal. Although most of these acute studies using TxA_2 synthetase inhibitors do not include data proving a reduction of renal TxA_2 during the entire study period, these experiments do support the concept that in induced forms of renal injury, inhibiting renal or urinary TxA_2 increases the renal blood flow and glomerular filtration rate[218,222,225,226,256-258] (Table 3.3). For example, a bolus i.v. administration of lipopolysaccharide endotoxin to rats caused a progressive fall in RBF and GFR without a fall in mean arterial pressure[5]. At this time renal cortical generation of TxB_2 in rats given endotoxin was increased over that of control rats. Pretreatment with the TxA_2 synthetase inhibitor UK 37.248 selectively abolished the LPS-induced rise in TxB_2 and preserved GFR. Thus, these observations point to a major role for TxA_2 in mediating renal functional impairments.

The macrophage: a source of thromboxane

What is the source of the increased intrarenal TxA_2? Several candidates emerge for the cellular source responsible for increasing renal TxA_2. Broadly, the cells could either be a component of the renal tissue or alternatively,

Table 3.3 TxA_2 synthetase inhibitors prevent loss of renal function in experimental rat models

	Reference
Immune mediated	
Acute allograft rejection	Coffmann et al. 1985 (220)
Antiglomerular basement membrane disease	Lianos et al. 1983 (218)
Non-immune mediated	
Hydronephrotic kidneys	Klotman et al. 1986 (257)
Adriamycin nephrosis	Remuzzi et al. 1985 (226)
Subtotal renal ablation	Purkerson et al. 1985 (225)
Glycerol-induced acute renal failure	Papanicolaou et al. 1986 (258)
Endotoxaemia	Badr et al. 1986 (282)

49

circulate into the kidney via the blood. Glomerular epithelial and mesangial cells and collecting tubules are the intrinsic elements capable of synthesizing TxA_2[259]. In murine lupus nephritis, there is an increase in mesangial cells and a broadening of glomerular epithelial foot processes[236,260]. Since these cell types are capable of synthesizing TxA_2, the intrarenal accumulation of this metabolite may be contributed to by these intrinsic components. However, since there is an increase in the medulla as well as the cortex, the glomerular changes cannot account exclusively for the total increase. This leaves the possibility of TxA_2 release by circulating cells, such as platelets and monocytes. The platelet can be eliminated. Although platelets secrete abundant amounts of TxA_2, it is unlikely that they are the source of increased intrarenal production because a dose of the cyclo-oxygenase inhibitor, ibuprofen, capable of blocking platelet TxA_2 formation, did not reduce renal levels or protect autoimmune mice from kidney injury[261]. Similarly, in human studies, the major metabolite of platelets, 2,3-dinor-TxB_2, is not elevated in the urine of lupus patients, making it unlikely that extrarenal platelet activation can account for enhanced urinary TxB_2 excretion in these patients [232]. Since monocytes/macrophages are abundant in the glomerulus and the interstitium of the cortex and medulla only in autoimmune mice with renal disease, it is probable that these cells, known to be instrumental in the pathogenesis of glomerulonephritis, are a major source of TxA_2 synthesis[252]. In fact, we have recently been able to isolate and clone invading macrophages from the cortex of MRL-*lpr* mice with renal disease. These macrophages express enhanced surface major histocompatability complex Ia antigens and are therefore considered to be activated[255]. While PGI_2 is the major eicosanoid elaborated by renal macrophages, they synthesize virtually no PGI_2 and less PGE_2 than unactivated cells. Thus, TxA_2 levels are proportionally increased. Stimulation of these cells with IL-1 greatly increased the amount of TxA_2 produced[255]. Thus, immunologically stimulated renal macrophages produce an abundance of TxA_2. This vasoconstrictor molecule is capable of inducing vasomotor changes important in renal injury.

The involvement of the macrophages in mediating renal injury is not restricted to immunologically mediated forms of renal injury. Mononuclear cells were implicated as the source of TxA_2 production in unilateral ureter obstruction in rabbits[230]. Stimulation of the obstructed kidney by endotoxin and bradykinin caused an exaggerated production of TxA_2 and PGE_2. Thus, since the monocyte/macrophage is present in immune and inflammatory forms of renal injury, eicosanoid production by this cell has the ability to regulate vasomotor events.

Dietary fatty acid in lupus nephritis

Studies altering dietary fatty acids have provided support that eicosanoid synthesis regulates immune-mediated forms of renal injury. A diet enriched with fish oil containing $\omega - 3$ polyunsaturated fatty acids (PUFA) protects murine strains with lupus nephritis from the formation of renal disease. These $\omega - 3$ fatty acids, such as eicosapentaenoic (EPA) and docosahexenoic acid

(DHA), are distinguished from the $\omega-6$ fatty acids, such as arachidonic acid, by the position of the first double bond counting from the methyl end of the molecule. The predominant fatty acids in most vegetable oils and meat belong to the $\omega-6$ class, whereas $\omega-3$ fatty acids are found exclusively in fish oil and some plants (linseed). PUFA are metabolized via cyclo-oxygenase and lipoxygenase pathways to yield eicosanoid products. $\omega-3$ fatty acids quantitatively and qualitatively alter eicosanoid synthesis. Studies primarily in platelets indicate that EPA is a poor substrate for cyclo-oxygenase with a high affinity for this enzyme[262,263]. This fatty acid functionally operates as a competitive inhibitor which decreases the level of cyclo-oxygenase metabolites. In addition, $\omega-3$ fatty acids are precursors for cyclo-oxygenase and lipoxygenase products containing an additional double bond. These more highly unsaturated molecules have different biological properties. For example, TxA_2 promotes the aggregation of platelets whereas TxA_3 does not appear to aggregate platelets. Thus, the fatty acids in fish oil reduce the quantity and change the profile of eicosanoid production.

Studies in our laboratory show that a basal diet composed of lipid exclusively from fish oil, instead of safflower oil, fed to autoimmune mice suppresses the progression of renal injury and prolongs survival. In MRL-*lpr* mice, the most aggressive model of lupus, a 20% fish oil diet suppresses the increase in proteinuria, the localization of immune complexes in the glomerulus and the development of renal pathology[264]. In the NZB $\times$ NZW mice with a less virulent form of this illness, a diet rich in fish oil can prevent renal injury when animals are started on it prior to the expression of renal disease and can arrest the progression and reduce mortality when treatment is delayed until the mice are mildly proteinuric[265-267]. These data suggest that a fish diet is not only prophylactically beneficial but also offers therapeutic promise.

How does the fish oil alter renal cyclo-oxygenase metabolites? Measurements of intrarenal cyclo-oxygenase products by competitive radioimmunoassays show a reduction in PGE_2, TxB_2 (stable breakdown product of TxA_2) and 6-keto-$PGF_{1\alpha}$ (stable breakdown product of PGI_2) in both the renal cortex and medulla[264]. Not only does the fish oil reduce the level of these metabolites but it also promotes the synthesis of approximately 20% of the trienoic series of molecules[264].

Is it necessary to eat a diet exclusive of fish in the absence of vegetable or beef oil to reduce the intrarenal cyclo-oxygenase metabolism? Studies show that a diet containing only 2.5% fish oil and 17.5% safflower oil is nearly as effective in lowering renal, cortical or medullary prostanoids as a diet limited to 20% fish oil (unpublished observation). Thus, a small proportion of fish oil in the presence of other lipid sources favourably competes and inhibits cyclo-oxygenase metabolite synthesis.

What is the fatty acid in fish oil responsible for lowering renal prostanoid metabolism? To determine whether EPA is responsible for reducing intrarenal prostanoid formation, mice were given a normal laboratory chow diet supplemented with pure EPA[268]. One group received 25 mg EPA daily by gavage while the control group was given phosphate-buffered saline. Ingesting EPA for six days reduced the TxA_2 synthesis in the renal cortex and medulla. This reduction in TxA_2 production by EPA was proportionally similar to the inhibition by fish oil in the diet containing a similar daily dose of EPA. Thus, the EPA in fish oil is at least partially responsible for the lower renal eicosanoid metabolism.

The action of fish oil is not limited to renal changes. In the MRL-*lpr* mice, studies show a suppression of lymphoproliferation, prevention of the enhanced expression of Ia on macrophages and inhibition in the levels of circulating antibodies of gp 70. The amount of gp 70 immune complexes is an excellent indicator of the severity of renal disease in these autoimmune mice. The antigen, which is the major envelope coat protein of a retrovirus, is considered a self antigen since it is vertically transmitted through the host's genome. All mice have gp 70 in their circulation, but only the autoimmune mice react to form antibodies to this protein[269]. Since fish oil affects cells of the immune system and not just renal tissue, these immune cells, which have been implicated in the development of renal disease, may be responsible for the protective effect of fish oil.

Essential fatty acid deficiency also provides protection from lupus nephritis. In NZB × NZW mice fed diets lacking essential fatty acids, survival increased and there was no evidence of histological glomerulonephritis[270]. In essential fatty acid deficiency, since arachidonic acid synthesis is reduced, there is a decrease in the dienoic cyclo-oxygenase metabolites. Since NZB × NZW mice have an enhanced synthesis of renal TxA_2, the protective mechanism of a EFA-deficient diet may be in part related to a reduction in this vasoconstrictor metabolite. EFA has also recently been reported to prevent the influx of macrophages into rat glomeruli after administration of nephrotoxic serum[271]. Thus, the reduction of arachidonate may alter macrophage chemotaxis and thereby protect from glomerular damage.

Dietary studies not only provide important means of dissecting the role of eicosanoids in renal injury, but offer an important approach to treatment of kidney disease.

Cyclosporine nephrotoxicity

Cyclosporine A (CyA) has proved to be an effective immunosuppressive agent, resulting in improved allograft survival in human transplantation[272,273]. However, acute renal dysfunction complicates the management of transplant patients and limits its usefulness in other immunological disorders[274]. Recent evidence suggests that altered renal haemodynamics are important in the pathogenesis of CyA-induced renal injury[275–277]. Studies in experimental models and man show that CyA reduces GFR in a dose-dependent manner and also increases TxA_2 synthesis[223,277–279]. In addition, vascular casting techniques demonstrate vasoconstriction in the afferent arteriolar proximal to the glomerulus by scanning electron microscopy. This finding provides a morphological correlate of the physiological finding that CyA reduces renal blood flow[280]. Furthermore, even though CyA causes proximal convoluted tubular damage, these studies do not support the concept that CyA causes any direct tubular damage.

TxA_2 may be responsible for CyA's vasoconstriction action. Experiments using fish oil rich in ω-3 fatty acids instead of the conventionally used olive oil, as a vehicle, to solubilize the hydrophobic CyA in a rodent given high doses of CyA $(50\,mg\,kg^{-1})$ show protection from renal nephrotoxicity by fish oil. These studies report that cyclosporine in olive oil increases renal TxA_2 levels and that fish oil prevents the increase in TxA_2, and protects from CyA-induced reduction in GFR and histological tubular damage. In addition, a recent report documents a selective rise in urinary TxB_2 in a similar rodent model which correlated with a decline in GFR[279]. Both urinary excretion of TxB_2 and GFR returned to normal values after withdrawal of the drug. Administration of a selective TxA_2 inhibitor, UK 38,485, caused a reduction in urinary excretion of TxB_2 accompanied by an increase in GFR. Thus, these studies suggest that the elevation in TxB_2 production induced by CyA plays an important role in nephrotoxicity and provides new approaches to reducing toxicity in patients being treated with this immunosuppressive molecule.

LEUKOTRIENES

Leukotrienes (LT), the products of lipoxygenase activation, have potent vasoactive properties and play a role in immunological and inflammatory reactions. LTC_4 has been shown to affect vascular smooth muscle, causing vasoconstriction and an increase in vascular permeability. Receptors for LTC_4 have been demonstrated in glomeruli[281]. Although LT have been shown to be potent mediators in many cell types, including endothelia, bronchial tissue and leukocytes, the effects of LT on renal function are in the early stages of investigation.

Studies in rats suggest that LT may modulate GFR. Infusion of LTC_4 produced a decrease in RBF, GFR, haemoconcentration (secondary to an increase in vascular permeability) and an increase in systemic and renal vascular resistances[282].

The role of LT in renal disease is unclear. Elevated production of 12-hydroxyeicosatetraenoic acid (12-HETE) and LTB_4 has been reported in renal cortical tissue from rejecting kidney allografts in dogs[221]. Although LTC_4 has been shown to release TxB_2 and PG from rat peritoneal macrophages, studies in our laboratory with renal macrophages do not show enhanced synthesis of TxB_2 with LT[255,283].

CONCLUSION

The pathophysiological effects of PG cannot readily be isolated from those of many other hormones and factors which regulate the haemodynamic, tubular and endocrine functions of the kidneys. It is clear that renal PG play a central role in water metabolism and renin release, whereas the effect of PG on transepithelial transport and the pathogenetic potential of other eicosanoids, such as leukotrienes, have not been fully explored. In addition, recent studies have supported the concept that enhanced generation of the vasoconstrictor, TxA_2, is prominent in many experimental models of immunologically induced and non-immune forms of renal injury. Detection of increased TxA_2 in human lupus and allograft rejection strengthens the concept that this metabolite is an important mediator of haemodynamic and immunological events important in inducing renal injury. Recent studies also introduce possible roles for LT in the induction of renal disease. Future studies evaluating eicosanoids action in renal damage will clarify the nature of their importance in diseases of the kidney.

ACKNOWLEDGEMENTS

This manuscript was supported in part by National Institutes of Health grants AM36149 and AM07199, the Gustavus and Louis Pfeiffer Research Foundation and the Pennsylvania Lupus Foundation. We wish to acknowledge the excellent secretarial assistance of Corinne Kennedy.

REFERENCES

1. Seyberth, H.W., Sweetman, B.J. and Frohlich, J.C. (1976). *Prostaglandins*, **13**, 1127–39
2. Frohlich, J.C., Walker, L., Rosenkranz, B., Falkner, F. and Robertson, G. (1984). Role of icosanoids in excretion of water and electrolytes. In Braquet, P., Garay, R.P., Frohlich, J.C. and Nicosia, S. (eds.) *Prostaglandins and Membrane Ion Transport*, pp. 241–251. (New York: Raven Press)
3. Orloff, J., Handler, J.S. and Bergstrom, S. (1965). Effect of prostaglandin (PGE) on the permeability response of the toad bladder to vasopressin, theophylline, and adenosine 3',5'-monophosphate. *Nature (London)*, **205**, 397–98
4. Grantham, J.J. and Orloff, J. (1968). Effect of prostaglandin E_1 on the permeability response of the isolated collecting tubule to vasopressin, adenosine 3',5'-monophosphate and theophylline. *J. Clin. Invest.*, **47**, 1154–61
5. Lipson, L.C. and Sharp, G.W. (1972). Effect of prostaglandin E_1 on sodium transport and osmotic water flow in toad bladder. *Am. J. Physiol.*, **220**, 1064–52
6. Ozer, A. and Sharp, G.W. (1972). Effect of prostaglandins and their inhibitors on osmotic water flow in the toad bladder. *Am. J. Physiol.*, **222**, 674–80
7. Urakabe, S., Takamitsu, Y., Shirai, D., Kimura, G., Orita, Y., Yuasa, S. and Abe, H. (1975). Effect of different prostaglandins on the permeability of the toad bladder. *Comp. Biochem. Physiol.* **52**, 1–4
8. Stokes, J.B. and Kokko, J.P. (1977). Inhibition of sodium transport by prostaglandin E_2 across the isolated, perfused rabbit collecting tubule. *J. Clin. Invest.*, **59**, 1099–1104
9. Iino, Y. and Imai, M. (1978). Effects of prostaglandins on Na transport in isolated collecting tubules. *Pflugers Arch.*, **373**, 125–32
10. Burch, R. M., Knapp, D.R. and Halushka, P.V. (1980). Vasopressin-stimulated water flow is decreased by thromboxane synthetase inhibition or antagonism. *Am. J. Physiol.*, **239**, F160–66
11. Burch, R.M. and Halushka, P.V. (1980). Thromboxane and stable prostaglandin endoperoxide analogs stimulate water permeability in the toad urinary bladder. *J. Clin. Invest.*, **66**, 1251–57
12. Holt, W.F. and Lechene, C. (1981). ADH–PGE_2 interactions in cortical collecting tubule. I. Depression of sodium transport. *Am. J. Physiol.*, **241**, F452–460
13. Patak, R.V., Mookergee, B.K., Bentzel, C.J., Hysert, P.E., Babej, M. and Lee, J.B. (1975). Antagonism of the effects of furosemide by indomethacin in normal and hypertensive man. *Prostaglandins*, **10**, 649–659
14. Fulgraff, G. and Meiforth, A. (1971). Effects of prostaglandin E_2 on excretion and reabsorption of sodium and fluid in rat kidneys (micropuncture studies). *Pflugers Arch.*, **330**, 243–56
15. Bartelheimer, H.K. and Senft, G. (1968). Zur Lokalisation der tubulaeren Wirkung einiger antirheumatisch wirkender Substanzen. *Arzneimittelforsch*, **18**, 567–79

16. Ganguli, M., Tobian, L., Azar, S. and O'Donnell, M. (1977). Evidence that prostaglandin synthesis inhibitors increase the concentration of sodium and chloride in rat renal medulla. *Circ. Res.*, **40**, *(suppl. 1)*, 135–139

17. Haylor, J. and Lote, C.J. (1980). Renal function in conscious rats after indomethacin. Evidence for a tubular action on endogenous prostaglandins. *J. Physiol.*, **298**, 371–381

18. Higashihara, E., Stokes, J.B., Kokko, J.P., Campbell, W.B. and DuBose, T.D. (1979). Cortical and papillary micropuncture examination of chloride transport in segments of the rat kidney during inhibition of prostaglandin production: a possible role for prostaglandins in the chloruresis of acute volume expansion. *J. Clin. Invest.*, **64**, 1277–87

19. Stoff, J.S., Rosa, R.M., Silva, P. and Epstein, F.H. (1982). Indomethacin impairs water diuresis in the DI rat: role of prostaglandins independent of ADH. *Am. J. Physiol.*, **241**, F231–37

20. Chang, L.C.T., Splawinski, J.A., Oates, J.A. and Nien, A.S. (1975). Enhanced renal prostaglandin production in the dog. II. Effects on intrarenal hemodynamics. *Circ. Res.*, **36**, 204–207

21. Larsson, C. and Anggard, E. (1974). Increased juxtamedullary blood flow on stimulation of prostaglandin biosynthesis. *Eur. J. Pharmacol.*, **25**, 327–34

22. Burch, R.M. and Halushka, P.V. (1982). Vasopressin stimulates prostaglandin and thromboxane synthesis in toad bladder epithelial cells. *Am. J. Physiol.*, **243**, F593–97

23. Zusman, T.R., Keiser, J.R. and Handler, J.S. (1977). Vasopressin-stimulated prostaglandin E biosynthesis in toad urinary bladder. *J. Clin. Invest.*, **60**, 1339–47

24. Beck, T.R., Hassid, A. and Dunn, M.J. (1980). Effect of arginine vasopressin and its analogues on the synthesis of PGE_2 by rat renal medullary interstitial cells in culture. *J. Pharmacol. Exp. Ther.*, **215**, 15–19

25. Kirschenbaum, M.A., Lowe, A.G., Trizna, W. and Fine, L.G. (1983). Regulation of vasopressin action by prostaglandin synthesis in the rabbit cortical collecting tubule. *J. Clin. Invest.* , **70**, 1193–1204

26. Dunn, M.J., Kinter, L.B., Beeuwkes, R., Shier, D., Greeley, H.F. and Valtin, H. (1980). Interaction of vasopressin and renal prostaglandins in the homozygous diabetes insipidus rat. In Samuelsson, B., Ramwell, P.W. and Paoletti, R. (eds.) *Advances in Prostaglandin and Thromboxane Research*, pp. 1009–1015. (New York: Raven Press)

27. Walker, L.A., Whorton, A.R., Smigel, R., France, R. and Frohlich, J.C. (1978). Antidiuretic hormone increases renal prostaglandin synthesis in vivo. *Am. J. Physiol.*, **235**, F180–185

28. Zusman, R.M. and Keiser, H.R. (1977). Prostaglandin biosynthesis by rabbit renomedullary interstitial cells in tissue culture. Stimulation by angiotensin II, bradykinin and arginine vasopressin. *J. Clin. Invest.*, **60**, 215–23

29. Schlondorff, D. (1984). Interaction of antidiuretic hormone and prostaglandin. In Braquet, P., Garay, M.D., Froelich, J.C. and Nicosia, S. (eds.) *Prostaglandins and Membrane Ion Transport*, pp. 343–47. (New York: Raven Press)

30. Stokes, J.B. (1979). Effect of prostaglandin E_2 on chloride transport across the rabbit thick ascending limb of Henle. *J. Clin. Invest.*, **64**, 495–502

31. Fine, L.G. and Trizna, W. (1977). Influence of prostaglandin on sodium transport of isolated medullary nephron segments. *Am. J. Physiol.*, **232**, F383–90

32. Lear, S. and Silva, P. (1985). Prostaglandin (PGE_2) inhibits chloride transport in medullary thick ascending limb (mTAL) cells. (abstract) *Kidney Int.*, **28**, 260

33. Culpepper, R.M. and Andreoli, T.E. (1983). Interactions among PGE_2, antidiuretic hormone and cyclic adenosine monophosphate in modulating Cl absorption in the single mouse medullary thick ascending limbs of Henle. *J. Clin. Invest.*, **71**, 1588–1600

34. Culpepper, R.M. and Andreoli, T.E. (1984). PGE_2, forskolin and cholera toxin interactions in modulating NaCl transport in mouse mTALH. *Am. J. Physiol.*, **247**, F784–92

35. Schlondorff, D., Yoo, P. and Alpert, B.E. (1978). Stimulation of adenylate cyclase in isolated glomeruli by prostaglandins. *Am. J. Physiol.*, **235**, F458–64

36. Whorton, A.R., Misono, K., Hollifield, J., Froelich, J.C., Inagami, T. and Oates, J.A. (1977). Prostaglandin and renin release. I. Stimulation of renin release from rabbit renal cortical slices by PGI_2. *Prostaglandins*, **14**, 1095–1104

37. Torikai, S. and Kurokawa, K. (1983). Effect of PGE_2 on vasopressin-dependent cell cAMP in isolated single nephron segments. *Am. J. Physiol.*, **245**, F58–66

38. Omachi, R.S., Robbie, D.E., Handler, J.S. and Orloff, J. (1974). Effects of ADH and other agents in cyclic AMP accumulation in toad bladder epithelium. *Am. J. Physiol.*, **226**, 1152–57

55

39. Pugliese, F., Sato, M., Williams, S., Aikawa, M., Hassid, A. and Dunn, M. (1983). Rabbit and rat renal papillary collecting tubule cells in culture: The interactions of arginine vasopressin, prostaglandins and cyclic AMP. In Samuelsson, B., Ramwell, P.W. and Paoletti, R. (eds.) *Advances in Prostaglandin, Thromboxane and Leukotriene Research*, pp.517–23. (New York: Raven Press)

40. Goldring, S.R., Sayer, J.M., Ausiello, D.A. and Krane, S.M. (1978). A cell strain cultured from porcine kidney increases cyclic AMP content upon exposure to calcitonin or vasopressin. *Biochem. Biophys. Res. Commun.*, **83**, 434–40

41. Grenier, F.C., Rollins, T.E. and Smith, W.L. (1981). Kinin-induced prostaglandin synthesis by renal papillary collecting tubule cells in culture. *Am. J. Physiol.*, **241**, F94–104

42. Edwards, R.M., Jackson, B.A. and Dousa, T.P. (1981). ADH-sensitive cAMP system in papillary collecting duct: Effect of osmolality and PGE_2. *Am. J. Physiol.*, **240**, F311–18

43. Jackson, B.A., Edwards, R.M. and Dousa, T.P. (1980). Vasopressin–prostaglandin interactions in isolated tubules from rat outer medulla. *J. Lab. Clin. Med.*, **96**, 119–28

44. Morel, F., Imbert-Teboul, M. and Chabardes, D. (1980). Cyclic nucleotides and tubule function. In Hamet, E. and Sands, H. (eds.) *Advances in Cyclic Nucleotide Research*, **12**, pp.301–313. (New York: Raven Press)

45. Halushka, P.V. and Burch, R.M. (1984). Effects of arachidonic acid metabolites on ^{45}Ca fluxes and intracellular calcium in epithelial cells from the toad urinary bladder. In Braquet, P. *et al.* (eds.) *Prostaglandin and Membrane Ion Transport*, pp.323–26. (New York: Raven Press)

46. McGiff, J.C., Crowshaw, K., Terragno, N.A. and Lonigro, A.J. (1970). Release of prostaglandin-like substance into renal venous blood in response to angiotensin II. *Circ. Res. (Suppl. 1)*, **26–27**, 121–30

47. Hsueh, W., Isakson, P.C. and Needleman, P. (1977). Hormone-selective lipase activation in the isolated rabbit heart. *Prostaglandins*, **13**, 1073–91

48. Dunn, M.J., Greely, H.P., Valtin, H., Kinter, L.B. and Beeuwkes, R. (1978). Renal excretion of prostaglandins E_2 and $F_{2\alpha}$ in diabetes insipidus rat. *Am. J. Physiol.*, **235**, E624–27

49. Levine, L. and Moskowitz, M.A. (1979). Alpha- and beta-adrenergic stimulation of arachidonic acid metabolism by cells in culture. *Proc. Natl. Acad. Sci. USA*, **76**, 6632–36

50. Gagnon, D.J., Gauthier, R. and Regoli, D. (1974). Release of prostaglandins from the rabbit perfused kidney: effects of vasoconstrictors. *Br. J. Pharmacol.*, **50**, 553–58

51. Needleman, P., Douglas, J.R. Jr. and Jakschik, B. (1974). Release of renal prostaglandin by catecholamines: relationship to renal endocrine function. *J. Pharmacol. Exp. Ther.*, **188**, 453–60

52. Craven, P.A., Briggs, R. and DeRubertis, F.R. (1980). Calcium-dependent action of osmolality on adenosine 3′,5′-monophophate accumulation in rat renal inner medulla: evidence for a relationship to calcium-responsive arachidonate release and prostaglandin synthesis. *J. Clin. Invest.*, **65**, 529–42

53. Flower, R.J. and Blackwell, G.J. (1976). The importance of phospholipase A_2 in prostaglandin biosynthesis. *Biochem. Pharmacol.*, **25**, 285–91

54. Craven, P.A. and DeRubertis, F.R. (1981). Effects of vasopressin and urea on Ca^{2+}-calmodulin-dependent renal prostaglandin E. *Am. J. Physiol.*, **241**, F649–58

55. Hassid, A.H. (1982). Regulation of prostaglandin biosynthesis in cultured cells. *Am. J. Physiol.*, **243**, C205–11

56. Dusing, R., Attallah, A.A., Prezyna, A.P. and Lee, J.B. (1978). Renal biosynthesis of prostaglandin E_2 and F_2: dependence on extracellular potassium. *J. Lab. Clin. Med.*, **92**, 669–77

57. Flower, R.J. and Blackwell, G.J. (1979). Anti-inflammatory steroids induce biosynthesis of phospholipase A_2 inhibitor which prevents prostaglandin generation. *Nature (London)*, **278**, 456–69

58. Morrison, A.R., Moritz, H. and Needleman, P. (1978). Mechanism of enhanced renal prostaglandin biosynthesis in ureter obstruction. Role of de novo protein synthesis. *J. Biol. Chem.*, **253**, 8210–12

59. Needleman, P., Wyche, A. and Bronson, S.D. (1979). Specific regulation of peptide-induced renal prostaglandin synthesis. *J. Biol. Chem.*, **254**, 9772–77

60. Zipser, R., Myers, S. and Needleman, P. (1980). Exaggerated prostaglandin and thromboxane synthesis in the rabbit with renal vein constriction. *Circ. Res.*, **47**, 231–37

61. Jacobson, H.R., Corona, S., Capdevila, J., Chacos, N., Manna, S., Womack, A. and Falck, J.R. (1984). Effects of epoxyicosatrienoic acids on ion transport in the rabbit cortical collecting tubule. In Braquet, P. et al. (eds.) Prostaglandins and Membrane Ion Transport, pp. 311–318. (New York: Raven Press)
62. Schwartzman, M., Ferreri, N.R., Carroll, M.A., Songu-Mize, E. and McGiff, J.C. (1985). Renal cytochrome P450-related arachidonate metabolite inhibits $(Na^+ + K^+)ATPase$. Nature (London), 314, 620–22
63. Cantley, L., Fuhro, R., Silva, P. and Epstein, F.H. (1986). Medullary thick ascending limb cells produce a transport inhibitor. Kidney Int., 29, 352
64. Smith, M.C. and Dunn, M.J. (1981). Renal kallikreins, kinins and prostaglandins in hypertension. In Brenner, B.M. and Stein, J.H. (eds.) Hypertension (Contemporary Issues in Nephrology, 8), pp. 168–202. (New York: Churchill Livingstone)
65. Dunn, M.J. (1983). Renal prostaglandins. In Dunn, M.J. (ed.) Renal Endocrinology, pp. 1–74. (Baltimore: Waverly Press Inc.)
66. Holland, O.B., Bhud, J.M. and Braunstein, H. (1980). Urinary kallikrein excretion in essential and mineralocorticoid hypertension. J. Clin. Invest., 65, 347–56
67. Lawton, W.J. and Fitz, A.E. (1980). Abnormal urinary kallikrein in hypertension is not related to aldosterone or plasma renin activity. Hypertension, 2, 787–93
68. Margolius, H.S., Pisano, J.J., Geller, R. and Sjoerdsma, A. (1971). Altered urinary kallikrein excretion in human hypertension. Lancet, 2, 1063–65
69. Abe, K., Seino, M., Yasujima, M., Chiba, S., Sakurai, Y., Irakawa, N., Miyazaki, S., Saito, K., Ito, T., Otsuka, Y. and Yoshinaga, K. (1977). Studies on renomedullary prostaglandin and renal kallikrein–kinin system in hypertension. Jpn. Circ. J., 41, 873–80
70. Abe, K., Yasujima, M., Chiba, S., Irakawa, N., Ito, T. and Yoshinaga, K. (1977). Effect of furosemide on urinary excretion of prostaglandin E in normal volunteers and patients with essential hypertension. Prostaglandins, 14, 513–21
71. Tan, S., Bravo, E. and Mulrow, R. (1978). Impaired renal prostaglandin E_2 biosynthesis in human hypertensive states. Prostagl. Med., 1, 76–85
72. Weber, P.C., Scherer, B., Held, E., Siess, W. and Stafel, H. (1979). Urinary prostaglandins and kallikrein in essential hypertension. Clin. Sci., 57, 259s–61s
73. Scherer, B., Held, E. and Lange, H-H. (1979). Erniedrigte renale Prostaglandin E_2-Ausscheidung and verminderte Stimulierbarkeit der Plasma Reninaktivitaet bei Patienten mit essentieller Hypertonie. Klin. Wochenschr., 57, 567–73
74. Grose, H.H., Lebel, M. and Gbeassor, F.M. (1980). Diminished urinary prostacyclin metabolite in essential hypertension. Clin. Sci., 59, 121s–23s
75. Lee, J., Kannegiesser, H., O'Toole, J. and Westura, E. (1971). Hypertension and the renomedullary prostaglandins: A human study of the anti-hypertensive effects of PGA_1. Ann. NY Acad. Sci., 180, 218–40
76. Lee, S.J., Johnson, J.G., Smith, C.J. and Hatch, F.E. (1972). Renal effects of prostaglandin A_1 in patients with essential hypertension. Kidney Int., 1, 254–62
77. O'Grady, J., Warrington, S. and Moti, M.J. (1980). Effects of intravenous infusion of prostacyclin (PGI_2) in man. Prostaglandins, 19, 319–32
78. Okada, F., Nukada, T., Yamauchi, Y. and Abe, H. (1974). The hypotensive effect of prostaglandin E_1 on hypertensive cases of various types. Prostaglandins, 7, 99–106
79. Smith, M.C., Danviriyasup, K., Cato, A.E., Crow, J.W. and Dunn, M.J. (1981). Prostacyclin substitution for heparin in hemodialysis. (abstract) Kidney Int., 19, 159
80. Gerhard, H. and Mulrow, P.J. (1974). The effect of acute renal failure on renal prostaglandin A (PGA). (abstract) Clin. Res., 22, 528A
81. Held, E., Weber, P. and Zatzkowski, I. (1975). Experimental oliguric acute renal failure: Protective effects of renomedullary autotransplants. Klin. Wochenschr., 53, 46–48
82. Torres, V.E., Romero, J.C., Strong, C.G. et al. (1974). Renal prostaglandin E during acute renal failure. Prostaglandins, 8, 353–60
83. Torres, V.E., Strong, C.G., Romero, J.C. and Wilson, C.M. (1975). Indomethacin enhancement of glycerol-induced acute renal failure in rabbits. Kidney Int., 7, 170–78
84. Mauk, R.H., Patak, R.V., Radem, S.Z. et al. (1977). Effect of prostaglandin E administration in a nephrotoxic and a vasoconstrictor model of acute renal failure. Kidney Int., 12, 122–30
85. Scherer, B., Schnermann, J., Sofronier, M. and Weber, P.C. (1978). Prostaglandin (PG) analysis in urine of humans and rats by different radioimmunoassays: Effect on PG

excretion by PG-synthetase inhibitors, laparotomy and furosemide. *Prostaglandins*, **15**, 255–66
86. Williamson, H.E., Bourland, W.A. and Marchand, G.R. (1975). Inhibition of furosemide-induced increase in renal blood flow by indomethacin. *Proc. Soc. Exp. Biol. Med.*, **148**, 164–70
87. DeTorrente, A., Miller, P.D., Cronin, R.F., Paulsen, P.E., Erickson, A.L. and Schrier, R.W. (1978). Effects of furosemide and acetylcholine in norepinephrine-induced acute renal failure. *Am. J. Physiol.*, **235**, F131–36
88. Patak, R.V., Fadem, S.Z., Lifschitz, M.D. and Stein, J.H. (1979). Study of factors which modify the development of norepinephrine-induced acute renal failure in the dog. *Kidney Int.*, **15**, 227–37
89. Bailey, R.R., Natale, R., Turnbull, D.I. and Linton, A.L. (1973). Protective effect of furosemide in acute tubular necrosis and acute renal failure. *Clin. Sci. Mol. Med.*, **45**, 1–17
90. Ufferman, R.C., Jaenike, J.R., Freeman, R.B. and Pabico, R.C. (1975). Effect of furosemide on low-dose mercuric chloride acute renal failure in the rat. *Kidney Int.*, **8**, 362–67
91. Thurau, K. and Schnermann, J. (1965). Die Natriumkonzentration an den Macula Densa-Zellen als regulierender Faktor fuer das Glomerulumfiltrat. *Klin. Wochenschr.*, **43**, 410–413
92. Wright, F.S. and Schnermann, J. (1974). Feedback control of glomerular filtration rate by furosemide, triflocin and cyanide. *J. Clin. Invest.*, **53**, 1695–1708
93. Donker, A.J., Arisz, L., Brentjens, J.R., VanderHem, G.K. and Hollemans, H.J. (1976). The effect of indomethacin on kidney function and plasma renin activity in man. *Nephron*, **17**, 288–96
94. Kimberly, R.P., Gill, J.R., Bowden, R.E., Keiser, H.R. and Plotz, P.H. (1978). Elevated urinary prostaglandins and the effects of aspirin on renal function in lupus erythematosus. *Ann. Intern. Med.*, **89**, 336–41
95. Berg, K.J. (1977). Acute effects of acetylsalicylic acid in patients with chronic renal insufficiency. *Eur. J. Clin. Pharmacol.*, **11**, 111–16
96. Kimberly, R.P. and Plotz, P.H. (1977). Aspirin-induced depression of renal function. *N. Engl. J. Med.*, **296**, 418–28
97. Kimberly, R.P., Bowden, R.E., Keiser, H.R. and Plotz, P.H. (1978). Reduction of renal function by newer non-steroidal anti-inflammatory drugs. *Am. J. Med.*, **64**, 804–07
98. Abe, K., Imai, Y. and Sato, M. (1981). Exaggerated fractional sodium excretion in hypertension with advanced renal disease: the role of renal prostaglandins and kallikrein. *Clin. Sci.*, **61**, 327s–30s
99. Ciabattoni, G., Cinotti, G.A., Pierucci, A., Simonetti, B.M., Manzi, M. and Pugliese, F. (1984). Effect of sulindac and ibuprofen in patients with chronic glomerular disease. Evidence for the dependence of renal function on prostacyclin. *N. Engl. J. Med.*, **310**, 279–83
100. Bowden, R.E., Gill, J.R. Jr., Radfar, N., Taylor, A.A. and Keiser, H.R. (1978). Prostaglandin synthetase inhibitors in Bartter's syndrome. *J. Am. Med. Assoc.*, **239**, 117–21
101. Arisz, L., Donker, A.J., Brentjens, J.R. and VanderHem, G.K. (1976). The effect of indomethacin on proteinuria and kidney function in the nephrotic syndrome. *Acta Med. Scand.*, **199**, 121–25
102. Bartter, F.C., Pronove, P., Gill, J.R. Jr. and McCardle, R.C. (1962). Hyperplasia of the juxtaglomerular complex with hyperaldosteronism and hypokalemic alkalosis. *Am. J. Med.*, **33**, 811–28
103. Zipser, R.D. and Rude, R.K., Zia, P.K. and Fichman, M.P. (1979). Regulation of urinary prostaglandins in Bartter's syndrome. *Am. J. Med.*, **67**, 263–67
104. Gullner, H-G., Cerletti, C., Bartter, F.C., Smith, J.B. and Gill, J.R. Jr. (1979). Prostacyclin overproduction in Bartter's syndrome. *Lancet*, **2**, 767–69
105. Fichman, M.P., Telfer, N. and Zia, P. (1976). Role of prostaglandins in the pathogenesis of Bartter's syndrome. *Am. J. Med.*, **60**, 785–97
106. Gill, J.R., Froelich, J.C., Bowden, R.E., Taylor, A.A., Keiser, H.R., Hannsjorg, W.S., Oates, J.A. and Bartter, F.C. (1976). Bartter's syndrome: A disorder characterized by high urinary prostaglandins and a dependence of hyperreninemia on prostaglandin synthesis. *Am. J. Med.*, **61**, 43–51

107. Halushka, P.V., Wohltmann, H., Privitera, P.J., Hurwitz, G. and Margolius, H.S. (1977). Bartter's syndrome: urinary prostaglandin E-like material and kallikrein; indomethacin effects. *Ann. Int. Med.*, **87**, 281–86

108. Sato, M., Abe, K. and Yasujima, M. (1980). Bartter's syndrome with normal urinary excretion of prostaglandin E: therapeutic effects of propanolol, spironolactone, indomethacin and potassium chloride. *Tohoku J. Exp. Med.*, **131**, 151–59

109. Lechi, A., Core, G., Lechi, C., Mantero, F. and Scuro, A. (1976). Urinary kallikrein excretion in Bartter's syndrome. *J. Clin. Endocrinol. Metab.*, **43**, 1175–78

110. Verbeckmoes, R., Van Damme, B. and Clement, J. (1976). Bartter's syndrome with hyperplasia of renomedullary cells: successful treatment with indomethacin. *Kidney Int.*, **9**, 302–307

111. McGiff, J.C. (1977). Bartter's syndrome results from imbalance of vasoactive hormones. *Ann. Int. Med.*, **87**, 369–72

112. Vinci, J.M., Gill, J.R. Jr., Bowden, R.E., Pisano, J.J., Izzo, J.L. Jr., Radfar, N., Taylor, A.A., Zusman, R.M. and Bartter, F.C. (1977). The kallikrein–kinin system in Bartter's syndrome and its response to prostaglandin synthetase inhibition. *J. Clin. Invest.*, **61**, 1671–82

113. Sasaki, H., Okumura, M., Asano, T. and Arakawa, K. (1977). Response of angiotensin II antagonist before and after treatment with indomethacin in Bartter's syndrome. *Br. Med. J.*, **2**, 995–96

114. Donker, A.H., deJong, P.E., Statius, van Eps, J.W., Brentjens, J.R., Bakker, K. and Doorenbos, H. (1977). Indomethacin in Bartter's syndrome. *Nephron*, **19**, 200–13

115. Veldhuis, J.D., Bardin, C.W. and Demers, L.M. (1979). Metabolic mimicry of Bartter's syndrome by covert vomiting. Utility of urinary chloride determination. *Am. J. Med.*, **66**, 361–63

116. Galvez, O.G., Bay, W.H., Roberts, B.W. and Ferris, T.F. (1978). The hemodynamic effects of potassium deficiency in the dog. *Circ. Res.*, **40**, (Suppl. 1), 11–16

117. Chan, J.C.M. (1980). Bartter's syndrome. *Nephron*, **26**, 155–62

118. Gill J.R. Jr. (1980). Bartter's syndrome. *Ann. Rev. Med.*, **31**, 405–19

119. Kurtzman, N.A. and Gutierrez, L.F. (1975). The pathophysiology of Bartter's syndrome. *J. Am. Med. Assoc.*, **234**, 758–59

120. Gill, J.R. and Bartter, F.C. (1978). Evidence for a prostaglandin-independent defect in chloride reabsorption in the loop of Henle as a proximal cause of Bartter's syndrome. *Am. J. Med.*, **65**, 766–72

121. Norby, L., Mark, A.L. and Kaloyanides, G.J. (1976). On the pathogenesis of Bartter's syndrome: report of studies in a patient with this disorder. *Clin. Nephrol.*, **6**, 404–13

122. Kurtz, I., Hernandez, R., Schambelan, M., Biglieri, E., Rector, F.C. Jr., Morris, R.C. Jr. and Sebastian, A. (1984). The results of tests of renal diluting ability do not support the hypothesis that NaCl transport in the loop of Henle is impaired in Bartter's syndrome. (abstract) *Kidney Int.*, **25**, 170

123. Garrick, R., Ziyadeh, F.M., Jorkasky, D. and Goldfarb, S. (1985). Bartter's Syndrome: a unifying hypothesis. *Am. J. Nephrol.*, **5**, 379–84

124. Cole, C.H. and O'Regan, S. (1981). Effects of treatment with prostaglandin synthetase inhibitors in the erythrocyte sodium transport abnormality in Bartter's syndrome. *Pediatr. Res.*, **15**, 926–29

125. Mongeau, J., Garay, R., DeMendonca, M., Broyer, M. and Meyer, P. (1983). Erythrocyte Na and K transport system in children with Bartter's syndrome: increase in passive sodium permeability. *Kidney Int.*, **23**, 530–35

126. Gallery, E.D.M., Koumantakis, G., Bean, C., Grigg, R. and Gyory, A.Z. (1984). Cellular electrolyte transport in Bartter's syndrome (abstract). *IXth International Congress of Nephrology*, Los Angeles

127. Brunois, J.P., Vistelle, R., Milcent, T., Toupance, O., Choisy, H. and Chanard, J. (1984). Erythrocyte Na and K transport systems in hypokalemia: only Bartter's syndrome is associated with increase in passive sodium permeability (abstract). *Kidney Int.*, **26**, 227

128. Ramos, E., Hall-Craggs, M. and Demers, L.M. (1980). Surreptitious habitual vomiting simulating Bartter's syndrome. *J. Am. Med. Assoc.*, **243**, 1070–72

129. Walker, R.M., Brown, R.S. and Stoff, J.S. (1981). Role of renal prostaglandins during antidiuresis and water diuresis in man. *Kidney Int.*, **21**, 365–70

130. Serros, E.R. and Kirschenbaum, M.A. (1981). Prostaglandin-dependent polyuria in hypercalcemia. *Am. J. Physiol.*, **241**, F224–30

131. Levison, S.P. and Levison, M.E. (1976). Effect of indomethacin and sodium meclofenamate on the renal concentrating defect in experimental enterococcal pyelonephritis in rats. *J. Lab. Clin. Med.*, **88**, 958–64
132. Kirschenbaum, M.A. and Serros, E.R. (1980). Effects of alterations in urine flow rate on prostaglandin E excretion in conscious dogs. *Am. J. Physiol.*, **238**, F107–11
133. Düsing, R., Attallah, A.A., Prezyna, A.P. and Lee, J.B. (1978). Renal biosynthesis of prostaglandin E_2 and F_{2a}: dependence on extracellular potassium. *J. Lab. Clin. Med.*, **92**, 669–77
134. Whinnery, M.A. and Kunau, R.T. (1979). Effect of potassium deficiency on papillary plasma flow in rat. *Am. J. Physiol.*, **237**, F226–31
135. Beck, N. and Shaw, J.O. (1981). Thromboxane B_2 and prostaglandin E_2 in the K^+-depleted rat kidney. *Am. J. Physiol.*, **240**, F151–57
136. Nadler, J.L., Lee, F.O., Hsueh, W. and Horton, R. (1986). Evidence of prostacyclin deficiency in the syndrome of hyporeninemic hypoaldosteronism. *N. Engl. J. Med.*, **314**, 1015–42
137. Scharschmidt, L.A. and Dunn, M.J. (1983). Prostaglandin synthesis by rat glomerular mesangial cells. Effects of angiotensin II and arginine vasopressin. *J. Clin. Invest.*, **71**, 1756–64
138. Garella, S. and Matarese, R.A. (1984). Renal effects of prostaglandins and clinical adverse effects of nonsteroidal anti-inflammatory agents. *Medicine*, **63**, 165–81
139. Flower, R.H. (1974). Drugs which inhibit prostaglandin biosynthesis. *Pharmacol. Rev.*, **26**, 33–50
140. Clive, D.M. and Stoff, J.S. (1984). Clinical nephrologic syndromes associated with the use of nonsteroidal anti-inflammatory drugs. *N. Engl. J. Med.*, **310**, 563–72
141. Dunn, M.J. and Zambraski, E.J. (1980). Renal effects of drugs that inhibit prostaglandin synthesis. *Kidney Int.*, **18**, 609–622
142. Ferreira, S.H. and Vane, J.R. (1974). New aspect of the mode of action of nonsteroidal anti-inflammatory drugs. *Ann. Rev. Pharmacol.*, **14**, 57–70
143. Rumpf, K.W., Frenzel, S., Lowitz, M.D. and Scheler, F. (1976). The effect of indomethacin on plasma renin activity in man. *Proc. Eur. Dial. Transplant Assoc.*, **12**, 299–301
144. Epstein, M., Lifschitz, M.D., Hoffman, D.S. and Stein, J.H. (1979). Relationship between renal prostaglandin E and renal sodium handling during water immersion on normal man. *Circ. Res.*, **45**, 71–80
145. Favre, L., Glasson, P. and Vallotton, M.B. (1982). Reversible acute renal failure from combined triamterene and indomethacin. A study in healthy subjects. *Ann. Int. Med.*, **96**, 317–20
146. Beeley, L. and Kendall, M.G. (1971). Effect of aspirin on renal clearance of ^{125}I-diatrozoate. *Br. Med. J.*, **1**, 707–08
147. Robert, M., Fillastre, J.P., Berger, H. and Malandain, H. (1972). Effect of intravenous infusion of acetylsalicylic acid on renal function. *Br. Med. J.*, **2**, 466–7
148. Berg, K.J. (1977). Acute effects of acetylsalicylic acid on renal function in normal man. *Eur. J. Clin. Pharmacol.*, **11**, 117–23
149. Muther, R.S. and Bennett, W.M. (1980). Effects of aspirin on glomerular filtration rate in normal humans. *Ann. Int. Med.*, **92**, 386–87
150. Muther, R.S., Potter, D.M. and Bennett, W.M. (1981). Aspirin-induced depression of glomerular filtration rate in normal humans – role of sodium balance. *Ann. Int. Med.*, **94**, 317–21
151. Oliver, J.A., Pinto, J., Sciacca, R.R. and Cannon, P.J. (1980). Increased renal secretion of norepinephrine and prostaglandin E_2 during sodium depletion in the dog. *J. Clin. Invest.*, **66**, 748–56
152. Oliver, J.A., Sciacca, R.R., Pinto, J. and Cannon, P.J. (1981). Participation of prostaglandin in the control of renal blood flow during acute reduction of cardiac output in the dog. *J. Clin. Invest.*, **67**, 229–37
153. Walshe, J.J. and Venuto, R.C. (1983). Acute oliguric renal failure induced by indomethacin: possible mechanism. *Ann. Intern. Med.*, **91**, 47–49
154. Boyer, T.D., Zia, P. and Reynolds, T.B. (1979). Effect of indomethacin and prostaglandin A_1 on renal function and plasma renin activity in alcoholic liver disease. *Gastroenterology*, **77**, 215–22

155. Attallah, A.A. (1979). Interaction on prostaglandins with diuretics. *Prostaglandins*, **18**, 369
156. Favre, L., Glasson, P.H., Riondel, A. and Vallotton, M.B. (1983). Interaction of diuretics and non-steroidal anti-inflammatory drugs in man. *Clin. Sci.*, **64**, 407–15
157. Mirouze, D., Zipser, R.D. and Reynolds, T.B. (1983). Effect of inhibitors of prostaglandin synthesis on induced diuresis in cirrhosis. *Hepatology*, **3**, 50–55
158. Tiggeler, R.G., Koene, R.A. and Wijdeveld, P.G. (1977). Inhibition of furosemide-induced natriuresis by indomethacin in patients with the nephrotic syndrome. *Clin. Sci. Mol. Med.*, **52**, 149–51
159. Williamson, H.E., Bourland, U.A. and Marchand, G.R. (1975). Inhibition of furosemide-induced increase in renal blood flow by indomethacin. *Proc. Soc. Exp. Biol. Med.*, **148**, 164–67
160. McCarthy, J.T., Torres, V.E. and Romero, J.C., Wochos, D.N. and Velosa, J.A. (1982). Acute intrinsic renal failure induced by indomethacin: Role of prostaglandin synthetase inhibition. *Mayo Clin. Proc.*, **57**, 289–96
161. Torres, V.E., Velosa, J.A., Holley, K.E., Frohnert, P.P., Zincke, H. and Sterioff, S. (1984). Meclofenamate treatment of recurrent idiopathic nephrotic syndrome with focal segmental glomerulosclerosis after renal transplantation. *Mayo Clin. Proc.*, **59**, 149–52
162. Velosa, J.A., Torres, V.E., Donadio, J.V. Jr., Wagoner, R.D., Holley, K.E. and Offord, K.P. (1985). Treatment of severe nephrotic syndrome with meclofenamate: an uncontrolled pilot study. *Mayo Clin. Proc.*, **60**, 586–92
163. Vriesendorp, R., Donder, A.J., deZeeus, D., deJong, P.E. and van der Hem, G.K. (1985). Antiproteinuric effect of naproxen and indomethacin. A double-blind crossover study. *Am. J. Nephrol.*, **5**, 236–42
164. Vriesendorp, R., de Zeeuw, D., de Jong, P.E., Donker, A.J., Pratt, J.J. and van der Hem, G.K. (1986). Reduction of urinary protein and prostaglandin E_2 excretion in the nephrotic syndrome by non-steroidal anti-inflammatory drugs. *Clin. Nephrol.*, **25**, 105–10
165. Usberti, M., Dechaux, M., Guillot, M., Seligmann, R., Pablovitch, H., Loirat, C., Sachs, C. and Broyer, M. (1980). Renal prostaglandin E_2 in nephrogenic diabetes insipidus: effects of inhibition of prostaglandin synthesis by indomethacin. *J. Pediatr.*, **97**, 476–78
166. Chevalier, R.L. and Rogol, A.D. (1980). Tolmetin sodium in the management of nephrogenic diabetes insipidus. *J. Pediatr.*, **101**, 787–89
167. Gross, P.A., Schrier, R.W. and Anderson, R.J. (1981). Prostaglandins and water metabolism: a review with emphasis on in vivo studies. *Kidney Int.*, **19**, 839–50
168. Zusman, R.M., Vinci, J.M., Bowden, R.E., Horwitz, D. and Keiser, H.R. (1979). Effect of indomethacin and adrenocorticotrophic hormone on renal function in man: an experimental model of inappropriate antidiuresis. *Kidney Int.*, **15**, 62–70
169. Goldszer, R.C., Coodley, E.L., Rosner, M.J., Simons, W.M. and Schwartz, A.M. (1980). Hyperkalemia associated with indomethacin. *Arch. Intern. Med.*, **141**, 802–04
170. Kutyrina, I.M., Androsova, S.O. and Tareyeva, I.E. (1979). Indomethacin-induced hyporeninemic hypoaldosteronism. *Lancet*, **1**, 785
171. Tan, S.Y., Shapiro, R., Stockard, H. and Mulrow, P.J. (1979). Indomethacin-induced prostaglandin inhibition with hyperkalemia. A reversible cause of hyporeninemic hypoaldosteronism. *Ann. Intern. Med.*, **90**, 783–85
172. Romero, J.C., Dunlap, C.L. and Strong, C.G. (1976). The effect of indomethacin and other anti-inflammatory drugs on the renin–angiotensin system. *J. Clin. Invest.*, **58**, 282–88
173. Bunning, R.D. and Werner, F.B. (1982). Sulindac: A potential renal-sparing non-steroidal anti-inflammatory drug. *J. Am. Med. Assoc.*, **248**, 2864–67
174. Ciabattoni, G., Pugliese, F., Cinotti, G.A. and Patrono, C. (1980). Renal effects of anti-inflammatory drugs. *Eur. J. Rheum. Inflam.*, **3**, 210–16
175. Brater, D.C., Anderson, S., Baird, B. and Campbell, W.B. (1985). The effect of ibuprofen, naproxen and sulindac on prostaglandins in men. *Kidney Int.*, **27**, 66–73
176. Steiness, E. and Waldorff, S. (1982). Different interactions of indomethacin and sulindac with thiazides in hypertension. *Br. Med. J.*, **285**, 1702–3
177. Whelton, A., Bender, W., Voghaiwalla, F., Hall-Craggs, M. and Solez, K. (1983). Sulindac and renal impairment (letters). *J. Am. Med. Assoc.*, **249**, 2892–93
178. Zipser, R., Hoefs, P., Speckart, P., Zia, P. and Horton, R. (1979). Evidence for a critical role of prostaglandins in renin release, vascular reactivity and renal function in liver disease. *J. Clin. Endocrinol. Metab.*, **48**, 895–900

179. Kleinknecht, C., Broyer, M., Gubler, M.C. and Palcoux, J.B. (1980). Irreversible renal failure after indomethacin in steroid-resistant nephrosis. *N. Engl. J. Med.*, **302**, 691–92

180. Zipser, R.D., Radvan, G.H., Kronborg, I.J., Duke, R. and Little, T.E. (1983). Urinary thromboxane B_2 and prostaglandin E_2 in the hepatorenal syndrome: Evidence for increased vasoconstriction and decreased vasodilator factors. *Gastroenterology*, **84**, 697–75

181. Lianos, E.A., Alavi, N. and Tobin, M. (1982). Angiotensin-induced sodium excretion patterns in cirrhosis: Role of renal prostaglandins. *Kidney Int.*, **21**, 70–77

182. Terragno, N.A., Terragno, D.A. and McGiff, J.C. (1977). Contribution of prostaglandins to the renal circulation in conscious, anesthetized and laparotomized dogs. *Circ. Res.*, **40**, 590–95

183. Itskovitz, H.D., Stemper, J., Pacholczyk, D. and McGiff, J.C. (1973). Renal prostaglandins: determinants of intrarenal distribution of blood flow in the dog. *Clin. Sci. Mol. Med.*, **45**, 321s–24s

184. Venuto, R.C., O'Dorisio, T., Ferris, T.F. and Stein, J.H. (1975). Prostaglandins and renal function: II. The effect of prostaglandin inhibition on autoregulation blood flow in the intact kidney of the dog. *Prostaglandins*, **9**, 817–28

185. Feigen, L.P., Klainer, E., Chapwick, B.M. and Kadowitz, P.J. (1976). The effect of indomethacin on renal function on pentobarbital-anesthetized dogs. *J. Pharm. Exp. Ther.*, **198**, 457–63

186. Pettinger, W.A., Tanaka, K., Keeton, K., Campbell, W.B. and Brooks, S.N. (1975). Renin release, an artifact of anesthesia and its implications in rats. *Proc. Soc. Exp. Biol. Med.*, **148**, 625–30

187. Kimberly, R.P., Sherman, R.L., Mouradian, J. and Lockshin, M.D. (1979). Apparent acute renal failure associated with therapeutic aspirin and ibuprofen administration. *Arthr. Rheum.*, **22**, 281–85

188. Fawaz-Estrup, F. and Ho, G. Jr. (1981). Reversible renal failure induced by indomethacin. *Arch. Int. Med.*, **141**, 1670–72

189. Findling, J.W., Beckstrom, D., Rawsthorne, L., Kozin, F. and Itskovitz, H. (1980). Indomethacin-induced hyperkalemia in three patients with gouty arthritis. *J. Am. Med. Assoc.*, **244**, 1127–28

190. Galler, M., Folkert, V.W. and Schlondorff, D. (1981). Reversible acute renal insufficiency and hyperkalemia following indomethacin therapy. *J. Am. Med. Assoc.*, **246**, 154–55

191. Tan, S.Y., Shapiro, R. and Kish, M.A. (1979). Reversible acute renal failure induced by indomethacin. *J. Am. Med. Assoc.*, **241**, 2732–33

192. Curt, B.A., Kaldany, A., Whitley, L.G. *et al.* (1980). Reversible rapidly progressive renal failure with nephrotic syndrome due to fenoprofen calcium. *Ann. Int. Med.*, **92**, 72–73

193. Carmichael, J. and Shankel, S.W. (1985). Effects of non-steroidal anti-inflammatory drugs on prostaglandins and renal function. *Am. J. Med.*, **78**, 992–1000

194. Bender, W.L., Whelton, A., Beschorner, W.E., Darwish, M.O., Hall-Craggs, M. and Solez, K. (1984). Interstitial nephritis, proteinuria, and renal failure caused by non-steroidal anti-inflammatory drugs. Immunologic characterization of the inflammatory infiltrate. *Am. J. Med.*, **76**, 1006–1012

195. Finkelstein, A., Fraley, D.S., Stachura, I., Feldman, H.A., Gandy, D.R. and Bourke, E. (1982). Fenoprofen nephropathy: lipoid nephrosis and interstitial nephritis. A possible T-lymphocyte disorder. *Am. J. Med.*, **72**, 81–87

196. Brezin, J.H., Katz, S.M., Schwartz, A.B. and Chinitz, J.L. (1979). Reversible renal failure and nephrotic syndrome associated with non-steroidal anti-inflammatory drugs. *N. Engl. J. Med.*, **301**, 1271–73

197. Wendland, M.L., Wagoner, R.D. and Holley, K.E. (1980). Renal failure associated with fenoprofen. *Mayo Clin. Proc.*, **55**, 103–107

198. Gary, N.E., Dodelson, R. and Eisinger, R.P. (1980). Indomethacin associated acute renal failure. *Am. J. Med.*, **69**, 135–136

199. Chatterjee, G. (1981). Nephrotic syndrome induced by tolmetin. *J. Am. Med. Assoc.*, **246**, 1589–90

200. Katz, S.M., Capaldo, R., Everts, E.A. and DiGregorio, J.G. (1981). Tolmetin: Association with reversible renal failure and acute interstitial nephritis. *J. Am. Med. Assoc.*, **246**, 243–45

201. Rennke, H.G., Roos, P.C. and Wall., S.G. (1980). Drug-induced interstitial nephritis with heavy glomerular proteinuria. *N. Engl. J. Med.*, **302**, 691–92
202. Fong, H.G. and Cohen, A.H. (1982). Ibuprofen-induced acute renal failure with acute tubular necrosis. *Am. J. Nephrol.*, **2**, 28–31
203. Levenson, D.J., Simmons, C.E. Jr. and Brenner, B.M. (1982). Arachidonic acid metabolism, prostaglandin and the kidney. *Am. J. Med.*, **72**, 354–74
204. Murray, T. and Goldberg, M. (1978). Analgesic-associated nephropathy in the USA: Epidemiologic, clinical and pathogenetic features. *Kidney Int.*, **13**, 64–71
205. Shelley, J.H. (1978). Pharmacologic mechanisms of analgesic nephropathy. *Kidney Int.*, **13**, 15–26
206. Nanra, R.S. and Kincaid-Smith, P. (1970). Papillary necrosis in rats caused by aspirin-containing mixtures. *Br. Med. J.*, **3**, 559–61
207. Kaump, D.H. (1966). Pharmacology of the fenamates. II. Toxicology in animals. *Ann. Phys. Med.*, **9**, 16–25
208. Emmerson, J.L., Gibson, W.R., Pierce, E.C. and Kiplinger, G.F. (1973). Preclinical toxicology of fenoprofen (abstract). *Toxicol. Appl. Pharmac.*, **25**, 444
209. Kincaid-Smith, P. (1970). Analgesic nephropathy. *Br. Med. J.*, **4**, 618
210. Morales, A. and Styn, J. (1971). Papillary necrosis following phenylbutazone ingestion. *Arch. Surg.*, **103**, 420–21
211. Husserl, F.E., Lange, R.K. and Kantrow, C.M. Jr. (1979). Renal papillary necrosis and pyelonephritis accompanying fenoprofen therapy. *J. Am. Med. Assoc.*, **242**, 1896–8
212. Caruana, R.J. and Semble, E.L. (1984). Renal papillary necrosis due to naproxen. *J. Rheumatol.*, **11**, 90–91
213. McDonald, F.D., Lazarus, G.S. and Campbell, W.L. (1967). Phenylbutazone anuria. *S. Med. J.*, **60**, 1318–20
214. Kimberly, R.P. and Brandstetter, R.D. (1978). Exacerbation of phenylbutazone-related renal failure by indomethacin. *Arch. Int. Med.*, **138**, 1711–12
215. Weisman, J.I. and Bloom, B. (1955). Anuria following phenylbutazone therapy. *N. Engl. J. Med.*, **252**, 1086–87
216. Zipsett, M.B. and Goldman, R. (1954). Phenylbutazone toxicity: report of a case of acute renal failure. *Ann. Int. Med.*, **41**, 1075–79
217. Kelley, V.E., Sneve, S. and Musinski, S. (1986). Increased renal thromboxane production in murine lupus nephritis. *J. Clin. Invest.*, **77**, 252–259
218. Lianos, E.A., Andres, G.A. and Dunn, M.J. (1983). Glomerular prostaglandin and thromboxane synthesis in rat nephrotoxic serum nephritis. *J. Clin. Invest.*, **72**, 1439–1448
219. Foegh, M.L., Winchester, J.F., Zmudka, M., Helfrich, G.B., Cooley, C., Ramwell, P.W. and Schreiner, G.E. (1981). Urine i-TxB$_2$ in renal allograft rejection. *Lancet*, **29**, 431–434
220. Coffman, T.M., Yarger, W.E. and Klotman, P.E. (1985). Functional role of thromboxane production by acutely rejecting renal allografts in rats. *J. Clin. Invest.*, **75**, 1242–1248
221. Mangino, M.J., Anderson, C.B., DeSchryver, K., Tyler, J.D., Sicard, G.A. and Turk, J. (1986). Eicosanoid synthesis associated with renal allograft rejection. *Transplant Proc.*, **18**, 63–70
222. Badr, K., Kelley, V.E., Rennke, H. and Brenner, B.M. (1986). Role for thromboxane A$_2$ and sulfidopeptide leukotrienes in endotoxin-induced acute renal failure. *Kidney Int.*, **30**, 474–480
223. Kawaguchi, A., Goldman, M.H., Shapiro, R., Foegh, M.L., Ramwell, P.W. and Lower, R.R. (1985). Increase in urinary thromboxane B$_2$ in rats caused by cyclosporine. *Transplantation*, **40**, 214–216
224. Elzinga, L., Kelley, V.E., Houghton, D.C. and Bennett, W.M. (1987). Fish oil as the vehicle for cyclosporine modifies experimental nephrotoxicity. *Transplantation*, **43**, 271–274
225. Purkerson, M.L., Joist, J.H., Yates, J., Valdis, A., Morrison, A. and Klahr, S. (1985). Inhibition of thromboxane synthesis ameliorates the progressive kidney disease of rats with subtotal renal ablation. *Proc. Natl. Acad. Sci.*, **82**, 193–197
226. Remuzzi, G., Imberti, L., Rossini, M., Marelli, C., Carminati, G., Cattaneo, M. and Bertani, T. (1985). Increased glomerular thromboxane synthesis as a possible cause of proteinuria in experimental nephrosis. *J. Clin. Invest.*, **75**, 94–101

227. Benabe, J.E., Klahr, S., Hoffman, M.K. and Morrison, A.R. (1980). Production of thromboxane A_2 by the kidney in glycerol-induced acute renal failure in the rabbit. *Prostaglandin*, **19**, 333–347
228. Sraer, J.D., Moulonquet-Doleris, L., Relarue, F., Sraer, J. and Ardaillou, R. (1981). Prostaglandin synthesis by glomeruli isolated from rats with glycerol-induced acute renal failure. *Circ. Res.*, **49**, 775–783
229. Morrison, A.R., Nishikawa, K. and Needleman, P. (1978). Thromboxane A_2 biosynthesis in the ureter obstructed isolated perfused kidney of the rabbit. *J. Pharmacol. Exp. Ther.*, **205**, 1–8
230. Okegawa, T., Jonas, P.E., DeSchryver, K., Kawasaki, A. and Needleman, P. (1983). Metabolic and cellular alterations underlying the exaggerated renal prostaglandin and thromboxane synthesis in ureter obstruction in rabbits. Inflammatory response involving fibroblasts and mononuclear cells. *J. Clin. Invest.*, **71**, 81–90
231. Konieczkowski, M., Dunn, M.J. Stork, J.E. and Hassid, A. (1982). Glomerular synthesis of prostaglandins and thromboxane in spontaneously hypertensive rats. *Hypertension*, **5**, 446–452
232. Patrono, C., Ciabattoni, G., Remuzzi, G., Gotti, E., Bombardieri, S., DiMunno, ·O., Tartarelli, G., Cinotti, G.A., Simonetti, B.M. and Pierucci, A. (1985). Functional significance of renal prostacyclin and thromboxane A_2 production in patients with systemic lupus erythematosus. *J. Clin. Invest.*, **76**, 1011–1018
233. Khirabadi, B.S., Foegh, M.L. and Ramwell, P.W. (1985). Urine immunoreactive thromboxane B_2 in rat cardiac allograft rejection. *Transplantation*, **39**, 6–8
234. Steinhauer, H.B., Wilms, H., Ruther, M. and Schollermeyer, P. (1986). Clinical experience with urine TxB_2 in acute renal allograft rejection. *Transplant Proc.*, **18**, 98–103
235. Kawasaki, A. and Needleman, P. (1982). Contribution of thromboxane to renal resistance changes in the isolated perfused hydronephrotic rabbit kidney. *Circ. Res.*, **50**, 486–490
236. Kelley, V.E., Winkelstein, A. and Izui, S. (1979). Effect of prostaglandin E on immune complex nephritis in NZB/W mice. *Lab. Invest.*, **41**, 531–537
237. Winkelstein, A. and Kelley, V.E. (1980). The pharmacologic effects of PGE_1 on murine lymphocytes. *Blood*, **55**, 437–443
238. Altman, A., Theofilopoulos, A.N., Weiner, R., Katz, D. and Dixon, F.J. (1981). Analysis of T cell function in autoimmune murine strains. Defects in production and responsiveness to interleukin 2. *J. Exp. Med.*, **154**, 791–808
239. Dauphinee, M.J., Kipper, S.B., Wofsy, D. and Talal, N. (1981). Interleukin 2 deficiency is a common feature of autoimmune mice. *J. Immunol.*, **127**, 2483–2487
240. Theofilopoulos, A.N. and Dixon, F.J. (1981). Etiopathogenesis of murine SLE. *Immunol. Rev.*, **55**, 179–216
241. Izui, S., McConahey, P.J. and Dixon, F.J. (1978). Increased spontaneous polyclonal activation of B lymphocytes in mice with spontaneous autoimmune disease. *J. Immunol.*, **121**, 2213–2219
242. Wofsy, D. and Seaman, W.E. (1985). Successful treatment of autoimmunity in NZB/NZW Fl mice with monoclonal antibody to L3T4. *J. Exp. Med.*, **161**, 378–391
243. Adelman, N.E., Watling, D.L. and McDevit, H.O. (1983). Treatment of (NZB × NZW) Fl disease with anti-IA monoclonal antibodies. *J. Exp. Med.*, **158**, 1350–1355
244. Theofilopoulos, A.N., Eisenberg, R.A., Bourdon, M., Crowell, J.S. and Dixon, F.J. (1979). Distribution of lymphocytes identified by surface markers in murine strains with systemic lupus erythematosus-like syndromes. *J. Exp. Med.*, **149**, 516–534
245. Morse, H.C. III, Davidson, W.F., Yetter, R.A., Murphy, E.D., Roths, J.B. and Coffman, R.L. (1982). Abnormalities induced by the mutant gene lpr: expression of a unique lymphocyte subset. *J. Immunol.*, **129**, 2612–2615
246. Wofsy, D., Hardy, R.R. and Seaman, W.E. (1984). The proliferating cells in autoimmune, MRL/lpr mice lack L3T4, an antigen on helper T cells that is involved in the response to class II major histocompatibility antigens. *J. Immunol.*, **32**, 2686–2689
247. Prud'homme, G.J., Park, C.L., Fiesar, T.M., Kofler, R., Dixon, F.J. and Theofilopoulos, A.N. (1983). Identification of a B cell differentiation factor(s) spontaneously produced by proliferating T cells in murine lupus strains of the lpr/lpr genotype. *J. Exp. Med.*, **157**, 730–742
248. Kelley, V.E., Winkelstein, A., Izui, S. and Dixon, F.J. (1981). Prostaglandin El inhibits T cell proliferation and renal disease in MRL/l mice. *Clin. Immunol. Immunopathol.*, **21**, 190–203

249. Wofsy, D., Ledbetter, J.A., Hendler, P.L. and Seaman, W.E. (1985). Treatment of murine lupus with monoclonal anti-T cell antibody. *J. Immunol.*, **134**, 852–857
250. Izui, S., Kelley, V.E., Masuda, K., Yoshida, H., Roths, J.B. and Murphy, E.D. (1984). Induction of various autoantibodies by mutant gene *lpr* in several strains of mice. *J. Immunol.*, **133**, 227–233
251. Kelley, V.E. and Roth, J. (1985). Interaction of mutant *lpr* gene with background strain influences renal disease. *Clin. Immunol. Immunopathol.*, **37**, 220–229
252. Romeo, L., Mazoujian, G. and Dolbashian, J. (1985). Enhanced renal Ia expression in murine autoimmunity. *Kidney Int.*, **29**, 289(a)
253. Davignon, J.L., Budd, R.C., Ceredig, R., Piguet, P.F., MacDonald, H.R., Cerottini, J.C., Vassalli, P. and Izui, S. (1985). Functional analysis of T cell subsets from mice bearing the lpr gene. *J. Immunol.*, **135**, 2423–2428
254. Dumont, F.J., Habbersett, R.C. and Coker, L.Z. (1985). Subsets of Lyt 2 + cells defined by differential expression of 9F3 antigen alterations in mice of the lpr/lpr genotype. *J. Immunol.*, **134**, 196–203
255. Altboum, I., Boswell, J. and Kelley, V.E. (1986). Thromboxane production by activated renal cortical macrophages. Presented at the *American Society of Nephrology*, December 7–10, Washington D.C.
256. Coffman, T.M., Schwertschag, U., Yarger, W.E., Pirotzky, E., Benveniste, J. and Klotman, P.E. (1986). Lipid mediators in acute renal allograft rejection. *Transplant. Proc.*, **18**, 94–97
257. Klotman, P.E., Smith, S.R., Volpp, B.D., Coffman, T.M. and Yarger, W.E. (1986). Thromboxane synthetase inhibition improves function of hydronephrotic rat kidneys. *Am. J. Physiol.*, **250**, F282–F287
258. Papanicolaou, N., Hatziatoniou, C. and Bariety, J. (1986). Selective inhibition of thromboxane synthesis partially protected while inhibition of angiotensin II formation did not protect rats against acute renal failure induced with glycerol. *Prostagl. Leuk. Med.*, **1**, 29–35
259. Dunn, M.J. (1983). Renal prostaglandins. In Klahr, S. and Massey, S.G. (eds). *Contemporary Nephrology*, pp. 145–191. (New York: Plenum Medical Books Co.)
260. Kelley, V.E., Winkelstein, A., Izui, S. and Dixon, F.J. (1981). Prostaglandin El inhibits T cell proliferation and renal disease in MRL/l mice. *Clin. Immunol. Immunopathol.*, **21**, 190–203
261. Kelley, V.E., Izui, S. and Halushka, P.V. (1982). Effect of ibuprofen, a fatty acid cyclooxygenase inhibitor in murine lupus. *Clin. Immunol. Immunopathol.*, **25**, 223–231
262. Culp, B.R., Titus, B.G. and Lands, W.E.M. (1979). Inhibition of prostaglandin biosynthesis by eicosapentaenoic acid. *Prostagl. Med.*, **3**, 269–275
263. Needleman, P., Raz, A., Munkes, M.S., Ferrendelli, J.A. and Sprecher, H. (1979). Triene prostaglandins: prostacyclin and thromboxane biosynthesis and unique biological properties. *Proc. Natl. Acad. Sci.*, **76**, 944–948
264. Kelley, V.E., Ferretti, A., Izui, S. and Strom, T.B. (1985). A fish oil diet rich in eicosapentaenoic acid reduces cyclooxygenase metabolites and suppresses lupus in MRL-lpr mice. *J. Immunol.*, **134**, 1914–1919
265. Prickett, J.D., Robinson, D.R. and Steinberg, A.D. (1981). Dietary enrichment with the polyunsaturated fatty acid eicosapentenoic acid prevents proteinuria and prolongs survival in NZB × NZW Fl mice. *J. Clin. Invest.*, **68**, 556–559
266. Prickett, J.D., Robinson, D.R. and Steinberg, A.D. (1983). Effects of dietary enrichment with eicosapentenoic acid upon autoimmune nephritis in female NZB × NZW/Fl mice. *Arthritis Rheum.*, **26**, 133–139
267. Robinson, D.R., Prickett, J.D., Polisson, R., Steinberg, A.D. and Levine, L. (1985). The protective effect of dietary fish oil on murine lupus. *Prostaglandins*, **30**, 51–75
268. Kelley, V.E. (1986). Dietary influence on the progression of autoimmune glomerulonephritis. In Carpenter, C.B. (ed.) *Clinics in Immunology and Allergy. Renal Immunology*, pp. 367–381. (London: W.B. Saunders Co.)
269. Izui, S., McConahey, P.J. and Dixon, F.J. (1978). Increased spontaneous polyclonal activation of B lymphocytes in mice with spontaneous autoimmune disease. *J. Immunol.*, **121**, 2213
270. Hurd, E.R., Johnston, J.M., Okita, J.R., MacDonald, P.C., Ziff, M. and Gilliam, J.N. (1981). Prevention of glomerulonephritis and prolonged survival in New Zealand Black/New

Zealand White Fl hybrid mice fed an essential fatty acid deficient diet. *J. Clin. Invest.*, **67**, 476–485
271. Schreiner, G. and Lefkowith, J. (1986). Essential fatty acid deficiency in rats regulates the localization of macrophages to the glomerular mesangium. Presented at the *American Society of Nephrology*, December 7–10, Washington D.C.
272. Starzl, T.E., Iwatsuki, S., Van Theil, D.H., Gartner, J.C., Zitelli, B.J. Malatrack, J.J., Schade, R.R., Shaw, B.W., Hakala, T.R. and Rosenthal, J.T. (1983). Report of Colorado-Pittsburgh liver transplantation studies. *Transplant. Proc.*, **15**, (Suppl. 1), 2582–2585
273. Reitz, B.A., Wallwork, J.L. and Hunt, S.A. (1982). Heart-lung transplantation. *N. Engl. J. Med.*, **306**, 557–564
274. Verani, R.R., Flechner, S.M., Van Buren, C.T. and Kahan, B.D. (1984). Acute cellular rejection of cyclosporine A nephrotoxicity? A review of transplant renal biopsies. *Am. J. Kidney Dis.*, **4**, 1985–1991
275. Myers, B.D., Ross, J., Newton, L., Leutscher, J. and Perbroth, M. (1984). Cyclosporine associated chronic nephropathy. *N. Engl. J. Med.*, **311**, 699–705
276. Hall, B.M., Tiller, D.J., Duggin, G.G., Horvath, J.S., Farnsworth, A., May, J., Robinson, J.R. and Sheil, A.G.R. (1985). Post-transplant acute renal failure in cadaver renal recipients treated with cyclosporine. *Kidney Int.*, **28**, 178–186
277. Murray, B.M., Paller, M.S. and Ferris, T.F. (1985). Effect of cyclosporine administration on renal hemodynamics in conscious rats. *Kidney Int.*, **28**, 767–774
278. Cohen, D.J., Loertscher, R., Rubin, M.F., Tilney, N.L., Carpenter, C.B. and Strom, T.B. (1984). Cyclosporine: A new immunosuppressive agent for organ transplantation. *Ann. Intern. Med.*, **101**, 667–682
279. Perico, N., Benigni, A., Zoja, C., Delaini, F. and Remuzzi, G. (1986). Functional significance of exaggerated renal thromboxane A_2 synthesis induced by cyclosporin A. *Am. J. Physiol.*, **251**, F581–F587
280. English, J., Evan, A., Houghton, D.C. and Bennett, W.M. (1987). Cyclosporine induced acute renal dysfunction in the rat: evidence for arteriolar vasoconstriction with preservation of tubular function. *Transplantation*, **44**, 135–141
281. Ballerman, B.J., Lewis, R.A., Corey, E.J., Austen, K.F. and Brenner, B.M. (1985). Identification and characterization of leukotriene C4 receptors in isolated rat renal glomeruli. *Circ. Res.*, **56**, 324–330
282. Badr, K.F., Baylis, C., Pfeffer, J.M., Pfeffer, M.A., Soberman, F.J., Lewis, R.A., Austen, K.F., Corey, E.J. and Brenner, B.M. (1984). Renal and systemic hemodynamic responses to intravenous infusion of leukotriene C4 in the rat. *Circ. Res.*, **54**, 492–499
283. Feuerstein, N., Foegh, M. and Ramwell, P.W. (1981). Leukotrienes C4 and D4 induce prostaglandin and thromboxane release from rat peritoneal macrophages. *Br. J. Pharmacol.*, **72**, 389–391

4
Eicosanoids and pulmonary injury

S. W. Chang and N. F. Voelkel

INTRODUCTION

The concept that eicosanoids might be involved in the pathogenesis of various forms of lung injury was most likely introduced in 1971 by Piper and Vane who reported that mechanical stimuli leading to lung-membrane deformations caused prostaglandin release by the lung[1]. The release of precursors from intracellular and membrane pools is one of the manifestations of membrane damage. Recent data provided new insight regarding the chemical association of arachidonic acid and lyso-PAF (platelet activating factor) (Figure 4.1). It is tempting to speculate that stimuli leading to membrane damage could affect 1-alkyl-2-arachidonyl-glycerophosphatidylcholine, thus paving the way for production of eicosanoids and of PAF[2]. This step may involve the activation of a phospholipase or may utilize yet-to-be-defined physiochemical membrane alterations. Whether membrane lipid derived mediators are instrumental in lung injury, whether they are mere, albeit sensitive, signals of injury or conceivably 'good guys', modulators of lung injury, is largely unclear. To examine the evidence for and against causal involvement of eicosanoids in lung injury is the purpose of this review. The bias of the investigator in this field may depend to a large degree on whether one perceives the real role of eicosanoids as being homeostatic or catastrophic and whether the arrow of evolution in Figure 4.2 is drawn from left to right or right to left. The greater picture may require that the role of eicosanoids is seen in context with neuro-endocrine control mechanisms[3]. Some of the eicosanoids are potent chemotactic agents and recent evidence which interfaces lymphokinins and eicosanoids[4] points towards a role for eicosanoids in immunoregulation and cell proliferation[5]. These latter aspects might come to play in chronic lung injury syndromes. In acute lung injury, which is defined as lung oedema associated with increased permeability of lung cell membranes to proteins, an intriguing problem has been to relate the mode of actions of the known eicosanoids to changes in lung haemodynamics[6,7] or to altered lung capillary permeability[8] observed in the human adult respiratory distress syndrome

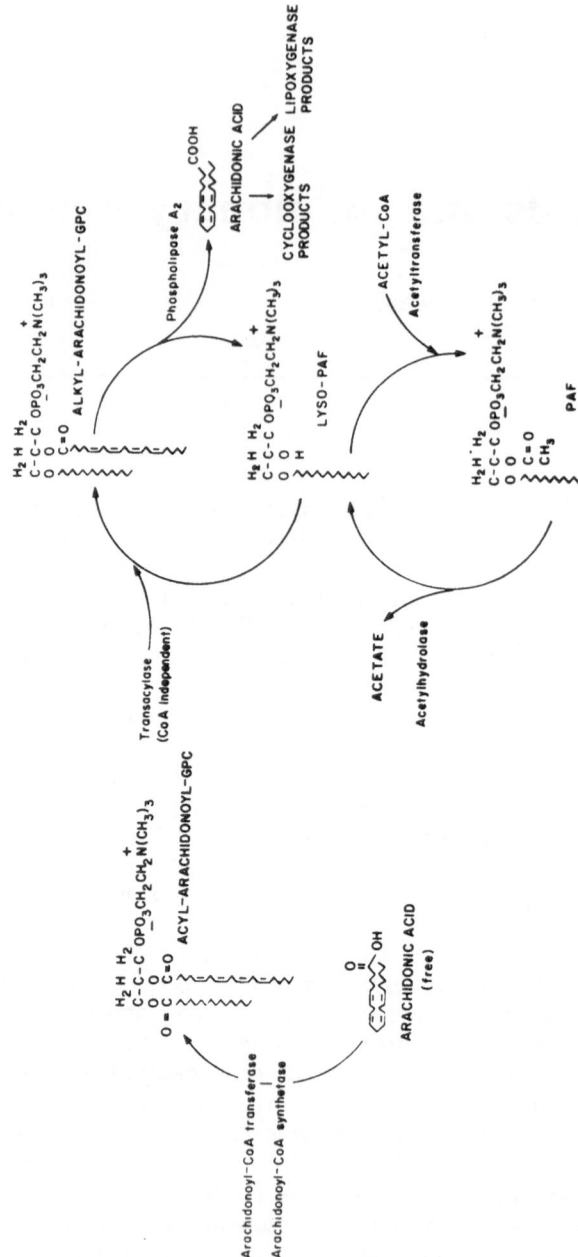

Figure 4.1 Proposed pathways for arachidonic acid metabolism and PAF production by the human neutrophil (with permission of *J. Biol. Chem.*, ref. 2)

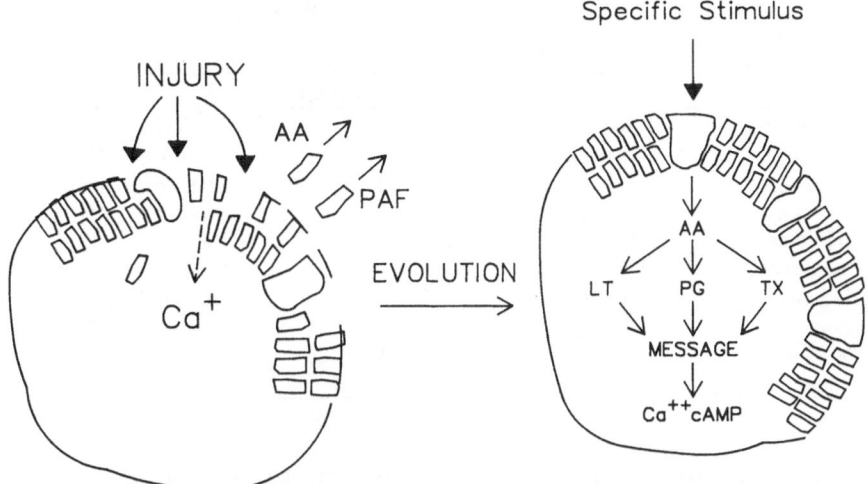

Figure 4.2 Evolution of arachidonic acid release from a response to catastrophic injury to an 'organized' signalling process

(ARDS)[9,10] or to the various animal models of lung injury which admittedly mimic aspects of the human conditions only incompletely.

Most workers in the field agree that non-cardiogenic pulmonary oedema is a consequence of generalized lung capillary injury. Effros recently suggested[11] the term 'inflammatory oedema' to express the widely held belief that inflammatory cells are pathogenetically important in at least some forms of ARDS[12,13]. Several animal studies provided compelling evidence for a crucial role of neutrophils in the development of acute lung vascular injury[14–18]. Heflin and Brigham[14] showed that granulocyte depletion prevented the increase in pulmonary vascular permeability in an endotoxin sheep model. Zimmerman et al.[15] described activation of circulating granulocytes in patients with ARDS. Shasby et al. demonstrated reduction of lung oedema due to active oxygen species by granulocyte depletion[16,17]. Till et al. demonstrated neutrophil dependency of complement-induced acute lung injury[18], and recently Chang in our laboratory showed a reduction of albumin leak from lungs of leukopenic rats in comparison with that in normal rats stimulated with endotoxin[19].

Recently, Shasby and co-workers demonstrated increased albumin transfer across endothelial monolayers when human granulocytes and arachidonic acid were applied in combination but not when arachidonic acid was applied alone[20], indicating that, in neutrophils, arachidonic acid had acted as a substrate in the metabolic production of a substance with permeability enhancing properties, or had unmasked an oedematogenic property of neutrophils.

The release of at least three different injurious species from activated neutrophils has been reported: lipid mediators of inflammation[21,22], proteolytic enzymes and cationic proteins[23,24], and oxygen radicals[25,26]. Following chemotaxis of neutrophils to the lung capillaries and adhesion to the endothelial

Table 4.1 Evidence for arachidonic acid metabolite synthesis or release in models of acute lung injury

Stimulus	Species	Arachidonic acid metabolites reported	Reference
Endotoxin	Rat	TxB_2, PGE_2	Cook et al.[30]
Endotoxin	Sheep	5-HETE	Ogletree et al.[31]
Endotoxin	Sheep	TxB_2, PGI_2	Ogletree et al.[32] McDonald et al.[33]
Endotoxin	Dog	PGI_2, TxB_2	Hales et al.[34]
Microembolism	Sheep	PGI_2, TxB_2	Demling et al.[35]
Air embolism	Sheep	TxB_2	Flick et al.[36]
Oxidants	Rabbit	TxB_2	Tate et al.[37]
Oxidants	Rat	PGI_2, PGF_2, TxB_2, 5-HETE	Burghuber et al.[38,39]

surface, local release of high concentrations of elastase and other oxygen-derived metabolites could result in pore or hole formation of the endothelial cells.

The mechanism of action and the injury potential of lipid mediators are still a matter of debate (Figure 4.3). Malik and co-workers recently reviewed the role of cellular and humoral mediators in pulmonary oedema[6] and concluded that few humoral factors act independently to increase capillary permeability and that these mediators might cause pulmonary venoconstriction and raise pulmonary capillary hydrostatic pressure. This concept is in agreement with results of Shasby et al.[20] which demonstrated that leukotriene C_4 applied directly to an endothelium monolayer did not accelerate albumin transfer across the monolayer. However, because the culture medium was rich in serum proteins (which avidly bind leukotrienes[27]), one cannot rule out a direct damaging effect to endothelial cells given access of the molecule to the endothelial cell.

A different mechanism of how mediators can promote protein leakage has been suggested for histamine. Miller and Sims[28] and Meyrick and Brigham[29] demonstrated contraction of the endothelium by histamine. Whether lipid mediators act via this direct contractile mechanism is unknown. Although

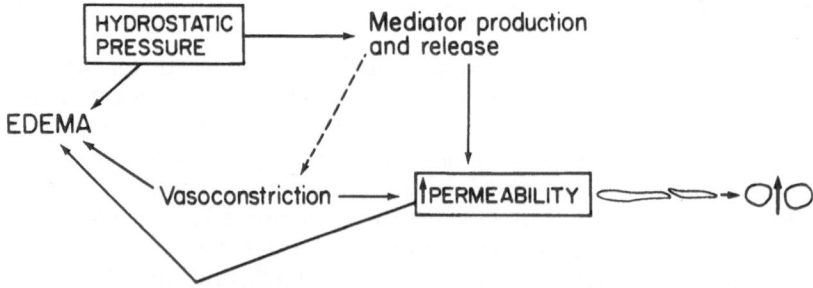

Figure 4.3 Schematic illustration of the interrelationship between pressure, mediator release and increase in vascular permeability

there is a great number of publications which describe a link between acute lung injury and lipid mediators (specifically via the arachidonic acid metabolism), the true pathogenetic importance of lipid mediators for the development of acute lung injury is still uncertain.

Table 4.1 lists some of the publications reporting evidence for arachidonic acid metabolite synthesis or release in models of acute lung injury.

IS THERE A ROLE FOR EICOSANOIDS IN THE PATHOGENESIS OF LUNG INJURY?

Human diseases

ARDS
Arachidonic acid-derived metabolites have been considered as potential mediators of ARDS (Figure 4.4). Lavage fluids obtained from patients with ARDS have been analysed by two different groups[40,41] yet the concentrations of LTC_4 found were small. It is difficult to assess from these studies whether or not leukotrienes are important in this disease. First, the data represent measurements of single lavage samples. Could different—in particular, higher—concentrations have occurred at different time points in the development of the syndrome? Clearly, serial lavage studies are lacking. Second, it is possible that the alveolar fluid represents an ideal milieu for rapid metabolism of leukotrienes. Since the metabolic pathways of the leukotrienes have not been completely elucidated, there is a chance that metabolites which signal the prior presence of leukotrienes have been missed.

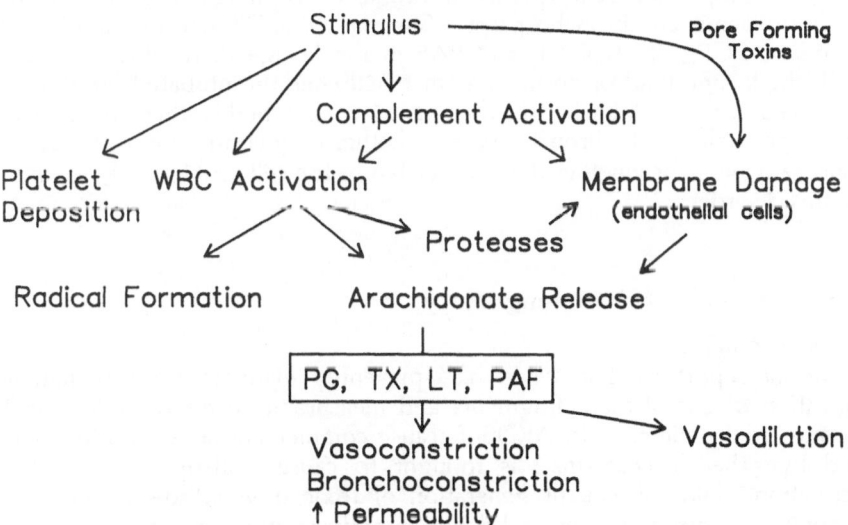

Figure 4.4 Schematic representation of the pathogenesis of ARDS on a cellular level

Evidence regarding a pathogenetic role of cyclo-oxygenase products in the development of ARDS is likewise sparse. Thromboxane plasma levels have been estimated[42,43], yet successful inhibition of thromboxane with dazoxiben in human sepsis and ARDS were virtually without therapeutic benefit[42]. The notion that arachidonic acid metabolites could be involved in the development of ARDS is largely based on the knowledge of the action profile of these mediators, and the expectation that these mediators could be released in a condition where activated neutrophils appear to lodge in capillaries and where lung membrane damage is known to occur.

One form of transient human lung injury, high altitude pulmonary oedema, has recently been examined in more detail. This usually patchy pulmonary oedema has features reminiscent of an inflammatory disorder. Schoene *et al.* studied the lavage fluid of young mountain climbers with this disorder which they obtained at high altitude using a bronchoscopic approach[44]. They found that the lavage fluid was protein rich (indicative of permeability oedema) and contained elevated levels of 6-Δ-*trans*-LTB$_4$, a metabolite of LTB$_4$. Whether LTB$_4$ is involved in this disorder as a chemotactic principle attracting neutrophils to the lung or whether alveolar fluid LTB$_4$ is a marker of activated alveolar neutrophils and macrophages is unclear at present.

Neonatal lung injury

Two serious disorders with frequent fatal outcome of the newborn have recently been reported to be characterized by elevated lung lavage eicosanoid levels. Stenmark and co-workers[45] reported the presence of LTC$_4$ in lavage samples from newborn children with persistent foetal pulmonary circulation syndrome. This syndrome is characterized by severe pulmonary hypertension, hypoxaemia and bronchospasm. It is tempting to associate some, if not all, of these disease manifestations with the actions of leukotrienes. In children with bronchopulmonary dysplasia – a chronic form of lung injury characterized by hypoxaemia and bronchospasm – Stenmark *et al.*[46] found increased levels of 6-keto-PGF$_{1\alpha}$, TxB$_2$, LTB$_4$ and PAF in the lavage fluid when compared with the lavage fluid of normal age-matched children intubated for surgery. It remains to be established in therapeutic trials whether these metabolites are responsible for the bronchospasm, whether they contribute to the airway mucosa oedema or whether they are related to the cell proliferative responses of this disorder.

Animal models of acute lung injury

Septic lung injury

A recent report by Parsons *et al.*[47] presented evidence for simultaneous elevation of complement fragments and measurable levels of endotoxin in plasma from patients with ARDS. Because complement activation by toxins and by other mechanisms[48] is thought to cause neutrophil and platelet activation[49] and subsequent generation of toxic oxygen species and eicosanoids[50,51], various strategies known to activate intravascular complement have been used to examine the role of eicosanoids in lung injury[52]. To

72

produce significant injury, it appears to be necessary that the complement activation is massive or repeated and it further appears that the process of complement activation is independent of cyclo-oxygenase products[52]. Yet following complement activation, significant amounts of eicosanoids are formed[34,53]. Drugs which inhibit cyclo-oxygenase activity prevent the development of hypoxaemia following complement activation[53]. The pulmonary pressor response and bronchoconstriction appear to be inconsistently affected by cyclo-oxygenase blockers. In sheep, neither meclofenamate[52] nor dazoxiben[53] blocked the pressor response to repeated bolus injections of zymosan-activated plasma, nor did they prevent the development of lung leak. However, ibuprofen did affect both parameters, the mechanism of action (most likely not due to its cyclo-oxygenase blocking qualities) remaining unclear[52]. The source of thromboxane generated subsequent to complement activation is probably not the platelet[34] but cells of the lung microcirculation[54].

The involvement and potential role of arachidonic acid-derived mediators in endotoxin–lung injury models has recently been reviewed[55,56]. Endotoxins can activate complement, either alone or – perhaps clinically more relevant both together[47], can promote a syndrome of moderate lung injury characterized by peripheral neutropenia and thrombocytopenia, sequestration of neutrophils in the lung circulation, initial pulmonary hypertension, bronchospasm and delayed vascular leak[36,57]. The thromboxane metabolite TxB_2 and the stable prostacyclin metabolite 6-keto-$PGF_{1\alpha}$ appear and peak early in the sequence of events following endotoxin infusion. Measurements have been performed in lymph[36,58], plasma[35,36,59,60], lung tissue[61] and recently in the bile of experimental animals[62,63]. This 'cyclo-oxygenase peak' has been shown in many studies using the sheep endotoxin model to be temporally related to a transient increase in pulmonary artery pressure[35,36,58]. In the sheep model, this is followed by a delayed second phase of increased lung vascular permeability characterized by elevated 5-HETE and 12-HETE lung lymph levels[32,64].

There is good experimental evidence that cyclo-oxygenase metabolites account for some of the manifestations of the endotoxin syndrome. Based on experiments with pretreatment of the animals with cyclo-oxygenase blockers, it is apparent that, at least in the sheep endotoxin model, bronchoconstriction, loss of lung compliance and initial pulmonary hypertension are caused by cyclo-oxygenase products[65]. An increase in vasodilator prostaglandins is responsible (at least in part) for the loss of hypoxic vasoconstriction which contributes to the hypoxaemia via impairment of ventilation–perfusion mismatch[35,61,66]. In addition, early studies[59] showed that cyclo-oxygenase inhibitors, such as aspirin and indomethacin, blocked endotoxic shock and prolonged survival in dogs. The protective effects of these drugs were probably due to inhibition of prostaglandin and thromboxane synthesis.

That endotoxin also activates the lipoxygenase pathways has been suspected and is now supported by experimental data[67]. In addition to the lymph measurements showing evidence for activation of the 5- and 12-lipoxygenase[32,64], Keppler and co-workers provided intriguing measurements of bile N-acetyl-LTE_4 concentrations during endotoxin shock in rats[63] and Westcott et al.[61] measured lung tissue 5-HETE, LTC_4 and LTB_4 (Figure 4.5)

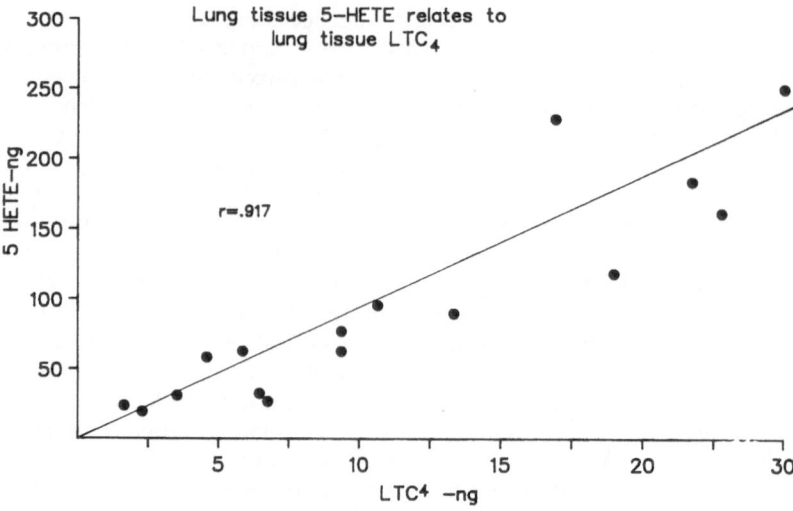

Figure 4.5 Measurements of 5-HETE by RIA and of LTC$_4$ (enzyme immunoassay) in rat lung extracts prepared at various tissue intervals following endotoxin injection

and found that these metabolites were only transiently increased; this observation is in agreement with the results of Keppler *et al.* who also reported a transient increase in the bile N-acetyl-LTE$_4$ (Figure 4.6). Thus, one might conclude that leukotrienes are formed during endotoxaemia in the lung and subsequently metabolized by the liver and excreted via the bile. Important questions remain. What triggers the leukotriene synthesis and why is it transient? Although leukotriene C$_4$ can contribute to lung oedema formation[68–70], whether leukotrienes are likely to be important in causing increased vascular permeability is uncertain, since they disappear rapidly from the lung tissue, whereas the increase in vascular permeability continues to persist.

Lipoxygenase inhibitors have been used in endotoxin lung injury models in the dog, sheep and rat. Diethylcarbamazine failed to influence lung vascular leak in the awake sheep[71] and anaesthetized dog[72], but increased (in high concentrations) survival in endotoxin treated rats (Figure 4.7) without protecting against lung injury (Chang, unpublished). Cook *et al.* studied the effects of the LTD$_4$/LTE$_4$ antagonist, LY 171883, in rats and found protection against endotoxin-induced neutropenia, hypotension and haemoconcentration[73]. The aspect of lung injury was not considered in this latter study.

Approaches other than the use of pharmacological inhibitors have also been tried. Dietary manipulations leading to essential fatty acid deficiency and various drug trials have led to inconclusive results. Cook and co-workers demonstrated decreased mortality from endotoxin shock in rats raised on an essential fatty acid-deficient diet[74]. Although the decreased mortality was associated with a failure of plasma TxB$_2$ levels to rise after endotoxin, one cannot conclude that thromboxane was instrumental in causing this syndrome since arachidonic acid deficiency may affect other metabolic pathways and

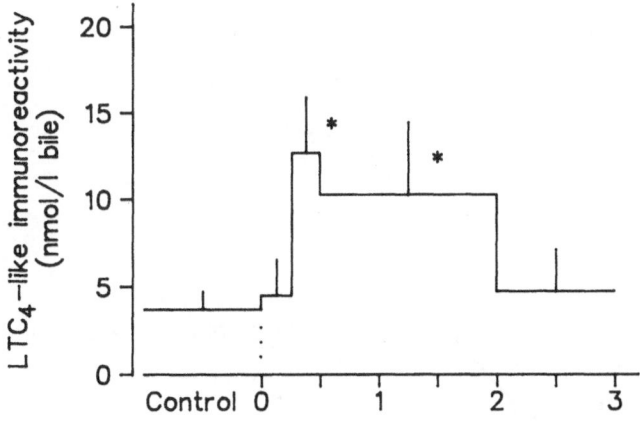

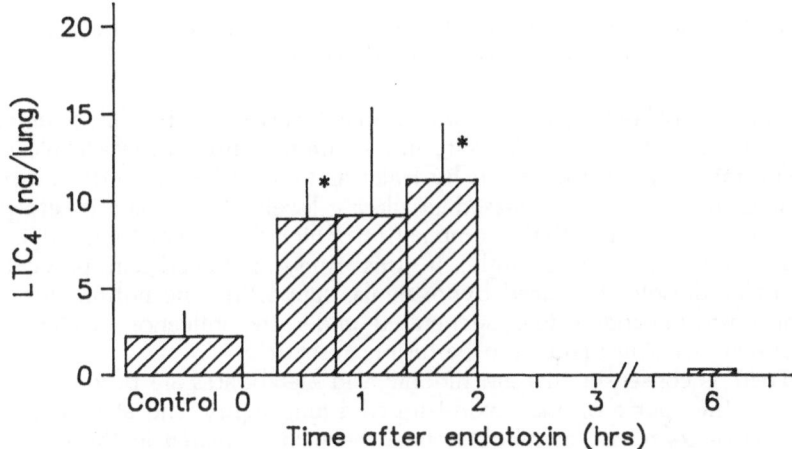

Figure 4.6 Comparison of bile LTE_4 measurement (taken from ref. 62) above and of lung tissue LTC_4 measured by enzyme immunoassay following HPLC separation

may decrease stimulated PAF synthesis and leukotriene synthesis[75,76]. The endotoxin-induced lung injury is probably not due to thromboxane since neither cyclo-oxygenase[77] nor thromboxane synthase blockade prevent lung injury in sheep[66,78] or in a rat model (Chang, unpublished). In a recent study, ibuprofen (12.5 mg kg^{-1}) was tested in dogs infused with live *Escherichia coli*. Ibuprofen prevented fever development in all experimental animals; yet two of the ibuprofen-treated animals died whereas none of the septic animals which had not received ibuprofen died[79]. Methylprednisolone, in high doses, attenuated the increased pulmonary vascular permeability and rise in lung lymph 12-HETE concentrations. Thus part of this steroid effect might be due

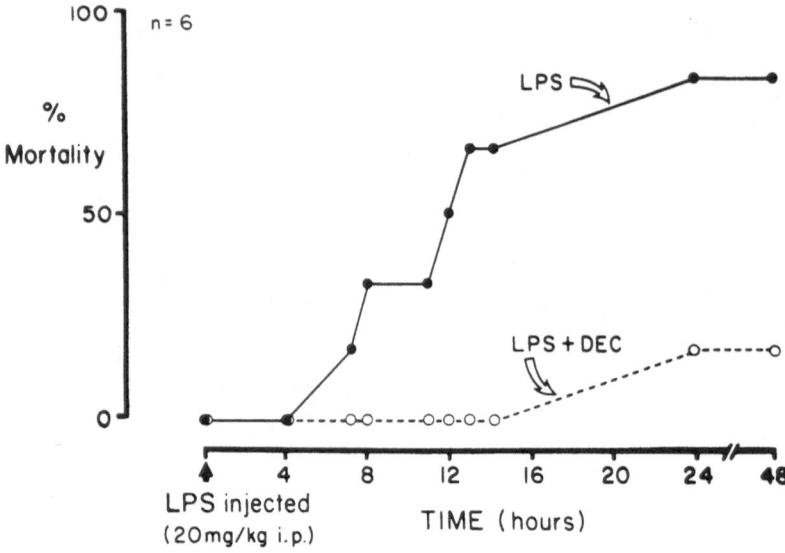

Figure 4.7 Intraperitoneal injection of diethylcarbamazine increased survival in rats treated with endotoxin (Morganroth and Voelkel, unpublished observation)

to inhibition of lipoxygenases or due to an influence on neutrophil accumulation in the lungs per se[64]. The difficulty in the interpretation of these 'clinical data' is illustrated by a recent report by Hales and co-workers who demonstrated, in anaesthetized dogs, increased circulating levels of TxB_2 and 6-keto-$PGF_{1\alpha}$ following treatment with the combination of high doses of methylprednisolone and endotoxin[80]. Interestingly, in this study, indomethacin prevented a methylprednisolone-induced hypoxaemia, supporting the notion that vaso-dilator prostaglandins were generated under the influence of the steroid treatment, causing ventilation/perfusion mismatch.

There is consensus that arachidonic acid metabolites are produced by the lung in the course of endotoxin-triggered lung injury, and at least some of the cyclo-oxygenase metabolites have been incriminated in the pulmonary vasomotor response to endotoxin. However, whether eicosanoids are causative for lung injury remains unclear. Recently, platelet activating factor has been suggested as an important mediator of endotoxic shock[81]. The evidence is as follows:

(1) Platelet activating factor increases in the plasma[19,83] and lung[19] of endotoxin treated rats.
(2) Administration of PAF to several animal species causes vascular collapse mimicking the haemodynamic effect of endotoxaemia[19,82–84], and
(3) Several PAF receptor antagonists blocked and reversed endotoxin-induced hypotension[19,83,85].

Recent studies by Chang et al.[19] strongly indicated that PAF, which acts in small concentrations as a pulmonary vasodilator[86,87], contributes to the

76

inhibition of hypoxic vasoconstriction in endotoxin-treated rats and may play an important role in the development of endotoxin-induced lung injury in rats (Figure 4.8). The extracellular origin of PAF during endotoxaemia remains to be established, although it is clear that neutropenia does not abolish lung PAF production[19]. Further studies are necessary to confirm the importance of PAF in endotoxin shock in other species.

At this time, it is difficult to reconcile the results from all the studies in the literature regarding the role of specific eicosanoids or PAF in the development of endotoxin-induced lung injury. The differences in results may be due to the use of inadequate or ineffective inhibitors, different doses and preparation of endotoxin, variable sensitivity of different species of animals to endotoxin effect and differences in eicosanoid metabolism in different species[88]. A final possibility is that perhaps none of the metabolites alone is adequate to cause injury, but mediator chain reactions and synergistic actions of several mediators are important. This might explain why interventions targeting a single mediator (thromboxane or leukotrienes) have so far met with limited success.

Since oxygen radicals are involved in complement-mediated lung injury and since endotoxin activates the complement cascade, one might expect involvement of oxygen radicals in endotoxin lung injury. There is indeed very little direct evidence that endotoxin treatment is associated with oxidant stress although the results from some published studies are consistent with this hypothesis. Neutrophils from patients with ARDS have been shown to be activated and are characterized by facilitated oxygen radical generation[89]. Traber et al.[90] demonstrated potentiation of lung vascular injury after endotoxin in sheep treated with superoxide dismutase, and suggested that increased concentration of hydrogen peroxide may be responsible. Bernard et al.[91] demonstrated a partial protective effect of N-acetyl cysteine on endotoxin-induced lung injury in sheep, although Wong et al.[92], in a similar model, failed to show protection against lung injury using the hydroxyl radical scavenger,

PAF- Induced Pulmonary Vasodilation is Independent of Prostaglandins

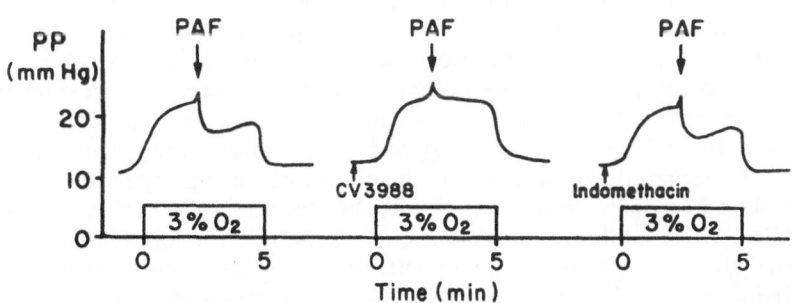

Figure 4.8 PAF (10 ng) bolus injection causes vasodilation in isolated rat lungs perfused with blood at constant flow. This vasodilation is inhibited by CV 3988 (10^{-4} mol L^{-1}) a PAF receptor antagonist but not by the cyclo-oxygenase inhibitor, indomethacin

dimethyl thiourea. A subsequent publication by this group demonstrated increased malondialdehyde in lung tissue following endotoxin administration[93]. However, the malondialdehyde reaction may not accurately reflect lipid peroxidation[94]. Recently, Chang et al.[95] demonstrated an increase in the plasma-oxidized glutathione of rats following injection of endotoxin. Moreover, pretreatment of the animals with BCNU, an inhibitor of glutathione reductase, greatly enhanced this signal, indicating an element of 'oxidant stress' in this model of acute lung injury[95].

Taken together, these data are consistent with the concept of several inflammatory principles (active oxygen species, cyclo-oxygenase and lipoxygenase products and PAF) working together to produce the manifestations of endotoxic shock and organ failure.

Oxidant-related lung injury

Hyperoxia causes injury to lung endothelial cells and active oxygen species have been shown to be involved in several lung injury animal models[96]. Injurious oxidants are generated by irradiation[97], paraquat[98], nitrofurantoin[99] and amiodarone[100]. The particular susceptibility of lung endothelial cells to oxidant injury[101] and the interaction between endothelial cells and neutrophils[102] makes the search for the mechanism of this injury important. Oxygen species can cause cell damage directly[103,104], yet because their known ability to stimulate lipid peroxidation[104-106], to activate phospholipase[107,108] and liberate arachidonic acid[104,109], it is conceivable that arachidonic acid metabolites might play a role in various forms of oxidant-induced lung injury[110]. Jacobson et al.[111] demonstrated recently that one hour of hyperbaric hyperoxia caused severe pulmonary hypertension and pulmonary oedema inhibited by indomethacin and a thromboxane synthesis inhibitor. Whereas in hyperoxia the endothelium produces increased amounts of oxygen metabolites and increased concentrations of prostacyclin[112], the source of thromboxane in the latter study is still unclear. Rat lungs perfused with cell-free solutions generate PGI_2 and thromboxane upon stimulation of H_2O_2 production by glucose-oxidase[39]. Rabbit lungs perfused with cell-free physiological salt solution generate thromboxane when stimulated via the xanthine–xanthine oxidase system[113] or t-butyl-hydroperoxide[114]. Similar results were obtained using phorbol myristate acetate in the isolated perfused dog lobe[115]. In the rabbit, the oxidant-induced vasoconstriction was inhibited by cyclo-oxygenase blockers[113,114,116], but, in the rat, no vasoconstriction was observed after the glucose oxidase addition unless indomethacin was present[38] suggesting that vasodilator prostaglandins were more important in the rat. The finding that indomethacin did not affect rat lung oedema following glucose oxidase led to the examination of a possible involvement of lipoxygenase-derived metabolites in oxidant-related lung injury. We found that BW 755C, Piriprost and FPL 55712, inhibitors of leukotriene synthesis or action, inhibited lung oedema after the glucose oxidase challenge and that this challenge had resulted in increased production of 5-HETE[39]. An interesting, albeit currently unexplained, aside of this study was the observation that meclofenamate was completely ineffective as a cyclo-oxgenase blocker in a milieu where H_2O_2 had been generated.

Others have demonstrated that hyperoxia altered cultured bovine pulmonary arterial endothelial cells in such a way that they released more 6-keto-$PGF_{1\alpha}$ and LTB_4 upon stimulation with Ca^{2+} ionophore[112]. Again it is unclear whether the ultrastructural changes of the endothelial cells (bleb formation, decreased membrane barrier) facilitates CA^{2+} influx and LTB_4 synthesis or whether stimulated lipid peroxidation primes the cells for leukotriene synthesis. Hyperoxia may also prime the lung tissue or the capillaries which appear to be more susceptible to exogenously added LTB_4[117] since LTB_4 resulted in generation of 6-keto-$PGF_{1\alpha}$ and in increased capillary permeability in lungs from rats exposed for 48 h to hyperoxia when compared with those from air-control animals. Krieger et al.[102] also concluded that hyperoxia affects the lung itself. The perfusate from hyperoxic lungs generated more chemotactic activity, perhaps LTB_4, than normal lungs. Indeed Taniguchi et al.[118] found that the lung lavage fluid from hyperoxic rats contained large amounts of LTB_4 and that there was a correlation between the number of neutrophils and the LTB_4 concentration. LTB_4, which is not metabolized by the lungs[119], may be generated by injured alveolar macrophages or endothelial cells and then be responsible for neutrophil chemotaxis.

Air embolism in unanaesthetized sheep causes increased permeability, lung oedema associated with oxidant stress[120] and increase in thromboxane and prostacyclin in lung lymph and plasma[121]. Whereas superoxide dismutase and heparin prevented the increase in lung vascular permeability[120], OKY-046, a thromboxane synthetase inhibitor, did not[121]. Therefore, it is conceivable that superoxide anion released from activated neutrophils is causative in this form of lung injury[120].

Microembolization
Thrombin injection in experimental animals causes the generation of fibrin, activation of neutrophils, platelet aggregation, leukostasis and an increase in pulmonary vascular permeability as measured by lymph flow and lymph to plasma protein concentration ratios[122]. Demling has measured prostaglandins in acute pulmonary microvascular injury[123], Garcia-Szabo and colleagues[124] found a protective effect of thromboxane synthase inhibition on lung vascular permeability in the sheep thrombin microembolism model, and Johnson and Malik demonstrated a protective effect of granulocytopenia on microemboli-induced lung injury[125]. Bizios et al.[126] found that vasoconstricting arachidonic acid metabolites (probably TxA_2) contribute 50% to the increase in pulmonary vascular resistance after thrombin-induced embolization and concluded that cyclo-oxygenase products generated via leukocyte activation may increase lung vascular permeability. BW 755 C, a combined cyclo-oxygenase and lipoxygenase inhibitor derived from the photosensitive antioxidant phenidone, prevented thrombin-induced and indomethacin-enhanced increases in lung lymph flow. The authors suggest that lipoxygenase metabolites might have been produced during cyclo-oxygenase blockade which may have been responsible for an increase in lung microvascular pressure and an increase in lung vascular surface area. Indeed, Voelkel et al. documented that LTC_4 and PAF caused increases in pulmonary microvascular pressure[7]. Thus leukotrienes could increase lung lymph flow via an increase in microvascular pressure,

whereas exogenous prostacyclin infused during thrombin microemboli challenge decreased the elevated lung lymph flow via lowering of lung microvascular pressure.

Oleic acid-induced acute lung injury
Intravenous injection of oleic acid (*cis*-9-octadecenoic acid) causes haemorrhagic lung oedema independent of platelet or neutrophil action[127]. Although corticosteroids have been reported to enhance animal survival after oleic acid[128] and Olanoff *et al.*[129] found increases in plasma TxB_2 levels after oleic acid, it appears that thromboxane is not causing the lung injury since neither ibuprofen[127] nor indomethacin[129] inhibited oleic acid-induced lung injury. Whether lipoxygenase products are involved in this particular lung injury model remains to be examined. Interestingly, Miyazawa *et al.*[130] reported that infusion of prostacyclin reversed oleic acid-induced lung injury. Again, it is unclear whether PGI_2 affected microvascular pressure or vascular permeability.

Models of chronic lung injury
One of the intensely investigated models of chronic pulmonary vascular injury is that observed after monocrotaline injection in young rats[131,132]. This pyrazolidine alkaloid causes early pulmonary vascular leak followed by later development of pulmonary hypertension and right ventricular hypertrophy. Chronic treatment with calcium entry blockers[133], but not with indomethacin[134,137] or dazmegrel, a thromboxane synthesis inhibitor[135], inhibit development of severe pulmonary hypertension. Stenmark and co-workers used chronic treatment with diethylcarbamazine – in high doses an inhibitor of lipoxygenase – and found that diethylcarbamazine inhibited the early injury phase after monocrotaline[137] as well as the development of severe pulmonary hypertension[134]. The latter finding is in agreement with the data of Morganroth *et al.*[138] who demonstrated protection against development of chronic hypobaric hypoxia-induced pulmonary hypertension after treatment with a combination of diethylcarbamazine administered interperitoneally and in drinking water. The lung injury caused by monocrotaline is felt by some[136] to resemble ARDS. It is of interest that, in Stenmark's study, there was an association between the number of inflammatory cells in lung lavage and lavage SRS-A-like activity as measured by guinea-pig ileum bioassay. A question currently unanswered is whether the diethylcarbamazine had affected the metabolism of monocrotaline to the active pyrrole[135,139], thus reducing the effective dose of the alkaloid, or whether inhibition of the lipoxygenase pathway was the important mechanism of diethylcarbamazine action. There can be no doubt that lung arachidonic acid metabolism is activated during monocrotaline injury, and that SRS-A-like material found in the lung lavage fluid, makes a contribution by the lipoxygenase pathway likely. To draw a firmer conclusion, one would like to see protective effects of several structurally unrelated lipoxygenase inhibitors and possibly synergistic protection if diethylcarbamazine and piriprost are used in combination[140].

Recently, Stenmark *et al.* measured eicosanoids and PAF in the lung lavage fluid from neonatal calves exposed to two weeks of high-altitude hypoxia. Prostacyclin, thromboxane and PAF were increased and accompanied by severe pulmonary hypertension and features of vascular injury[141,142]. It is not clear at present whether the increased levels of inflammatory mediators in this model of severe neonatal pulmonary hypertension are causes or effects.

MEASUREMENT OF EICOSANOIDS IN LUNG INJURY

Several aspects regarding the measurement of eicosanoids in states of lung injury are worth highlighting. First, it appears that the route of entry of the injurious stimulus determines where in the lung one can find mediators elevated and also what pattern of mediator interactions one can expect. Injury to the airways, as in aspiration of hydrochloric acid or after SO_2 inhalation, may remain restricted to the airways. Metabolites may or may not be detectable in the lung lymph draining the interstitium or in the lung effluent. Noxious stimuli entering via the blood stream may not lead to mediator production measurable in the lung lavage. In a recent study using endotoxin-treated rats, PAF was found to be elevated in the blood and in the lung parenchyma but not in the lung lavage fluid[19]. Alternatively, alveolar hypoxia may lead to measurable increases in lavage leukotrienes[143] not accompanied by a rise in lung perfusate leukotriene levels (Voelkel, unpublished). The reasons for this mediator compartmentalization are several. Most importantly, the different compartments in the lung contain different cell types which produce different metabolites, and secondly, airway cells metabolize PAF[144] and LTC_4 but not LTB_4[119] whereas lung vascular cells do not metabolize PGI_2[145] nor PAF[144]. It follows that the variety of mediator constellations reported in different lung injury models not only depends on the species under investigation[88] but also on the dominant cell type involved in synthesis and metabolism of the particular mediator.

The timing of the measurements is also important. The endotoxin models teach us that the eicosanoids appear in various body fluids, but they also disappear[146]. The measurement of the eicosanoids and of PAF in complex biological fluids may be difficult and interpretation without validation of the method and without the rigorous use of good internal standards may be fraught with error[61]. Lastly, there may be a problem with the signal to noise ratio of some of the mediators measured which should make one cautious in interpreting small percentage differences which may be of statistical but not of biological significance.

ARE EICOSANOIDS MODULATORS OF LUNG INJURY?

Arachidonic acid metabolite accumulation in body fluids may be a sign of injury rather than its cause or even – the authors apologize for their teleology – the organism's attempt to restore homeostasis.

Because the lung capillary endothelium when stimulated produces prostacyclin – a potent vasodilator and antiaggregatory substance – it was hypothesized that endogenous PGI_2 production may comprise part of the lung's defence system against injury. Prostacyclin formation can be stimulated by endotoxin[147], bradykinin[148], angiotensin II[149], thrombin[150] and LTC_4[151,152] to name just a few of the compounds which may be produced in close proximity to endothelium during injury. If endogenous prostacyclin is important as a defense against lung injury, then inhibition of PGI_2 synthesis should increase lung injury and treatment with PGI_2 should decrease or prevent injury. The schematic representation below summarizes the concept of PGI_2 action:

$$PGI_2 \rightarrow \uparrow adenylate\ cyclase \rightarrow \uparrow [cAMP_i] \rightarrow \downarrow [Ca^{2+}]$$
$$\rightarrow relaxation\ of\ smooth\ muscle + \downarrow in\ mediator\ synthesis$$

There is some evidence that indomethacin, an inhibitor of the cyclo-oxygenase enzyme, worsens lung vascular permeability. Ogletree and Brigham[153] showed this in the sheep endotoxin lung injury model. Whether this effect is related to the absence of PGI_2 or whether there is a shunting of arachidonic acid substrate into the lipoxygenase pathway is unclear. On the other hand, there are several reports indicating a beneficial effect of prostacyclin infusion in the sheep endotoxin[154] and sheep thrombin[155] lung injury models. Perlman et al.[155] interpreted their findings of a decreased pulmonary vascular permeability as an effect of PGI_2 infusion on pulmonary–capillary pressure. As stated above, it is tempting to suggest that a link between PGI_2 action or microvascular pressure might be the inhibition of action or synthesis of vasoconstrictors.

TREATMENT OF HUMAN LUNG INJURY BASED ON MANIPULATIONS OF THE EICOSANOID METABOLISM

The rationale for this approach is based on the belief that eicosanoids play a central part in the development and the maintenance of the injury state and that some eicosanoids are 'bad guys' and others 'good guys'. Garrett and Thomas were able to show that meclofenamate decreased the shunt fraction in dogs with lobar atelectasis[156,157]; Light[158] demonstrated a reduction in intrapulmonary shunt in experimental pneumoccal pneumonia with aspirin or indomethacin. Whether such a strategy is beneficial in human lung injury remains to be evaluated because the effect of cyclo-oxygenase blockade is complex and the ramifications of such a manoeuvre, and the consequences on cell functions, are incompletely understood. A study by Shasby et al. investigated the interactive effects of neutrophils in the presence of arachidonic acid on cultured endothelial cell monolayers[20]. Neither component alone caused endothelial cell injury as measured by albumin transfer and the injury due to neutrophils in the presence of arachidonic acid was blocked by aspirin or indomethacin pretreatment of the neutrophils but not by piriprost – a lipoxygenase inhibitor[20]. The authors concluded that arachidonic acid stimulated a neutrophil activity rather than being metabolized to an oedemagenic compound. Interestingly, piriprost appeared to increase neutrophil PGE_2 production, a finding consistent with shunting of substrate towards the cyclo-oxygenase pathway. The opposite shunting, to favour lipoxygenase metabolism, has been discussed as a potential side effect of cyclo-oxygenase blockers and might occur in the lung[159]. Although steroids could potentially

82

inhibit phospholipase A_2 and therefore limit the availability of arachidonic acid, whether steroids inhibit eicosanoid production in injured lungs is a question which is currently being investigated. With the exception of the prophylactic treatment with steroids in a subgroup of patients with ARDS due to fat embolism[160], the clinical impressions regarding steroids as a successful treatment modality in ARDS patients have been equivocal at best[161].

Two uncontrolled clinical studies attempted to manipulate pulmonary haemodynamics in patients with ARDS with infusions of PGE_1[162,163]. Although PGE_1 beneficially affected lung vascular injury in sheep due to complement activation[164], PGE_1 caused an increase in mortality in paraquat-treated rats[165]. A reduction in pulmonary artery pressure and increase in cardiac output with increased oxygen transport were found in these studies. No reports are available on studies in man utilizing prostacyclin infusion or agents which are known to stimulate endogenous prostacyclin production. Given the complex nature of the adult respiratory distress syndrome with the potential involvement of complement activation, cell activation and mediator release, a single drug treatment is probably doomed to fail. The mediators most likely form a network[166], and the eicosanoids are part of it – possibly integrating messages originating from the neuroendocrine system[3]. Norepinephrine, angiotensin II and acetylcholine all stimulate vascular prostacyclin synthesis[149,167-169,171]. The immunosurveillance system may 'use' eicosanoids to transmit inflammatory signals. Pathways may lead from endothelial cells via interleukin and LTB_4 formation to chemotaxis of neutrophils and macrophages[170]. PGE_2 released from fibroblasts due to stimulation by interleukin I may inhibit lung fibrosis[172].

SUMMARY

Eicosanoids and PAF are thought to play an important role in acute lung injury. Most of the evidence is circumstantial. Cause and effect relationships are often unclear due to the lack of specific inhibitors, multiple cell and mediator interactions and due to differences in the models and species used. If a broader view is taken, and the eicosanoids (including those remaining to be discovered) are studied as part of a large mediator network with input from neuroendocrine signals and connections with the immune surveillance system, new insights into the pathophysiology of lung injuries can be expected. These will lead to new treatment strategies.

Supported in part by grants from the National Institutes of Health (PPG HL-14985 and CIA HL 01966-01 to Dr Chang) and the American Lung Association (Career Development Award to Dr Voelkel).

REFERENCES

1. Piper, P. and Vane, J. (1971). The release of prostaglandins from lung and other tissues. Ann. NY Acad. Sci., 180, 363–385
2. Chilton, F.H. and Murphy, R.C. (1986). Remodeling of arachidonate-containing phosphoglycerides within the human neutrophil. J. Biol. Chem., 261, 7771–7777

3. Lands, W.E.M. (1987). Biochemical and cellular actions of membrane lipids. *Am. Rev. Respir. Dis.*, **136**, 200–204
4. Gately, C.L., Wahl, S.M. and Oppenheim, J.J. (1983). Characterization of hydrogen peroxide-potentiating factor, a lymphokine that increases the capacity of human monocytes and monocyte-like cell lines to produce hydrogen peroxide. *J. Immunol.*, **131**, 2853–2858
5. Albrightson, C.R., Baenziger, N.L. and Needleman, P. (1985). Exaggerated human vascular cell prostaglandin biosynthesis mediated by monocytes: role of monokines and interluekin-1. *J. Immunol*, **135**, 1872–1877
6. Malik, A.B., Selig, W.M. and Burhop, K.E. (1985). Cellular and humoral mediators of pulmonary edema. *Lung*, **163**, 193–219
7. Voelkel, N.F., Chang, S., Sakai, A. and Harris, A. (1986). The importance of pulmonary vasoconstriction in the LTC$_4$ and PAF-induced lung edema. Presented at the *6th International Conference on Prostaglandins and Related Compounds*, Florence, Italy
8. Staub, N.C. (1984). Pathophysiology of pulmonary edema. In Staub, N.C. and Taylor, A.E. (eds.) *Edema*, pp. 719–746. (New York: Raven Press)
9. Ashbaugh, D.G., Bigelow, D.B., Petty, T.L. and Levine, B.E. (1967). Acute respiratory distress in adults. *Lancet*, **88**, 319–323
10. Fowler, A.A., Hamman, R.F., Good, J.T., Benson, K.N., Baird, M., Eberle, D.J., Petty, T.L. and Hyerst, M. (1983). Adult respiratory distress syndrome: risk with common predispositions. *Ann. Intern. Med.*, **98**, 593–597
11. Effros, R.M. and Mason, G.R. (1986). An end to ARDS. *Chest*, **89**, 162–163
12. Petty, T.L. (1982). Adult respiratory distress syndrome: definition and historical perspective. *Clin. Chest Med.*, **3**, 3–7
13. Hyers, T.M. and Fowler, A.A. (1986). Adult respiratory distress syndrome: causes, morbidity, and mortality. *Fed. Proc.*, **45**, 25–29
14. Heflin, A.C. and Brigham, K.L. (1981). Prevention by granulocyte depletion of increased vascular permeability of sheep lung following endotoxemia. *J. Clin. Invest.*, **68**, 1253–1260
15. Zimmerman, G.A., Renzetti, A.D. and Hill, H.R. (1983). Functional and metabolic activity of granulocytes from patients with adult respiratory distress syndrome. *Am. Rev. Respir. Dis.*, **127**, 290–300
16. Shasby, D.M., Fox, R.B., Harada, R.M. and Repine, J.E. (1982). Reduction of edema of acute hyperoxic lung injury by granulocyte depletion. *J. Appl. Physiol.*, **52**, 1237–1244
17. Shasby, D.M., VanBenthuysen, K.M., Tate, R.M., Shasby, S.S., McMurtry, I.F. and Repine, J.E. (1982). Granulocytes mediate acute edematous lung injury in rabbits and in isolated rabbit lungs perfused with phorbol myristate acetate: Role of oxygen radicals. *Am. Rev. Respir. Dis.*, **125**, 443–447
18. Till, G.O., Johnson, K.J., Kundel, R. and Ward, P.A. (1982). Intravascular activation of complement and acute lung injury: Dependency on neutrophils and toxic oxygen metabolites. *J. Clin. Invest.*, **69**, 1126–1135
19. Chang, S.W., Feddersen, C.O., Henson, P.M. and Voelkel, N.F. (1987). Platelet activating factor mediates hemodynamic changes and lung injury in endotoxin-treated rats. *J. Clin. Invest.*, **69**, 1498–1509
20. Shasby, D.M., Shasby, S.S. and Peach, M.J. (1985). Polymorphonuclear leukocyte: arachidonate edema. *J. Appl. Physiol.*, **59**, 47–55
21. Goldyne, M.E., Burrish, G.F., Poubelle, P. and Borgeat, P. (1984). Arachidonic acid metabolism among human mononuclear leukocytes: Lipoxygenase-related pathways. *J. Biol. Chem.*, **259**, 8815–8819
22. Lewis, R.A., Lee, C.W., Krilis, S., Corey, E.J. and Austen, K.F. (1984). C-6-sulfidopeptide leukotrienes: potential roles in inflammatory disease. *Adv. Inflamm. Res.*, **7**, 17
23. Janoff, A. and Scherer, J. (1968). Mediators of inflammation in leukocyte lysosomes. IX. Elastinolytic activity in granules of human polymorphonuclear leukocytes. *J. Exp. Med.*, **128**, 1137–1151
24. Camussi, G., Tetta, C., Bussolinio, F., Caligaris-Cappaio, F., Coda, R., Masera, C. and Segoloni, G. (1980). Mediators of immune complex-induced aggregation of polymorphonuclear leukocytes. I. C5a anaphylatoxin, neutrophil cationic proteins and their cleavage fragments. *Int. Arch. Allergy Appl. Immunol.*, **62**, 1–15

25. Babior, B.M., Kipnes, R.S. and Curnutte, J.T. (1973). The production by leukocytes of superoxide, a potential bactericidal agent. *J. Clin. Invest.*, **52**, 741–744
26. Tauber, A.I. and Baboir, B.M. (1985). Neutrophil oxygen reduction: the enzymes and the products. *Adv. Free Radical Biol. Med.*, **1**, 265–307
27. Voelkel, N.F., Stenmark, K.R., Reeves, J.T., Mathias, M.M. and Murphy, R.C. (1984). Actions of lipoxygenase metabolites in isolated rat lungs. *J. Appl. Physiol.*, **57**, 860–867
28. Miller, F.N. and Sims, D.E. (1986). Contractile elements in the regulation of macromolecular permeability. *Fed. Proc.*, **45**, 84–88
29. Meyrick, B. and Brigham, K.L. (1984). Increased permeability associated with dilatation of endothelial cell junctions caused by histamine in intimal explants from bovine pulmonary artery. *Exp. Lung Res.*, **6**, 11–25
30. Cook, J.A., Wise, W.C. and Halushka, P.V. (1980). Elevated thromboxane levels in the rat during endotoxic shock. *J. Clin. Invest.*, **65**, 227–230
31. Ogletree, M.L., Dates, J.A., Brigham, K.L. and Hubbard, W.C. (1982). Evidence for pulmonary release of 5-hydroxyeicosatetraenoic acid (5-HETE) during endotoxemia in unanesthetized sheep. *Prostaglandins*, **23**, 459–468
32. Ogletree, M.L., Hutchison, A.A., Snapper, J.R. and Brigham, K.L. (1982). Effects of alveolar hypoxia and endotoxin on lung lymph prostacyclin and thromboxane metabolites in unanesthetized sheep. *Fed. Proc.*, **41**, 1686
33. McDonald, J.W.D., Ali, M., Morgan, E., Townsend, E.R. and Cooper, J.D. (1983). Thromboxane synthesis by sources other than platelets in association with complement-induced pulmonary leukostasis and pulmonary hypertension in sheep. *Circ. Res.*, **52**, 1–6
34. Hales, C.A., Sonne, L., Peterson, M., Kong, D., Miller, M. and Watkins, W.D. (1981). Role of thromboxane and prostacyclin in pulmonary vasomotor changes after endotoxin in dogs. *J. Clin. Invest.*, **68**, 497–505
35. Demling, R.H., Smith, M., Gunther, R., Flynn, J.T. and Gee, M.H. (1981). Pulmonary injury and prostaglandin production during endotoxemia in conscious sheep. *J. Appl. Physiol.*, **240**, H348–H353
36. Flick, M.R., Perel, A. and Staub, N.C. (1981). Leukocytes are required for increased lung microvascular permeability after microembolization in sheep. *Circ. Res.*, **48**, 344–351
37. Tate, R.M., VanBenthuysen, K.M., Shasby, D.M., McMurtry, I.F. and Repine, J.E. (1982). Oxygen radical mediated permeability edema and vasoconstriction in isolated perfused rabbit lungs. *Am. Rev. Respir. Dis.*, **126**, 802–806
38. Burghuber, O., Mathias, M.M., McMurtry, I.F., Reeves, J.T. and Voelkel, N.F. (1984). Lung edema due to hydrogen peroxide is independent of cyclooxygenase products. *J. Appl. Physiol.*, **56**, 900–905
39. Burghuber, O.C., Strife, R., Zirrolli, J., Mathias, M.M., Henson, P., Henson, J., Reeves, J.T., Murphy, R.C. and Voelkel, N.F. (1985). Leukotriene inhibitors attenuate H_2O_2-induced lung injury. *Am. Rev. Respir. Dis.*, **131**, 778–785
40. Matthay, M.S., Escenbacker, W.L. and Goethe, E.J. (1984). Elevated concentration of leukotriene D_4 in pulmonary edema fluid of patients with adult respiratory distress syndrome. *J. Clin. Immunol.*, **4**, 479–483
41. Hyers, T.M., Fowler, A.A., Stephenson, A.H., Dettenmeir, P.A., Fisher, B. and Webster, R.O. (1985). The appearance of neutrophils and metabolites of arachidonic acid in bronchial fluid of patients at risk for ARDS. *Am. Rev. Respir. Dis.*, **131**, A135
42. Reines, H.D., Halushka, P.V., Cook, J.A., Wise, W.C. and Rambo, W. (1982). Plasma thromboxane concentrations are raised in patients dying with septic shock. *Lancet*, **2**, 174–175
43. Lamy, M., Deby-Dupont, G., Pincemail, J., Braun, M., Duchateau, J., Deby, C., Van Erck, J., Bodson, L., Damas, P. and Franchimont, P. (1985). Biochemical pathways of acute lung injury. *Bull. Eur. Physiopathol. Respir.*, **21**, 221–229
44. Schoene, R.B., Hackett, P.H., Henderson, W.R., Sage, E.H., Chow, M., Roach, R.C., Mills, W.J. Jr. and Martin, T.R. (1986). High altitude pulmonary edema. Characteristics of lung lavage fluid. *J. Am. Med. Assoc.*, **256**, 63–69
45. Stenmark, K.R., James, S.L., Voelkel, N.F., Reeves, J.T. and Murphy, R.C. (1983). Recovery of leukotriene C_4 and D_4 from the airways of newborn infants with hypoxemia and pulmonary hypertension. *N. Engl. J. Med.*, **309**, 77 80
46. Stenmark, K.R., Eyzaguirre, M., Remigio, L., Seccombe, J. and Henson, P.M. (1985). Recovery of platelet activating factor and leukotrienes from infants with severe

85

bronchopulmonary dysplasia: clinical improvement with cromolyn treatment. *Am. Rev. Respir. Dis.*, **131**, A236 (Abstract)
47. Parsons, P.E., Tate, R.M., Worthen, G.S. and Henson, P.M. (1986). Endotoxin and complement fragments (C5f) in plasma, but not elevated C5f levels alone, correlate with the development of ARDS. *Am. Rev. Respir. Dis.*, **133**, A277
48. Craddock, P.R., Fehr, J., Dalmasso, A.P., Brigham, K.L. and Jacob, H.S. (1977). Hemodialysis leukopenia. Pulmonary vascular leukostasis resulting from complement activation by dialyzer cellophane membranes. *J. Clin. Invest.*, **59**, 879–888
49. Tvedten, H.W., Till, G.O. and Ward, P.A. (1985). Mediators of lung injury in mice following systemic activation of complement. *Am. J. Pathol.*, **119**, 92–100
50. Cooper, J.D., McDonald, J.W.D., Ali, M., Menkes, E., Masterson, J. and Klement, P. (1980). Prostaglandin production associated with the pulmonary vascular response to complement activation. *Surgery*, **88**, 215–221
51. Perkowski, S.Z., Havill, A.M., Flynn, J.T. and Gee, M.H. (1983). Role of intrapulmonary release of eicosanoids and superoxide anion as mediators of pulmonary dysfunction and endothelial injury in sheep with intermittent complement activation. *Circ. Res.*, **53**, 574–585
52. Gee, M.H., Perkowski, S.Z., Tahamont, M.V. and Flynn, J.T. (1985). Arachidonate cyclooxygenase metabolites as mediators of complement-initiated lung injury. *Fed. Proc.*, **44**, 46–52
53. Gee, M.H., Perkowski, S.Z., Tahamont, M.V., Flynn, J.T. and Wasserman, M.A. (1986). Thromboxane as a mediator of pulmonary dysfunction during intravascular complement activation in sheep. *Am. Rev. Respir. Dis.*, **133**, 269–273
54. Egan, T.M., Saunders, N.R., Dubois, P., Choiniere, L., McDonald, J.W.D. and Cooper, J.D. (1985). Contribution of circulating formed elements to prostanoid production in complement-mediated lung injury in sheep. *Surgery*, **98**, 350–358
55. Brigham, K.L. and Meyrick, B. (1986). Endotoxin and lung injury. *Am. Rev. Respir. Dis.*, **133**, 913–927
56. Ball, H.A., Cook, J.A., Wise, W.C. and Halushka, P.V. (1986). Role of thromboxane, prostaglandins and leukotrienes in endotoxic and septic shock. *Intens. Care Med.*, **12**, 116–126
57. Brigham, K.L., Bowers, R.E. and Haynes, J. (1979). Increased sheep vascular permeability caused by E. coli endotoxin. *Circ. Res.*, **45**, 292–297
58. Brigham, K.L. (1985). Metabolites of arachidonic acid in experimental lung vascular injury. *Fed. Proc.*, **44**, 43–45
59. Fletcher, J.R. and Ramwell, P.W. (1977). Modification, by aspirin and indomethacin, of the haemodynamic and prostaglandin releasing effects of E. Coli endotoxin in the dog. *Br. J. Pharmacol.*, **61**, 175–181
60. Bult, H., Bettens, J. and Herman, A.G. (1980). Blood levels of 6-oxo-prostaglandin $F_{1\alpha}$ during endotoxin-induced hypotension in rabbits. *Eur. J. Pharmacol.*, **63**, 47–56
61. Westcott, J.Y., Chang, S., Balazy, M., Stene, D.O., Pradelles, P., Maclouf, J., Voelkel, N.F. and Murphy, R.C. (1986). Analysis of 6-keto-PGF$_{1\alpha}$, 5-HETE and LTC$_4$ in rat lung: Comparison of GC/MS, RIA and EIA. *Prostaglandins*, **32**, 857–873
62. Hagmann, W., Fritz, M.M. and Keppler, D. (1983). Leukotrienes and endotoxin lethality. In Piper, P.J. (ed.) *Leukotrienes and Other Lipoxygenase Products*, pp. 128–133. (Chichester: John Wiley and Sons)
63. Hagmann, W., Denzlinger, C. and Keppler, D. (1984). Role of peptide leukotrienes and their hepatobiliary elimination in endotoxin action. *Circ. Shock*, **14**, 223–235
64. Ogletree, M.L., Begley, C.J., King, G.A. and Brigham, K.L. (1986). Influence of steroidal and nonsteroidal anti-inflammatory agents on the accumulation of arachidonic acid metabolites in plasma and lung lymph after endotoxemia in awake sheep. *Am. Rev. Respir. Dis.*, **133**, 55–61
65. Snapper, J.R., Hutchinson, A.A., Ogletree, M.L. and Brigham, K.L. (1983). Effects of cyclooxygenase inhibitors on the alterations in lung mechanics caused by endotoxemia in the unanesthetized sheep. *J. Clin. Invest.*, **72**, 63–76
66. Weir, E.K., Mlczoch, J., Reeves, J.T. and Grover, R.F. (1976). Endotoxin and prevention of hypoxic pulmonary vasoconstriction. *J. Lab. Clin. Med.*, **88**, 975–983
67. Bremm, K.D., Konig, W., Spur, B., Crea, A. and Galanos, C. (1984). Generation of slow-reacting substance (leukotrienes) by endotoxin and lipid A from human polymorphonuclear granulocytes. *Immunology*, **53**, 229–304

68. Seeger, W., Radinger, H. and Neuhof, H. (1984). Increase in the capillary filtration coefficient in isolated rabbit lungs due to non-cyclooxygenase pathway of arachidonic acid. *Microcirc. Clin. Exp.*, **3**, 351

69. Farrukh, I.S., Sciuto, A.M., Spannhake, E.W., Gurtner, G.H. and Michael J.R. (1986). Leukotriene D$_4$ increases pulmonary vascular permeability and pressure by different mechanisms in the rabbit. *Am. Rev. Respir. Dis.*, **134**, 229–232

70. Noonan, T.C., Garcia-Szabo, R.R. and Malik, A.B. (1983). Pulmonary microcirculatory effects of leukotriene C$_4$ (LTC$_4$) and D$_4$ (LTD$_4$). *Fed. Proc.*, **42**, 731

71. Zadoff, A.D., Kobayashi, T., Brigham, K.L. and Newman, J.H. (1986). Diethylcarbamazine on pulmonary vascular response to endotoxin in awake sheep. *J. Appl. Physiol.*, **60**, 1380–1385

72. Welsh, C.H., Voelkel, N.F. and Weil, J.V. (1985). Diethylcarbamazine fails to prevent endotoxin lung injury. *Am. Rev. Respir. Dis.*, **131**, 414 (Abstract)

73. Cook, J.A., Wise, W.C. and Halushka, P.V. (1985). Protective effect of a selective leukotriene antagonist in endotoxemia in the rat. *J. Pharm. Exp. Ther.*, **235**, 470–474

74. Cook, J.A., Wise, W.C. and Halushka, P.V. (1980). Elevated thromboxane levels in the rat during endotoxic shock. *J. Clin. Invest.*, **65**, 227–230

75. Ramesha, C.S. and Pickett, W.C. (1986). Platelet activating factor and leukotriene biosynthesis is inhibited in polymorphonuclear leukocytes depleted of arachidonic acid. *J. Biol. Chem.*, **261**, 7592–7595

76. Morganroth, M.L., Pickett, W.C., Worthen, S., Mathias, M., Reeves, J.T. and Voelkel, N.F. (1986). Decreased pulmonary vascular responsiveness in rats raised on an essential fatty acid deficient diet. *Prostaglandins*, **33**, 181–197

77. Ogletree, M.L. and Brigham, K.L. (1982). Effects of cyclooxygenase inhibitors on pulmonary vascular responses to endotoxin in unanesthetized sheep. *Prostaglandins*, **8**, 489–502

78. Ogletree, M.L. and Brigham, K.L. (1981). Imidazole, a selective inhibitor of thromboxane synthesis, inhibits pulmonary vascular responses to endotoxin in awake sheep . *Am. Rev. Respir. Dis.*, **123**, 247–253

79. Hulton, N.R., Johnson, D.J. and Wilmore, D.W. (1985). Limited effects of prostaglandin inhibitors in E. coli sepsis. *Surgery*, **98**, 291–297

80. Hales, C.A., Brandstter, R.D., Neely, C.F., Peterson, M.B., Kong, D. and Watkins, W.D. (1986). Methylprednisolone on circulating eicosanoids and vasomotor tone after endotoxin. *J. Appl. Physiol.*, **61**, 185–191

81. Terashita, Z., Imura, Y., Nishikawa, K. and Sumida, S. (1985). Is platelet activating factor (PAF) a mediator of endotoxin shock? *Eur. J. Pharmacol.*, **109**, 257–261

82. Hamasaki, Y., Mojarad, M., Saga, T., Tai, H. and Said, S.I. (1984). Platelet-activating factor raises airway and vascular pressures and induces edema in lungs perfused with platelet-free solution. *Am. Rev. Respir. Dis.*, **129**, 742–746

83. Doebber, T.W., Wu, M.S., Robbins, J.C., Choy, B.M., Chang, M.N. and Shen, T.Y. (1985). Platelet activating factor (PAF) involvement in endotoxin-induced hypotension in rats. Studies with PAF-receptor antagonist kadsurenone. *Biochem. Biophys. Res. Commun.*, **127**, 799–808

84. Burhop, K.E., van der Zee, H., Bizios, R., Kaplan, J.E. and Malik, A.B. (1986). Pulmonary vascular response to platelet-activating factor in awake sheep and the role of cyclooxygenase metabolites. *Am. Rev. Respir. Dis.*, **134**, 548–554

85. Handley, D.A., Van Valen, G., Melden, M.K., Flury, S., Lee, M.L. and Saunders, R.N. (1986). *Immunopharmacology*, **12**, 11–16

86. McMurtry, I.F. and Morris, K.G. (1986). Platelet-activating factor causes pulmonary vasodilation in the rat. *Am. Rev. Respir. Dis.*, **134**, 757–762

87. Voelkel, N.F., Chang, S., Pfeffer, K., McMurtry, I.F. and Henson, P.M. (1986). PAF antagonists: different effects on platelets, neutrophils, guinea pig ileum and isolated rat lung. *Prostaglandins*, **32**, 359–372

88. Voelkel, N.F. (1985). Species variation in lung arachidonic acid metabolism. *Prostaglandins*, **29**, 867–889

89. Zimmerman, G.A., Renzetti, A.D. and Hill, H.R. (1983). Functional and metabolic activity of granulocytes from patients with adult respiratory distress syndrome. *Am. Rev. Respir. Dis.*, **127**, 290–300

90. Traber, D.L., Adams, T. Jr., Sziebert, L., Stein, M. and Traber, L. (1985). Potentiation of lung vascular response to endotoxin by superoxide dismutase. *J. Appl. Physiol.*, **58**, 1005–1009

91. Bernard, G., Lucht, W., Nerdermeyer, M., Snapper, J., Ogletree, M. and Brigham, K. (1984). Effect of *n*-acetylcysteine on the pulmonary response to endotoxin in the awake sheep and upon in vitro granulocyte function. *J. Clin. Invest.*, **73**, 1772–1784

92. Wong, C., Fox, R. and Demling, R.H. (1985). Effect of hydroxyl radical scavenging on endotoxin-induced lung injury. *Surgery*, **97**, 300–306

93. Demling, R.H., Lalonde, C., Jin, L.J., Ryan, P. and Fox, R. (1986). Endotoxemia causes increased lung tissue lipid peroxidation in unanesthetized sheep. *J. Appl. Physiol.*, **60**, 2094–2100

94. Mead, J.F., Alfin-Glater, R.B., Houston, D.R. and Popjak, G. (1986). *Lipids, Chemistry, Biochemistry and Nutrition*, Chapter 6, pp. 88. (New York, London: Plenum Press)

95. Chang, S.W., Lauterburg, B.H. and Voelkel, N.F. (1986). Plasma but not lung tissue oxidized glutathione (GSSG) is increased in endotoxin-treated rats. *Fed. Proc.*, **46**, 663

96. Deneke, S.M. and Fanburg, B.L. (1982). Oxygen toxicity of the lung: an update. *Br. J. Anaesth.*, **54**, 737–749

97. Petkau, A., Kelly, K., Chelack, W.S., Pleskach, S.D., Barefoot, C. and Meeker, B.E. (1975). Radioprotection of bone marrow stem cells by superoxide dismutase. *Biochem. Biophys. Res. Commun.*, **67**, 1167–1173

98. Bus, J. and Gibson, J.E. (1984). Paraquat: Model for oxidant-initiated toxicity. *Environ. Health Perspect.*, **55**, 37–46

99. Martin, W.J. II. (1983). Nitrofurantoin: evidence for the oxidant injury of lung parenchymal cells. *Am. Rev. Respir. Dis.*, **127**, 482–496

100. Kennedy, T.P., Paky, A., McShane, A., Sciuto, M., Atkinson, N.F. and Gurtner, G.H. (1986). Inhibitors of arachidonate metabolism protect from amiodarone lung injury. *Am. Rev. Respir. Dis.*, **133**, A24

101. Lee, S., Douglas, W.H.J., Deneke, S.M. and Fanburg, B.C. (1983). Ultrastructural changes in bovine pulmonary artery endothelial cells exposed to 80% O_2 in vitro. *In Vitro*, **19**, 714–722

102. Krieger, B.P., Loomis, W.H., Czer, G.T. and Spragg, R.G. (1985). Mechanisms of interaction between oxygen and granulocytes in hyperoxic lung injury. *J. Appl. Physiol.*, **58**, 1326–1330

103. Fantone, J.C. and Ward, P.M. (1982). Role of oxygen-derived radicals and metabolites in leukocyte-dependent inflammatory reactions. *Am. J. Pathol.*, **107**, 397–418

104. Freeman, B.A. and Crapo. J.D. (1982). Biology of disease: free radicals and tissue injury. *Lab. Invest.*, **67**, 412–426

105. Halliwell, B. (1978). Biochemical mechanism accounting for the toxic action of oxygen on living organism: the key role of superoxide dismutase. *Cell. Biol. Int. Rep.*, **2**, 113–128

106. Kellogg, E.W. and Fridovich, I. (1977). Liposome oxidation and erythrocyte lysis by enzymatically generated superoxide and hydrogen peroxide. *J. Biol. Chem.*, **752**, 6721–6728

107. Del Maestro, R.F. (1980). An approach to free radicals in medicine and biology. *Acta Physiol. Scand. Suppl.*, **692**, 153–168

108. Del Maestro, R.F., Bjork, J. and Arfors, K.E. (1981). Increase in microvascular permeability induced by enzymatically generated free radicals. II. Role of superoxide anion radical, hydrogen peroxide, and hydroxyl radical. *Microvasc. Res.*, **22**, 255–270

109. Chan, P.M., Yurko, M. and Fishman, R.A. (1982). Phospholipid degradation in cellular edema induced by free radicals in brain cortical slices. *Neurochemistry*, **38**, 525–531

110. Gurtner, G.H., Knoblauch, P., Smith, L., Sies, H. and Adkinson, N.F. (1983). Oxidant- and lipid-induced pulmonary vasoconstriction mediated by arachidonic acid metabolites. *J. Appl. Physiol.*, **55**, 949–954

111. Jacobson, J.M., Michael, J.R., Bradley, M.B. and Gurtner, G.H. (1986). Inhibition of thromboxane synthesis prevents hyperbaric oxygen-induced pulmonary damage. *Am. Rev. Respir. Dis.*, **135**, A283

112. Jackson, R.M., Chandler, D.B. and Fulmer, J.D. (1986). Production of arachidonic acid metabolism by endothelial cells in hyperoxia. *J. Appl. Physiol.*, **61**, 584–591

113. Tate, R.M., Van Benthuysen, K.M., Shasby, D.M., McMurtry, I.F. and Repine, J.E. (1982). Oxygen radical mediated permeability edema and vasoconstriction in isolated perfused rabbit lungs. *Am. Rev. Respir. Dis.*, **126**, 802–806

114. Farrukh, I.S., Michael, J.R., Summer, W.R., Adkinson, N.F. Jr. and Gurtner, G.H. (1985). Thromboxane-induced pulmonary vasoconstriction: involvement of calcium. *J. Appl. Physiol.*, **58**, 34–44

115. Allison, R.C., Marble, K.T., Hernandez, E.M., Townsley, M.I. and Taylor, A.E. (1986). Attenuation of permeability lung injury after phorbol myristate acetate by verapamil and OKY-046. *Am. Rev. Respir. Dis.*, **134**, 93–100

116. Seeger, W., Wolf, H., Stahler, G., Neuhof, H. and Roka, L. (1982). Increased pulmonary vascular resistance and permeability due to arachidonate metabolism in isolated rabbit lungs. *Prostaglandins*, **23**, 157–173

117. Jackson, R., Chandler, D. and Fulmer, J. (1986). Effects of leukotriene B_4 on permeability and thromboxane and prostacyclin production of isolated, perfused rat lungs. *Am. Rev. Respir. Dis.*, **135**, A283

118. Taniguchi, H., Taki, F., Takagi, K., Satake, T., Sugiyama, S. and Ozawa, T. (1986). The role of leukotriene B_4 in the genesis of oxygen toxicity in the lung. *Am. Rev. Respir. Dis.*, **133**, 805–808

119. Harper, T.W., Westcott, J.Y., Voelkel, N. and Murphy, R.C. (1984). Metabolism of leukotrienes B_4 and C_4 in the isolated perfused rat lung. *J. Biol. Chem.*, **259**, 14437–14440

120. Flick, M.R., Hoeffel, J.M. and Staub, N.C. (1983). Superoxide dismutase with heparin prevents increased lung vascular permeability during air emboli in sheep. *J. Appl. Physiol.*, **55**, 1284–1291

121. Fukushima, M. and Kobayashi, T. (1986). Effects of thromboxane synthase inhibition on air emboli lung injury in sheep. *J. Appl. Physiol.*, **60**, 1828–1833

122. Malik, A.B. (1983). Pulmonary microembolism. *Physiol. Rev.*, **63**, 1114–1207

123. Demling, R.H. (1982). Role of prostaglandins in acute pulmonary microvascular injury. *NY Acad. Sci.*, **384**, 517–533

124. Garcia-Szabo, R.R., Peterson, M.B., Watkins, W.D., Bizios, R., Kong, D.L. and Malik, A.B. (1983). Thromboxane generation after thrombin. *Circ. Res.*, **53**, 214–222

125. Johnson, A. and Malik, A.b. (1980). Effect of granulocytopenia on extravascular lung water content after microembolization. *Am. Rev. Respir. Dis.*, **122**, 561–566

126. Bizios, R., Minnear, F.L., van der Zee, H. and Malik, A.B. (1983). Effects of cyclooxygenase and lipoxygenase inhibition on lung fluid balance after thrombin. *J. Appl. Physiol.*, **55**, 462–471

127. Julien, M., Hoeffel, J.M. and Flick, M.R. (1986). Oleic acid lung injury in sheep. *J. Appl. Physiol.*, **60**, 433–440

128. Kries, W.R., Lindenauer, S.M. and Dent, T.L. (1983). Corticosteroids in experimental fat embolization. *J. Surg. Res.*, **14**, 238–246

129. Olanoff, L.S., Reines, H.D., Spicer, K.M. and Halushka, P.V. (1984). Effects of oleic acid on pulmonary capillary leak and thromboxanes. *J. Surg. Res.*, **36**, 597–605

130. Miyazawa, T., Hiramoto, M. and Nishida, O. (1982). Reversal of oleic acid-induced respiratory distress by PGI_2. *Respir. Physiol.* **47**, 351–364

131. Meyrick, B., Gamble, W. and Reid, L. (1980). Development of crotalaria pulmonary hypertension: hemodynamic and structural study. *Am. J. Physiol.*, **239**, H692–702

132. Sugita, T., Hyers, T.M., Dauber, I.M., Wagner, W.W., McMurtry, I.F. and Reeves, J.T. (1983). Lung vessel leak precedes right ventricular hypertrophy in monocrotaline-treated rats. *J. Appl. Physiol.*, **54**, 371–374

133. Stanbrook, H.S., Morris, K.G. and McMurtry, I.F. (1984). Prevention and reversal of hypoxic pulmonary hypertension by calcium antagonists. *Am. Rev. Respir. Dis.*, **130**, 81–85

134. Stenmark, K.R., Morganroth, M.L., Remigio, L.K., Voelkel, N.F., Murphy, R.C., Henson, P.M., Mathias, M.M. and Reeves, J.T. (1985). Alveolar inflammation and arachidonate metabolism in monocrotaline-induced pulmonary hypertension. *Am. J. Physiol.*, **248**, H859–866

135. Roth, R.A. and Ganey, P.E. (1987). Arachidonic acid metabolites and the mechanisms of monocrotaline pneumotoxicity. *Am. Rev. Respir. Dis.* (In press)

136. Langleben, D., Carvalho, A.C.A. and Reid, L.M. (1986). The platelet thromboxane inhibitor, dazmegrel, does not reduce monocrotaline-induced pulmonary hypertension. *Am. Rev. Respir. Dis.*, **133**, 789–791

137. Stenmark, K.R., Fasules, J.W., Morris, K.G., Voelkel, N.F. and Reeves, J.T. (1986). Diethylcarbamazine (DEC) but not indomethacin (INDO) prevents the early lung leak and late pulmonary hypertension in monocrotaline treated rats. *Am. Rev. Respir. Dis.*, **133**, A277 (Abstract)

138. Morganroth, M.L., Stenmark, K.R., Morris, K.G., Murphy, R.C., Mathias, M.M., Reeves, J.T. and Voelkel, N.F. (1985). Diethylcarbamazine inhibits acute and chronic hypoxic pulmonary hypertension in awake rats. *Am. Rev. Respir. Dis.*, **131**, 488–492

139. Huxtable, R.J. (1979). New aspects of the toxicology and pharmacology of pyrrolizidine alkaloids. *Biochem. Pharmacol.*, **10**, 159–167

140. Bach, M.K. and Brashler, J.R. (1986). Inhibition of the leukotriene synthetase of rat basophil leukemia cells by diethylcarbamazine, and synergism between diethylcarbamazine and piriprost, a 5-lipoxygenase inhibitor. *Biochem. Pharmacol.*, **35**, 425–433

141. Stenmark, K.R., Fasules, J., Voelkel, N.F., Henson, J., Tucker, A., Hyde, D.M., Wilson, H. and Reeves, J.T. (1987). Severe pulmonary hypertension and arterial adventitial changes in newborn calves at 4300 m. *Am. J. Physiol.*, **62**, 821–830

142. Fasules, J., Stenmark, K.R., Henson, P.M., Voelkel, N.F., Tucker, A. and Reeves, J.T. (1986). Platelet activating factor (PAF) in lung lavage of chronically hypoxic neonatal calves. *Am. Rev. Respir. Dis.*, **133**, A227

143. Morganroth, M.L., Stenmark, K.R., Zirrolli, J.A., Mauldin, R., Mathias, M., Reeves, J.T., Murphy, R.C. and Voelkel, N.F. (1984). Leukotriene C_4 production during hypoxic pulmonary vasoconstriction in isolated rat lung. *Prostaglandins*, **28**, 867–875

144. Haroldsen, P.E., Voelkel, N.F., Henson, J.E., Henson, P.M. and Murphy, R.C. (1987). Metabolism of platelet activating factor (PAF) in the isolated perfused rat lung. *J. Clin. Invest.*, **79**, 1860–1867

145. Gryglewski, R.J., Korbut, R. and Ocetkiewica, A. (1978). Generation of prostacyclin by lungs in vivo and its release into the arterial circulation. *Nature (London)*, **273**, 765–767

146. Westcott, J.Y., Clay, K.L. and Murphy, R.C. (1984). Decomposition of leukotriene C_4. *J. Allerg. Clin. Immunol.*, **74**, 363–368

147. Meyrick, B.O. (1986). Endotoxin-mediated pulmonary endothelial cell injury. *Fed. Proc.*, **45**, 19–24

148. Folco, G.C., Omini, C., Vigano, T. and Berti, F. (1981). Pharmacology of leukotriene C_4 in guinea-pig. In Berti, F., Folco, G.C. and Velo, G.P. (eds.) *Leukotrienes and Prostaglandins* pp. 107–124 (New York; London: Plenum Press)

149. Voelkel, N.F., Gerber, G.J., McMurtry, I.F., Nies, A.S. and Reeves, J.T. (1981). Release of vasodilator prostaglandin, PGI_2, from isolated rat lung during vasoconstriction. *Circ. Res.*, **48**, 207–213

150. Weksler, B.B., Ley, C.W. and Jaffe, E.A. (1978). Stimulation of endothelial cell prostacyclin production by thrombin, trypsin, and the ionophore A 23187. *J. Clin. Invest.*, **62**, 923–930

151. Cramer, E.B., Pologe, L., Pawlowski, N.A., Cohn, Z.A. and Scott, W.A. (1983). Leukotriene C_4 promotes prostacyclin synthesis by human endothelial cells. *Proc. Natl. Acad. Sci. USA*, **80**, 4109–4113

152. Pologe, L.G., Cramer, E.B., Pawlowski, N.A., Abraham, E., Cohn, Z.A. and Scott, W.A. (1984). Stimulation of human endothelial cell prostacyclin synthesis by select leukotrienes. *J. Exp. Med.*, **160**, 1043–1053

153. Ogletree, M.L. and Brigham, K.L. (1979). Indomethacin augments endotoxin-induced increased lung vascular permeability in sheep. *Am. Rev. Respir. Dis.*, **119**, A303 (Abstract)

154. Demling, R.H., Smith, M., Gunther, R., Gee, M. and Flynn, J. (1981). The effect of prostacyclin infusion on endotoxin-induced lung injury. *Surgery*, **90**, 257–263

155. Perlman, M.B., Lo, S.K. and Malik, A.B. (1986). Effect of prostacyclin on pulmonary vascular response to thrombin in awake sheep. *J. Appl. Physiol.*, **60**, 546–553

156. Garrett, R.C. and Thomas, H.M. III. (1983). Meclofenamate uniformly decreases shunt fraction in dogs with lobar atelectasis. *J. Appl. Physiol.*, **54**, 284–289

157. Garrett, R.C. and Thomas, H.M. III. (1985). Relation of prostanoids to strength of hypoxic vasoconstriction in dogs with lobar atelectasis. *J. Appl. Physiol.*, **59**, 72–77

158. Light, R.B., (1986). Indomethacin and acetylsalicylic acid reduce intrapulmonary shunt in experimental pneumococcal pneumonia. *Am. Rev. Respir. Dis.*, **134**, 520–525
159. Voelkel, N.F., Morganroth, M., Stenmark, K.R., Fedderson, O.C., Murphy, R.C. and Reeves, J.T. (1983). Leukotrienes in the lung circulation: actions and interactions. In *Hypoxia, Exercise and Altitude. Proceedings of the 3rd Banff International Hypoxia Symposium*, pp. 141–152. (New York: Liss)
160. Schoenfeld, S.A., Ploysongsang, Y., Dilisio, R., Crissman, J., Miller, E., Hammerschmidt, D.E. and Jacob, H.S. (1983). Fat embolism prophylaxis with corticosteroids – a prospective study in high risk patients. *Ann. Int. Med.*, **99**, 438–443
161. Flick, M.R. and Murray, J.F. (1984). High dose corticosteroid therapy in the adult respiratory distress syndrome. *J. Am. Med. Assoc.*, **251**, 1054–1056
162. Holcroft, J.W., Vassar, M.J. and Weber, C.J. (1986). Prostaglandin E_1 and survival in patients with the adult respiratory distress syndrome. *Ann. Surg.*, **90**, 371–383
163. Shoemaker, W.C. and Appel, P.L. (1986). Effects of prostaglandin E_1 in adult respiratory distress syndrome. *Surgery*, **99**, 275–282
164. Tahamont, M.V., Gee, M.H., Flynn, J.T. and Cox, J. (1985). Prostaglandin E_1 prevents lung injury during intravascular complement activation in sheep. *Am. Rev. Respir. Dis.*, **131**, A281 (Abstract)
165. Williams, J.H., Fairshter, R.D., Chen, M., Crosby, S., Chun, L., Ulich, T. and Vaziri, N. (1985). Prostaglandin E_1 analog effects on the lungs of normal and paraquat injured rats. *Am. Rev. Respir. Dis.*, **131** A281 (Abstract)
166. Murphy, R.C. and Henson, P.M. (1985). Mediator network. *Ann. Inst. Pasteur./Immunol.*, **136D**, 219–221
167. Brand, R., Dembinski-Kiec, A., Korbut, R., Gryglewski, R.J. and Novak, R.J. (1984). Release of prostacyclin from the human pulmonary vascular bed in response to cholinergic stimulation. *Naunyn-Schmeidebergs Arch. Pharmacol.*, **325**, 69–75
168. Feddersen, C.O., Mathias, M.M., McMurtry, I.F. and Voelkel, N.F. (1986). Acetylcholine induces vasodilation and prostacyclin synthesis in rat lungs. *Prostaglandins*, **31**, 973–987
169. Förstermann, U., Hertting, G. and Neufang, B. (1986). The role of endothelial and non-endothelial prostaglandins in the relaxation of isolated blood vessels of the rabbit induced by acetylcholine and bradykinin. *Br. J. Pharmac.* **87**, 521–532
170. Kato, K., Koshihara, Y. and Murota, S. (1986). Contribution of lipoxygenase metabolites to IL-2 production in the early phase of lymphocyte activation. *Prostaglandins*, **22**, 301–311
171. Stewart, D., Pountney, E. and Fitchett, D. (1983). Norepinephrine-stimulated vascular prostacyclin synthesis. Receptor-dependent calcium channels control prostaglandin synthesis. *Can. J. Physiol. Pharmacol.*, **62**, 1341–1347
172. Elias, J., Gustilo, K., Rossman, M. and Daniele, R. (1985). Blood monocyte and alveolar macrophage inhibition of lung fibroblast growth: relationship to interleukin-1. Presented to the *28th Aspen Lung Conference*

5
Eicosanoids in sepsis and its sequelae

J. A. Cook, G. E. Tempel, H. A. Ball, W. C. Wise, G. Matera,
H. D. Reines and P. V. Halushka

INTRODUCTION

Circulatory shock resulting from sepsis continues to be a major clinical problem with 100 000 to 300 000 cases reported yearly in the United States alone[1]. In spite of the introduction of specific antibiotics, careful monitoring, aggressive surgical intervention and intravenous hyperalimentation, mortality from septic shock still exceeds 50%[2,3]. A major complication of sepsis is adult respiratory distress syndrome (ARDS)[4,5]. This form of pulmonary injury can also be elicited by unrelated etiological factors, such as trauma, inhalation injury and fat embolism[6,7]. Despite this diversity in origin, the major underlying pathophysiological alterations are similar. Diffuse alveolar and capillary endothelial injury, increased microvascular permeability, an inflammatory cell infiltrate, and hypoxaemia characterize this condition[6,7].

The specific cellular and biochemical mechanisms mediating septic shock and ARDS are undefined. Current concepts favour inflammatory mediators, a number of which have been implicated in experimentally induced sepsis and ARDS. These include oxygen free radicals, endogenous opiates, kinins, angiotensin, histamine, serotonin and catecholamines[8,9].

In recent years, considerable interest has arisen concerning another group of inflammatory mediators, the eicosanoids. Eicosanoids are arachidonic acid (AA) products derived from metabolism via the cyclo-oxygenase or lipoxygenase pathways. A variety of stimuli are known to activate phospholipase A_2 leading to the release of arachidonic acid. Further metabolism by fatty acid cyclo-oxygenase results in the formation of several products, including thromboxane A_2 (TxA_2), PGE_2, $PGF_{2\alpha}$ and prostacyclin (PGI_2). TxA_2 is a potent vasoconstrictor and proaggregatory substance whereas PGI_2 is a vasodilator and inhibitor of platelet aggregation[10-12]. Since tissue ischaemia, systemic hypotension and disseminated intravascular coagulation are frequent manifestations in both patients and laboratory animals with sepsis, it has been proposed that an imbalance in the synthesis of TxA_2 and PGI_2 contributes to these shock sequelae.

The other major pathway of arachidonic acid metabolism gives rise to the lipoxygenase products[13]. Two classes of leukotrienes are derived from enzymatic conversion of the LTA_4 precursor: the sulphidopeptide leukotrienes, LTC_4, LTD_4 and LTE_4, and the non-peptide metabolite, LTB_4. These lipoxygenase products exert a variety of inflammatory actions and haemodynamic effects that mimic features of circulatory shock. LTB_4, for example, promotes leukostasis, chemokinesis of neutrophils and macrophages, and stimulates the release of lysosomal hydrolases, all of which potentiate microvascular injury[14,15]. The sulphidopeptide leukotrienes cause reductions in cardiac output and more potent vasoconstrictors in coronary, mesenteric, renal, pulmonary and skeletal muscle vascular beds in certain species[16–20]. These leukotrienes also promote bronchoconstriction and increase microvascular permeability[16,21]. In recent years, the development of highly selective leukotriene antagonists and 5-lipoxygenase inhibitors has provided the means to investigate the potential involvement of leukotrienes in experimental models of endotoxaemia, sepsis and forms of acute lung injury[22–24]. This chapter focuses on selected aspects of involvement of eicosanoid products in these conditions.

ROLE OF CYCLO-OXYGENASE PRODUCTS IN ENDOTOXAEMIA AND SEPSIS

Evidence for increased synthesis of cyclo-oxygenase products

Administration of purified preparations of bacterial endotoxin, an extract from the cell wall of Gram-negative bacteria, produces circulatory shock characterized by reductions in mean arterial pressure, cardiac output, tissue perfusion and the release of inflammatory mediators[25]. The first evidence implicating cyclo-oxygenase products in endotoxic shock derived from the observations of Northover and Subramanian[26], Hinshaw et al.[27], and Erdos et al.[28]. These investigators found that pretreatment of dogs with aspirin and other non-steroidal anti-inflammatory compounds significantly improved the altered haemodynamics, as well as survival, following endotoxin. The subsequent demonstration that non-steroidal anti-inflammatory drugs inhibit fatty acid cyclo-oxygenase prompted measurements of various cyclo-oxygenase products in plasma of several animal models of sepsis[29–36]. These earlier studies demonstrated increased levels of PGE_2 and $PGF_{2\alpha}$ which correlated temporally with the systemic hypotension and pulmonary hypertension.

Increased plasma TxB_2, the stable immunoreactive (i) metabolite of TxA_2, and i6-keto-$PGF_{1\alpha}$, the stable metabolite of PGI_2, were demonstrated in rats administered bolus injection of *Salmonella enteritidis* endotoxin[37]. As shown schematically in Figure 5.1, plasma iTxB_2 levels rise within 5 min following induction of endotoxaemia, subsequently subsiding over a 2–3 h period. Plasma i6-keto-$PGF_{1\alpha}$ levels are lower in the early stages of shock but increase to higher levels. iPGE_2 levels are intermediate between iTxB_2 and i6-keto-$PGF_{1\alpha}$. This basic profile of release of these cyclo-oxygenase products in response to bolus endotoxin injection has been subsequently observed in a large number of other species, including sheep[38,39], baboons[40,41], ponies[42], goats[43,44], pigs[45], cats[46] and rabbits[47].

The profile of eicosanoid release is influenced by both the route and time course of the endotoxin administration. In contrast to the acute paradigm of bolus endotoxin, infusion of low doses of endotoxin in rats produces comparatively small increases in plasma iTxB$_2$ with less severe cardiopulmonary abnormalities[48]. This may be due, in part, to the reduced plasma levels of iTxB$_2$[49]. Demling et $al.$[50] compared the effects of intravenous and subcutaneous tissue injection of endotoxin in sheep. With intravenous injections, lung lymph and aortic plasma levels of iTxB$_2$ and i6-keto-PGF$_{1\alpha}$ were significantly higher than tissue lymph. Subcutaneous injections produced higher iTxB$_2$ and i6-keto-PGF$_{1\alpha}$ in venous plasma and tissue lymph. The pulmonary hypoxaemia and hypertension seen in both groups were prevented by ibuprofen pretreatment. This suggests that localized tissue eicosanoid synthesis can impair function of distant organs, such as the lung[50].

Repeated sublethal intraperitoneal injection of endotoxin in rats over several days results in lower plasma iTxB$_2$ and i6-keto-PGF$_{1\alpha}$ upon subsequent administration of a much higher dose[51]. In ponies, repeated administration of bacterial endotoxin also induces[52,53] progressive reductions in endotoxin-stimulated increases in plasma iTxB$_2$. Thus, it appears that cellular or metabolic changes occur during chronic endotoxaemia which render the host less responsive to endotoxin challenge.

The clinical relevance of the use of purified preparations of bacterial endotoxin to induce shock has been questioned because of the acute nature of the insult. Eicosanoid production has therefore been assessed in septic models where the septic process is presumably slower in onset and occurs over a more sustained period. Induction of faecal peritonitis in rats produces minimal, but sustained, increases in plasma iTxB$_2$ over a 6 h period[54] (Figure 5.2). In this model of shock, plasma i6-keto-PGF$_{1\alpha}$ greatly exceeds the increases in iTxB$_2$ throughout the course of sepsis and appears to parallel the shock severity. Using yet a different model, Fink et $al.$[55] demonstrated increased plasma levels of i6-keto-PGF$_{1\alpha}$ but no significant changes in plasma iTxB$_2$ in rats subjected to sepsis by caecal ligation and puncture. Similar increases in plasma i6-keto-PGF$_{1\alpha}$ have been observed in rats following peritonitis induced by abdominal implantation of gauze innoculated with $Escherichia$ $coli$ bacteria[56]. Increased plasma iTxB$_2$ levels were observed in this model but were comparable to the levels seen in sham controls. Thus, surgery and implantation of sterile gauze pads are sufficient to induce a moderate rise in iTxB$_2$. Different effects on cyclo-oxygenase metabolism are seen in response to sepsis in other species. Proportionally greater amounts of plasma iTxB$_2$ are produced relative to i6-keto-PGF$_{1\alpha}$ in the early phase of $E.$ $coli$ infusion in goats[44] or $Aeromonas$ $hydrophilia$ in pigs[57], whereas higher levels of i6-keto-PGF$_{1\alpha}$ have been reported in baboons and rabbits with $E.$ $coli$ sepsis[58,59].

Tissue and cellular sources of eicosanoids

Since the major organ sources of AA metabolites during endotoxaemia and sepsis were unknown in the rat, studies were designed to determine the contribution of the kidneys, hepatosplanchnic region and extremities to plasma

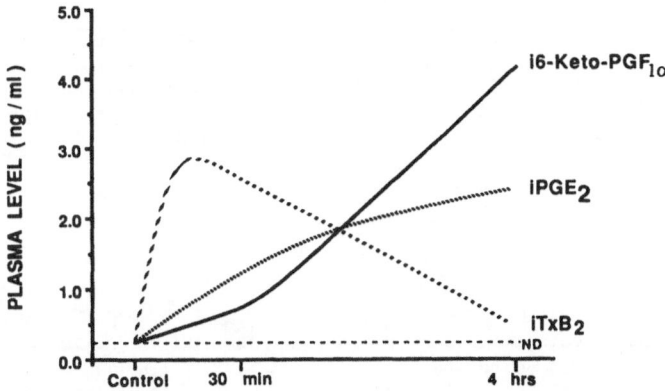

Figure 5.1 Schematic representation of changes in venous plasma immunoreactive (i) TxB_2, i6-keto-$PGF_{1\alpha}$ and iPGE_2 levels in rats after *S. enteritidis* endotoxin ($20\,mg\,kg^{-1}$ i.v.). N.D. = non-detectable

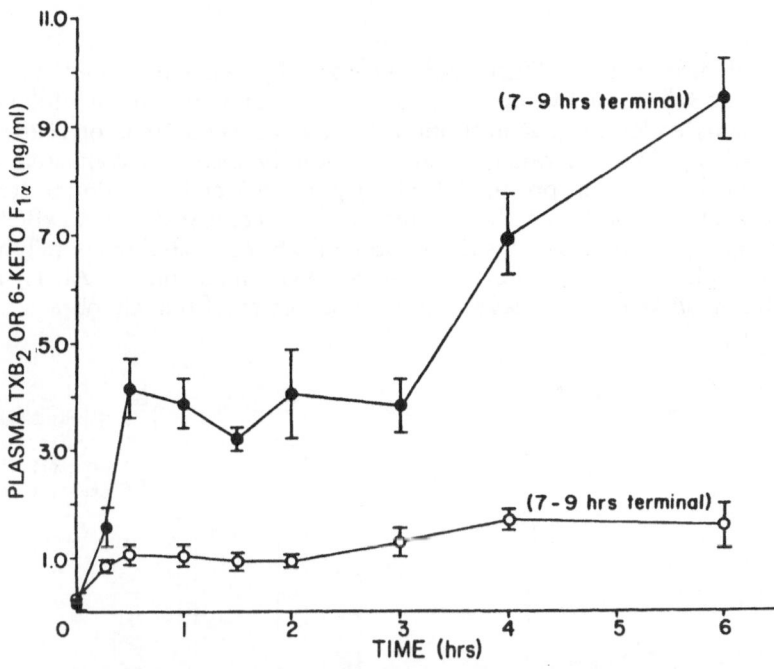

Figure 5.2 Time course of plasma iTxB_2 (○) and i6-keto-$PGF_{1\alpha}$(●) during intra-abdominal sepsis in rats. Sepsis was produced by instillation of a faecal suspension in the peritoneal cavity. Data expressed as mean ± SEM. From Cook *et al.*[151], reprinted by permission of W.B. Saunders Co.

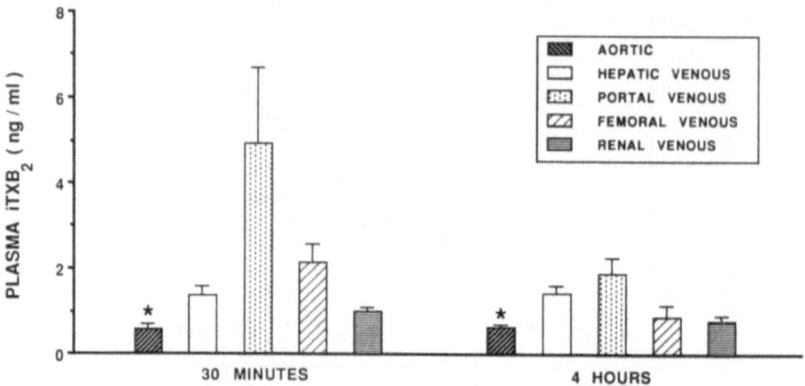

Figure 5.3 Plasma iTxB$_2$ at 30 min and 4 h following i.v. *S. enteritidis* endotoxin (20 mg kg^{-1}) from aortic and designated organ venous sources. All venous plasma iTxB$_2$ levels were increased ($p < 0.05$) relative to aortic levels ($n = 12$) at 30 min. Hepatic venous ($n = 5$) and portal venous ($n = 15$) were increased ($p < 0.05$) relative to aortic levels ($n = 22$) at 4 h. Data expressed as mean $\pm$ SEM

levels of eicosanoids[60]. iTxB$_2$ and i6-keto-PGF$_{1\alpha}$ were measured in renal, hepatic, portal, femoral venous and aortic plasma at 30 min and 4 h following intravenous endotoxin administration. Venous concentrations of iTxB$_2$ and i6-keto-PGF$_{1\alpha}$ from all organs were significantly increased compared with aortic levels at 30 min post-endotoxin (Figures 5.3 and 5.4). Portal venous iTxB$_2$ levels demonstrated the greatest increase compared with iTxB$_2$ from other organs (Figure 5.3). This rise in portal iTxB$_2$ correlated temporally with reduced splanchnic blood flow and small bowel infarction[61,62]. At 4 h after endotoxin, i6-keto-PGF$_{1\alpha}$ levels in venous plasma from all organs were

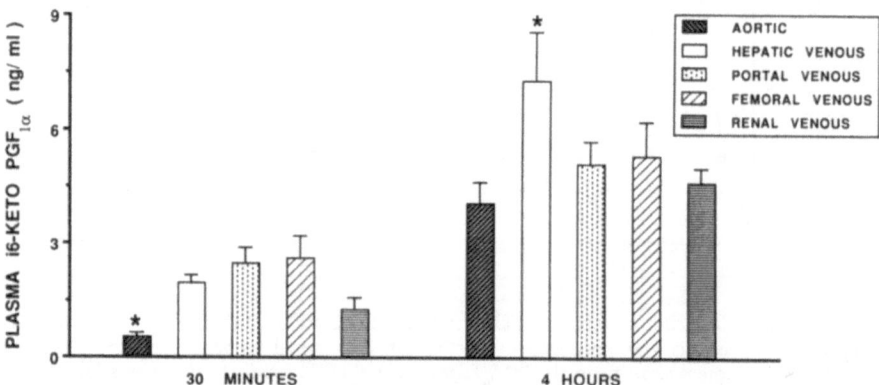

Figure 5.4 Plasma i6-keto-PGF$_{1\alpha}$ at 30 min and 4 h following i.v. *S. enteritidis* endotoxin (20 mg kg^{-1}) from aortic and designated venous organ sources. All venous plasma i6-keto-PGF$_{1\alpha}$ were increased ($p < 0.05$) relative to aortic levels ($n = 12$) at 30 min. Hepatic venous levels ($n = 16$) were increased ($p < 0.05$) relative to aortic levels ($n = 22$) at 4 h. Data expressed as mean $\pm$ SEM

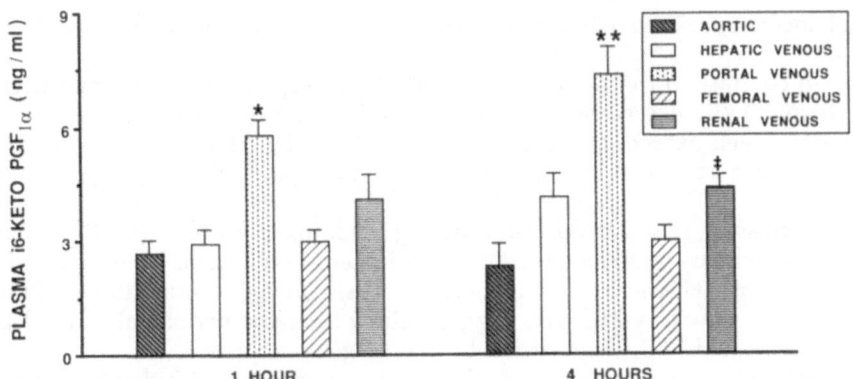

Figure 5.5 Plasma i6-keto-PGF$_{1\alpha}$ at 1 h and 4 h following acute faecal peritonitis from aortic and designated venous organ sources. Portal venous levels ($n = 7$) were increased ($p < 0.05$) vs aortic levels ($n = 6$) at both time periods. Renal venous levels ($n = 5$) were increased vs. aortic levels at 4 h.
Data expressed as mean $\pm$ SEM

significantly increased compared with 30 min values, with hepatic venous concentration demonstrating the greatest increase (Figure 5.4).

Similar studies have been conducted in rats subjected to acute faecal peritonitis. At 1 h and 4 h following the onset of sepsis, portal venous i6-keto-PGF$_{1\alpha}$ values were increased approximately two fold compared with aortic levels (Figure 5.5). Portal venous iTxB$_2$ concentrations were also increased but not to the extent observed in venous i6-keto-PGF$_{1\alpha}$ (Figure 5.6). These studies have identified the hepatosplanchnic circulation as a region

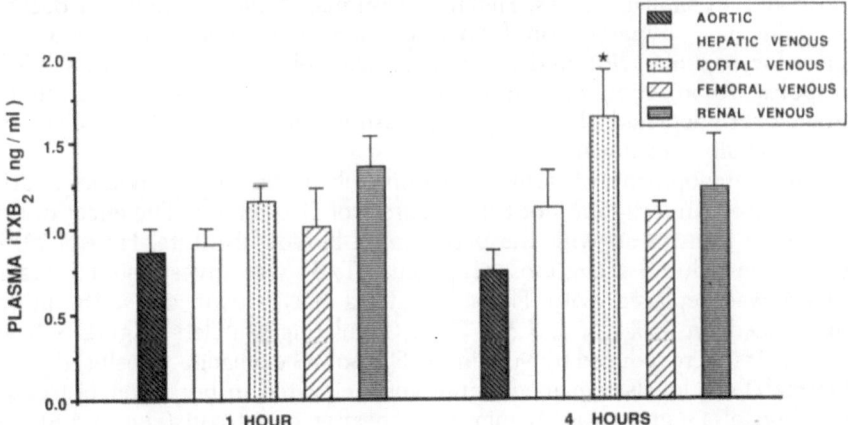

Figure 5.6 Plasma iTxB$_2$ at 1 h and 4 h following acute faecal peritonitis from aortic and designated venous organ sources. Portal venous iTxB$_2$ levels ($n = 8$) were increased ($p < 0.05$) relative to aortic levels ($n = 5$) at 4 h.
Data expressed as mean $\pm$ SEM

97

of increased eicosanoid production during endotoxaemia and sepsis in the rat.

In contrast to the rat, endotoxaemic sheep respond with systemic arterial plasma iTxB$_2$ exceeding pulmonary arterial plasma levels, and pulmonary lymph levels exceeding those of blood[39,63,64]. Similar arterial increases in iTxB$_2$ have been reported in a porcine model of sepsis[57]. This transpulmonary gradient of iTxB$_2$ suggests that, in these species, the lung is a source of increased iTxB$_2$ production during endotoxaemia or sepsis[57]. Similar transpulmonary gradients for increased i6-keto-PGF$_{1\alpha}$ have been reported in the sheep[64]. However, during porcine sepsis, mixed venous i6-keto-PGF$_{1\alpha}$ levels are more elevated. This suggests either increased peripheral PGI$_2$ release or accelerated PGI$_2$ degradation by the lung[57].

Specific cellular sources of iTxB$_2$ have not been elucidated in either endotoxaemia or sepsis. Since platelets are potentially a rich source of iTxB$_2$ synthesis[10], the effect of platelet depletion on pulmonary alterations and plasma increases in eicosanoids have been investigated. Snapper et al.[64] depleted circulating platelets in sheep using anti-sheep platelet antibodies. Pulmonary hypertension and lung lymph concentrations of iTxB$_2$ increased significantly in platelet-depleted sheep given endotoxin, suggesting iTxB$_2$ release from other sources. Similar results supporting other cellular sources have been obtained with sheep infused with activated complement[65], a stimulus which also increases eicosanoid metabolism. Increases in plasma iTxB$_2$ induced by complement peptides in thrombocytopenic sheep were comparable to iTxB$_2$ in sheep with normal circulating platelet levels.

Studies have also shown[66] that bacterial endotoxin stimulates granulocyte synthesis of iTxB$_2$. Huttemeir et al.[67] assessed the effect of granulocytopenia on pulmonary responses to endotoxin in sheep. In granulocyte-depleted sheep, pulmonary hypertension and absolute iTxB$_2$ levels decreased but a positive transpulmonary gradient of iTxB$_2$ during endotoxaemia was still observed. In similar studies, Heflin and Brigham[68] did not detect a decrease in pulmonary hypertension following endotoxin infusion in sheep made granulocytopenic with hydroxyurea. Finally, plasma increases of iTxB$_2$ in response to injection of zymosan-activated plasma are not attenuated in granulocyte-depleted sheep[69]. These observations suggest that cells other than granulocytes are sources of TxA$_2$.

The development of artificial blood substitutes has provided another approach for investigation of tissue sources of eicosanoids. The effect of total exchange transfusion with the perfluorated blood substitute, Fluosol-43, on endotoxin-induced elevations of plasma iTxB$_2$ was investigated in rats[70]. Blood was replaced with Fluosol-43 to a haematocrit of $< 3\%$ in rats maintained on 95% O$_2$ and 5% CO$_2$. Circulating platelets (Figure 5.7) and leukocytes were reduced by 90% in the Fluosol-43 exchange-transfused group. Plasma iTxB$_2$ levels remained significantly elevated in both the control and the Fluosol-43 groups at 30 min and 2 h after endotoxin (Figure 5.8). It is noteworthy that the increase in iTxB$_2$ in response to endotoxin between these two groups was not significantly different. Furthermore, Fluosol-43 from exchange-transfused rats incubated with the calcium ionophore, A23187, stimulated synthesis of iTxB$_2$ ex vivo to only 1.6% that of whole blood[70].

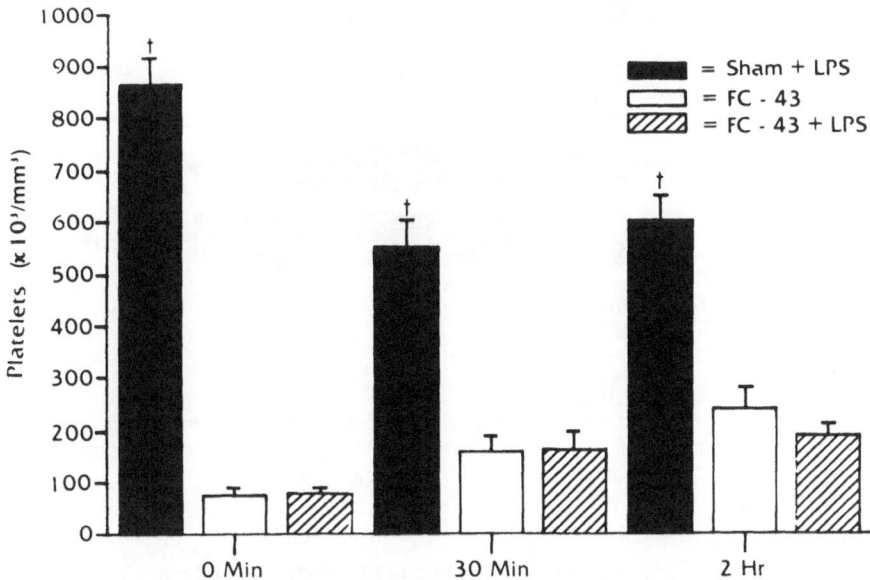

Figure 5.7   Platelet counts in sham and Fluosol-43 exchange transfused rats prior to (0 min) $n = 17–21$, and at 30 min, $n = 14–20$, or 2 h, $n = 8–11$, after endotoxin (LPS).† Sham + LPS vs FC-43 or FC-43 + LPS ($p < 0.01$). From Cook et al.[70], reprinted with permission of Alan R. Liss, Inc.

These observations suggest that circulating blood components are not the major source of iTxB$_2$ during endotoxaemia in the rat.

The macrophage is both a major site of endotoxin sequestration *in vivo* and a major source of endotoxin-induced mediators[71,72]. A potential role of macrophage-derived arachidonic acid metabolites in the sequelae of endotoxic shock is supported by studies demonstrating direct *in vitro* endotoxin stimulated synthesis of iPGE$_2$[73–75], iPGF$_{2\alpha}$[74], iTxB$_2$ and i6-keto-PGF$_{1\alpha}$[76,77] by monocytes or peritoneal macrophages. The potential importance of macrophages as a source of cyclo-oxygenase products is further supported by the studies of Bowers et al.[78]. Increasing doses of endotoxin *in vitro* enhanced Kupffer cell synthesis of iPGE$_2$ and iTxB$_2$. It was concluded that Kupffer cell-derived eicosanoids, in particular TxA$_2$, may be important mediators of some pathophysiological manifestations of acute endotoxaemia[78]. Previous studies have also noted a correlation between a lack of prostaglandin release by macrophages and endotoxin resistance in non-responder C3H/HeJ mice[79]. It has thus been postulated that the macrophage may be a significant source of arachidonic acid metabolites in endotoxic shock. Agents which modulate reticuloendothelial (RE) function and endotoxin susceptibility should also affect arachidonic acid metabolism if this hypothesis is tenable.

Pretreatment with glucan, a potent RE phagocytic stimulant, sensitizes rats to endotoxic shock induced by *S. enteritidis* endotoxin (0.1 mg kg^{-1}) and its

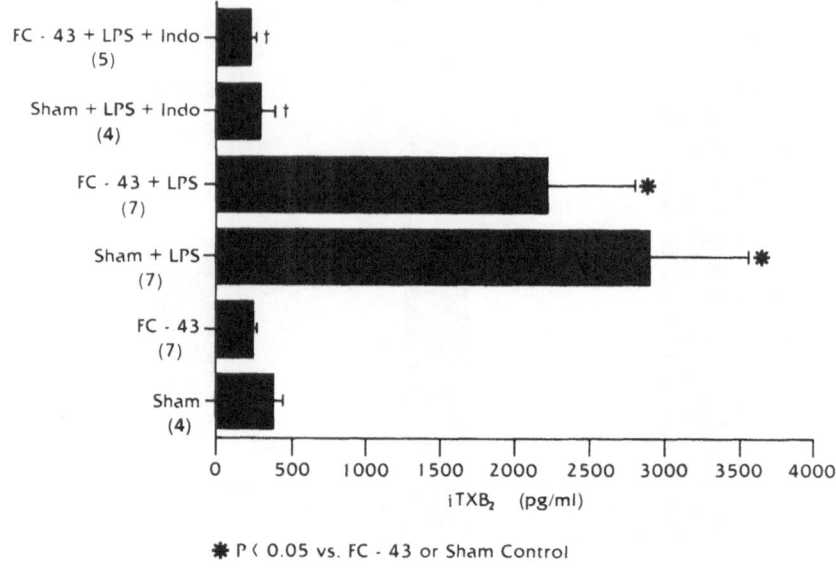

* P < 0.05 vs. FC - 43 or Sham Control

† P < 0.05 vs. FC - 43 + LPS or Sham + LPS; ( ) = N

Figure 5.8   iTxB$_2$ levels 30 min after endotoxin in sham and Fluosol-43 exchange transfused rats prior to endotoxin or rats pretreated 30 min with indomethacin (Indo, 2 mg kg^{-1}). iTxB$_2$ levels 30 min after LPS in sham and FC-43 exchange transfused rats were not significantly different from each other. Numbers in parentheses = n. *Sham or FC-43 vs sham + LPS or FC-43 + LPS ($p < 0.002$). Sham + LPS or FC-43 + LPS + Indo ($p < 0.004$). From Cook *et al.*[70], reprinted with permission of Alan R. Liss, Inc.

associated sequelae (hypoglycaemia, lysosomal labilization and disseminated intravascular coagulopathies)[80]. In contrast, pretreatment with methyl palmitate, a RE phagocytic depressant, confers resistance to the pathophysiological sequelae induced by larger doses of endotoxin (15 mg kg^{-1})[80]. Plasma levels of iTxB$_2$ and i6-keto-PGE$_{1\alpha}$ were measured after endotoxin in these animals with altered RE function. Plasma iTxB$_2$ and i6-keto-PGF$_{1\alpha}$ were synergistically increased in rats pretreated with glucan following endotoxin (0.1 mg kg^{-1}) compared with control groups given glucan or endotoxin alone[80]. By contrast, pretreatment with methyl palmitate markedly attenuated plasma elevations in iTxB$_2$ and i6-keto-PGF$_{1\alpha}$. Parallel *in vitro* studies[80] demonstrated that glucan activated macrophages exhibit both enhanced basal and endotoxin-stimulated levels of iTxB$_2$ and i6-keto-PGF$_{1\alpha}$. Peritoneal macrophages taken from methyl palmitate-pretreated rats exhibited reduced synthesis of these cyclo-oxygenase products. Similar effects of endotoxin on plasma iTxB$_2$ and i6-keto-PGF$_{1\alpha}$ after RES stimulation with glucan in rats have been observed by Bowers *et al.*[81].

The effect of glucan on survival time and eicosanoid synthesis in the rat faecal peritonitis (LD$_{100}$) model has also been assessed[82]. A high dose of glucan decreased survival time from 11.5 ± 0.4 h to 7.3 ± 0.5 h during sepsis

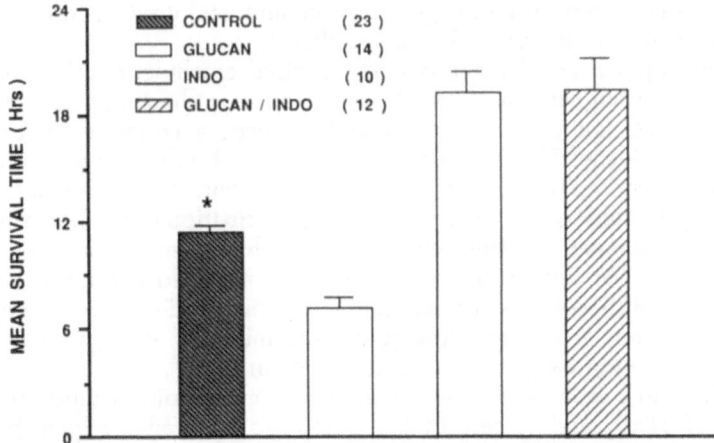

Figure 5.9 Effect of glucan on survival time in rats subjected to acute faecal peritonitis (LD_{100}). Glucan (40 mg kg^{-1} i.p., for 5 days prior) decreased survival time ($p < 0.001$) compared with shock controls. Indomethacin (Indo), 10 mg kg^{-1} ip. 30 min before peritonitis improved survival time ($p < 0.001$) compared with glucan-treated and shock control groups. From Wise et al.[82], with permission

(Figure 5.9). Plasma levels of both i6-keto-PGF$_{1\alpha}$ and iTxB$_2$ 4 h after induction of faecal peritonitis were significantly increased (2–3 fold) in glucan-treated rats compared with controls (Figure 5.10). Indomethacin pretreatment significantly improved survival time to 19 h, suggesting that the increased cyclo-oxygenase products are pathogenic mediators in this model. Thus,

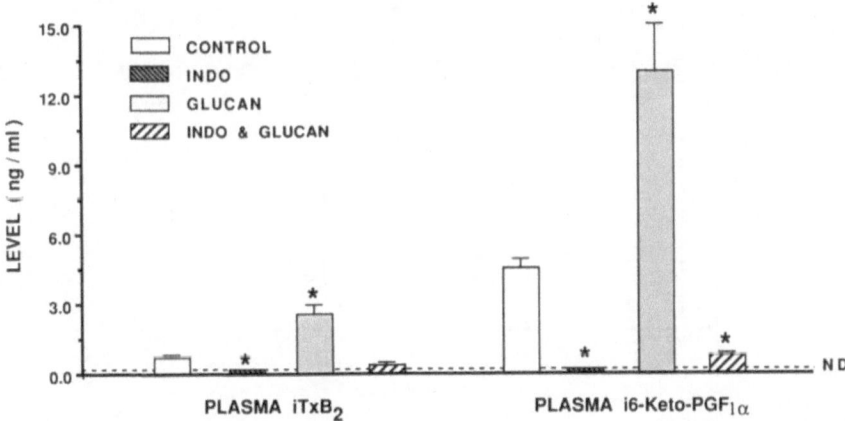

Figure 5.10 Effect of glucan on plasma iTxB$_2$ and i6-keto-PGF$_{1\alpha}$ at 4 h in rats subjected to acute faecal peritonitis (LD_{100}). Glucan (40 mg kg^{-1} for 5 days prior, $n = 14$) increased ($p < 0.05$) plasma iTxB$_2$ and 6-keto PGF$_{1\alpha}$ compared with shock controls ($n = 23$). Indomethacin (Indo), 10 mg kg^{-1} 30 min before peritonitis inhibited synthesis of these products in both glucan-treated and shock control groups. From Wise et al.[82], with permission

agents which alter macrophage function and endotoxin sensitivity affect plasma $iTxB_2$ and $i6$-keto-$PGF_{1\alpha}$ in parallel.

Knowledge of cellular sources of increased arachidonic acid metabolites and other pathogenic mediators during endotoxic shock has been advanced through investigations of 'endotoxin tolerance', a condition of endotoxin hyporesponsiveness[83,84]. It has been known for years that sublethal administration of endotoxin renders experimental animals and human subjects refractory to subsequent challenge[83]. The participation of tissue macrophages in the development of this refractory state has been of interest since the observation that administration of agents which block reticuloendothelial function abolish endotoxin tolerance[85]. Previous studies have demonstrated that production of the macrophage-derived mediator, endogenous pyrogen, is reduced during early endotoxin tolerance in mice[86].

Endotoxin tolerance also results in altered eicosanoid metabolism. Plasma levels of $iTxB_2$ and $i6$-keto-$PGF_{1\alpha}$ were measured after administration of endotoxin at normally lethal ($15\ mg\ kg^{-1}$) and supralethal ($50\ mg\ kg^{-1}$) doses[51]. In contrast to marked elevations of plasma $iTxB_2$ and $i6$-keto-$PGF_{1\alpha}$ after endotoxin administration in non-tolerant control rats, levels in tolerant rats were significantly reduced. Tolerant rats also demonstrated enhanced

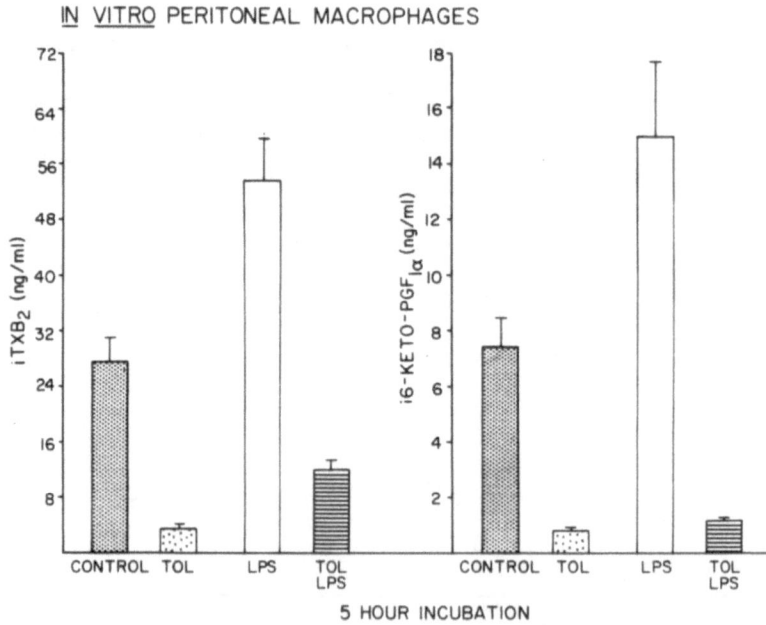

IN VITRO PERITONEAL MACROPHAGES

5 HOUR INCUBATION

Figure 5.11 Culture media levels of immunoreactive (i)TxB_2 and $i6$-keto-$PGF_{1\alpha}$ ($ng\ ml^{-1}$) 5 h after *in vitro* incubation of adherent peritoneal cells (1×10^6/ml) from tolerant (TOL) and non-tolerant (control) Long–Evans rats with and without *S. enteritidis* endotoxin ($50\ \mu g\ ml^{-1}$) (LPS). Values are presented as mean $\pm$ SEM with 5 animals per group. All values are significantly ($p < 0.01$) different from the control values. Reproduced from Wise *et al.*[51], by permission of Alan R. Liss, Inc.

survival even at the supralethal doses[51]. The *in vitro* ability of platelets to synthesize iTxB$_2$ was not significantly different between tolerant and non-tolerant rats suggesting other sites of altered iTxB$_2$ synthesis.

Reduced basal and endotoxin-stimulated synthesis of iTxB$_2$ and i6-keto-PGF$_{1\alpha}$ were demonstrated in peritoneal macrophages from tolerant compared to non-tolerant rats (Figure 5.11). This attenuation is similar to the results of Rietschel *et al.*[75] who reported decreased iPGE$_2$ and iPGF$_2$ synthesis by peritoneal macrophages from endotoxin-tolerant mice. Macrophages from tolerant rats also produced significantly lower levels of cyclo-oxygenase products than did non-tolerant cells in response to glucan, a phagocytic stimulus[87]. This suggests that the altered arachidonic acid metabolism of endotoxin tolerance is not due to an endotoxin-specific phenomenon, such as increased detoxification, nor is it an endotoxin receptor-mediated event alone. Unlike endotoxin and glucan, calcium ionophore (A23187) was a potent stimulus, increasing arachidonic acid metabolism in cells from both tolerant and non-tolerant rats[87] (Figure 5.12). Although levels of stimulated iTxB$_2$ by the two groups of cells were not significantly different, iPGE$_2$ production in cells from tolerant rats were 2-fold higher while i6-keto-PGF$_{1\alpha}$ synthesis was significantly decreased (Figure 5.12). These observations demonstrate that the reduced synthesis of cyclo-oxygenase products associated with endotoxin tolerance is not the result of arachidonic acid substrate depletion. Alterations in the events involved in signal transduction and/or changes in compartmentalization or storage pools of arachidonic acid may thus occur during chronic endotoxin exposure, accounting for tolerance. Similar shifts in the profile of

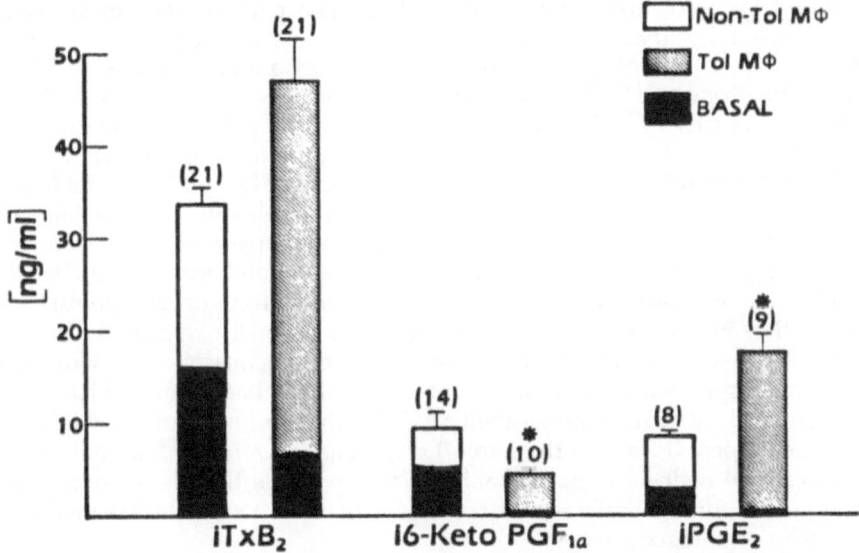

Figure 5.12 A23187-stimulated (1 μmol L^{-1}) iTxB$_2$, i6-keto-PGF$_{1\alpha}$, and iPGE$_2$ production by control and tolerant macrophages. Bars represent mean $\pm$ SEM. Numbers in parenthesis represent numbers of plates per group. Cells were diluted in RPMI to 1×10^6/ml and incubated for 3 h with A23187 *($p < 0.01$). From Rogers *et al.*[87], with permission

arachidonic acid metabolism by macrophages occur in cells stimulated by *Corynebacterium parvum*[88] or infected with *Listera monocytogenes*[89]. Collectively, these data suggest that macrophages are an important source of arachidonic acid metabolites during endotoxaemia and sepsis.

Other cell types obviously participate in the increased eicosanoid metabolism. Vascular endothelium is a significant source of PGI_2 synthesis[10]. A variety of agents which reduce vascular injury during endotoxaemia also reduce plasma increases in i6-keto-$PGF_{1\alpha}$[90]. Increased *in vitro* PGI_2 synthesis occurs in response to endotoxin-induced vascular injury[91,92]. This effect of endotoxin may be exacerbated *in vivo* through activation of complement and inflammatory cells[91]. It has been suggested that i6-keto-$PGF_{1\alpha}$ may be a sensitive marker of endothelial injury since its release *in vitro* and *in vivo* occurs prior to other indicators of cellular injury, such as lactate dehydrogenase release[91].

Effect of thromboxane synthetase inhibitors and receptor antagonists

The role of TxA_2 in the pathogenesis of endotoxaemia and sepsis has been studied extensively using Tx synthetase inhibitors and Tx receptor antagonists. A variety of Tx inhibitors, e.g. imidazole[93–96], 7-IHA[62,95], dazoxiben[44,61,97,98], pyridine derivatives[99], OKY-046[100,101], and OKY 1581[40,100] ; and Tx receptor antagonists, e.g. 13-azaprostanoic acid[37], trans-13-APT[102], U63577A[103], AH23848[104], BM13.177[105] and EP092[106] have been tested. Pretreatment with these compounds in rats and mice attenuates many of the sequelae of shock induced by bolus endotoxin administration. The pathophysiological events ameliorated by these pharmacological agents include reductions in mortality[37,44,95,98–100,105], plasma lysosomal and hepatic transaminase levels[61,95,99,100], thrombocytopenia[61,95,100,102], renal fibrin deposition and plasma fibrin degradation products[61,95,98–100]. Improvement in cardiac output and tissue perfusion have also been observed during the acute phase of endotoxic shock[62]. In the baboon[40], sheep[93,94,101,103,106], and cat[104,106], selective Tx synthetase inhibitors or receptor antagonists have been shown to ameliorate cardiopulmonary dysfunction in endotoxic shock, reducing pulmonary hypertension and improving cardiac output, systemic arterial pressure and arterial $P O_2$. Several studies have indicated that Tx synthetase inhibitors or antagonists are ineffective in preventing endotoxin-induced pulmonary microvascular permeability associated with the later phase of endotoxaemia[43,44,101,103]. However, certain Tx synthetase inhibitors or antagonists have been reported to reduce the delayed increase in permeability[93,107,108]. Since infusion of prostaglandin cyclic endoperoxides[109] or the stable TxA_2 mimetic, U46619[108], do not induce permeability oedema in normal animals, it is possible that these compounds may have additional salutary actions independent of Tx synthetase inhibition or receptor antagonism.

Tx synthetase inhibitors have been uniformly unsuccessful in improving survival in septic neonatal rats[110], adult rats[111,112], and in the baboon model of endotoxaemia[40]. The lack of protection afforded by these agents in these models may be, in part, a consequence of different profiles of eicosanoid synthesis. Arachidonic acid metabolism in the septic rat induced by acute peritonitis, is characterized by high plasma i6-keto-$PGF_{1\alpha}$ to iTxB_2 ratios. Therefore, eicosanoids, such as PGI_2 or other mediators, may dominate the extent of pathophysiological sequelae contributing to mortality.

Nevertheless, TxA_2 may potentiate some of the acute manifestations of sepsis. Truog et al.[113] studied the effects of the thromboxane synthetase inhibitor, Dazmegral (UK 38,485), on pulmonary gas exchange and haemodynamics in septic newborn piglets. Inhibition of TxA_2 synthetase resulted in preservation of normal pulmonary gas exchange and delayed the decrease in pulmonary blood flow. Based upon findings with a Tx antagonist (SQ 29,548) in graded porcine bacteraemia, Slotman et al.[108] concluded that TxA_2 was necessary and sufficient for the development of pulmonary hypertension and impaired alveolar-capillary oxygen diffusion.

In vitro studies with Tx synthetase inhibitors have shown that these compounds cause rediversion of endoperoxide metabolism to i6-keto-$PGF_{1\alpha}$[61,99]. This has led to speculation that the beneficial action of these pharmacological agents in vivo may, in part, be derived from this shunting to PGI_2. However, while certain studies with TxA_2 inhibition have shown augmentation of plasma i6-keto-$PGF_{1\alpha}$ during endotoxaemia[40,43,94], others have shown little or no evidence of shunting[100,114]. Studies have also reported reduced plasma i6-keto-$PGF_{1\alpha}$ formation with Tx synthetase inhibitors[61,98,99] or TxA_2 antagonists[102]. The latter results may be a consequence of reduced tissue ischaemia and vascular injury by inhibition of TxA_2 which lessen the stimulus for enhanced PGI_2 synthesis. Evidence that TxB_2 may directly stimulate PGI_2 synthesis is supported by observations that the Tx mimetic, U46619, stimulates i6-keto-$PGF_{1\alpha}$ synthesis from cultured smooth muscle cells[115].

Non-steroidal anti-inflammatory drugs (NSAIDs)

There are numerous studies substantiating positive effects of NSAIDs in endotoxaemia. The compounds tested in experimental endotoxic shock include aspirin[26,27,34,116-118], flurbiprofen[119-120], ibuprofen[121-124], meclofenamate[36], indomethacin[28,34,35,37,125-128], flunixin meglumine[42,129,130] and benoxaprofen[131,132]. NSAIDs in endotoxaemia generally improve survival or survival time, reduce cardiopulmonary dysfunction and improve indices of tissue ischaemia. These compounds do not, however, reduce the late-phase increase in microvascular permeability measured by increases in protein-rich lymph or extravascular lung water[43,133-136]. The latter may be a result of shunting of arachidonic acid to the lipoxygenase pathway[137,138].

Unlike Tx synthetase inhibitors and receptor antagonists, NSAIDs given alone or with other adjunctive therapy (discussed below) improve survival or survival time in the rat model of sepsis[54,82,110,112,139]. The beneficial action of the cyclo-oxygenase inhibitors in these sepsis models must therefore be attributed to inhibition of other prostanoid metabolites, e.g. PGE_2, $PGF_{2\alpha}$ and PGI_2. As indicated earlier, i6-keto-$PGF_{1\alpha}$ levels are markedly increased in acute faecal peritonitis in the rat[54]. PGI_2 has strong vasodilating actions on pulmonary vessels[140], particularly when vascular tone is increased[141]. This increase in PGI_2 may worsen the ventilation–perfusion mismatch and thus hypoxaemia[101] and may also be deleterious by promoting a reduction in peripheral vascular resistance resulting in systemic hypotension[11]. In a canine model of hyperdynamic sepsis, cyclo-oxygenase inhibitors improved systemic vascular resistance[142]. Cyclo-oxygenase inhibition also significantly improved the haemodynamics and arterial P O_2 in rabbits subjected to *Streptococcal* sepsis[143].

Diminished pressor responses to exogenous norepinephrine and angiotensin II occur in rats made septic by caecal ligation[144]. Since indomethacin restored responsiveness to both chemically dissimilar pressors, it was concluded that the sepsis-induced vascular hyporesponsiveness is prostaglandin mediated. Both PGI_2 and PGE_2 have also been shown to regulate sympathetic adrenergic activity by presynaptic inhibition of norepinephrine release[145]. Whether this negative modulation of adrenergic nerve activity by prostaglandins contributes to the altered circulatory dysfunction of endotoxaemia and sepsis is uncertain. For example, indomethacin pretreatment in endotoxaemic cats reduced, rather than increased, circulating catecholamines[128].

Vasolidating prostaglandins may play a beneficial role in moderating renal function. In certain pathological conditions, NSAIDs markedly alter renal function in patients through their negative effects on both renal blood flow and glomerular filtration rate[146]. Compromised renal blood flow has been observed following NSAID treatment in experimental septic shock[147]. It remains to be determined if this adverse effect of NSAIDs in septic patients, who may already have compromised renal function, will outweigh their beneficial actions.

Prostaglandins have also been suggested as important regulators of skeletal muscle protein breakdown. Enhanced protein catabolism and synthesis of PGE_2 is seen in skeletal muscle of rats injected with endotoxin[148]. Indomethacin reduced leukocyte-pyrogen-induced proteolysis of skeletal muscle *in vitro*[149]; however, in a canine model of *E. coli* sepsis, ibuprofen had minimal effects on protein catabolism[150].

Essential fatty acid deficiency

The involvement of arachidonic acid metabolites in endotoxic and septic shock is further supported by studies with essential fatty acid-deficient (EFAD) rats[151]. Rats raised on a diet deficient in arachidonic acid become depleted of this substrate necessary for eicosanoid formation. Studies have shown that EFAD rats are significantly more resistant to lethal endotoxic shock than normal rats[37] and do not exhibit plasma elevations in $iTxB_2$ in response to endotoxin[151]. This impaired $iTxB_2$ synthesis may be attributed to a depletion of arachidonic acid from phospholipid pools or an increase in $(\omega-9)$-eicosatrienoic acid. The latter increases in EFA deficiency and has been reported to inhibit fatty acid cyclo-oxygenase[152]. This possibility is, however, unlikely. Ethyl arachidonic acid supplementation restored the ability of EFAD rats to synthesize $iTxB_2$ in response to endotoxin[153,154]. These deficient rats

106

also became more sensitive to lethal endotoxaemia following supplementation with ethyl arachidonate.

EFAD rats also exhibit prolonged survival time to acute intra-abdominal sepsis compared with normal rats[112,151]. Additionally, conjoint therapy with the aminoglycoside antibiotic, gentamicin, of EFAD rats following faecal peritonitis resulted in an improvement in overall survival at 48 h that was not seen with the antibiotic or EFA-deficiency alone. These observations and the beneficial actions of cyclo-oxygenase inhibitors suggest a deleterious effect of these arachidonic acid metabolites in endotoxaemia and sepsis.

Effect of corticosteroids and combination therapy with NSAIDs

Corticosteroids are used in the treatment of both inflammation and shock, pathological processes associated with increased eicosanoid synthesis. Gryglewski et al.[155], Kantrowitz et al.[156] and Tashjian et al.[157] were the first to report suppression of prostaglandin synthesis by hydrocortisone and other synthetic anti-inflammatory steroids. These independent investigators demonstrated an effect at low doses in different in vitro systems. This effect was suggested to involve a decrease in available substrate for fatty acid cyclo-oxygenase, and not a direct action on the enzyme or the transport of its products across membranes.

These findings were supported and extended by the studies of Floman et al.[158,159]. They suggested that pharmacological doses of corticosteroids which stabilize lysosomes inhibit phospholipase release, preventing its action on membrane phospholipids. This reduced the amount of free AA available for eicosanoid synthesis. Danon and Assouline[160], Flower and Blackwell[161] and Carnuccio et al.[162] presented evidence that inhibition of phospholipase A_2 by anti-inflammatory steroids is via induction of synthesis of a protein or polypeptide which inhibits phospholipase A_2. These findings all suggest that the use of steroids in shock and associated acute lung injury should decrease eicosanoid synthesis and prove beneficial. Indeed, reports have supported improvement in both cardiovascular and respiratory function as well as improved survival in animals treated with high doses of steroids[25,163].

More recently, however, it has become clear that extrapolation from results of in vitro studies to in vivo responses in sepsis is not possible. Brigham et al.[164] studied the pulmonary vascular responses to endotoxaemia with chronically instrumented unanaesthetized sheep. Inhibition of fatty acid cyclo-oxygenase prevented the pulmonary hypertension seen with endotoxaemia in this model. They found that methylprednisolone, given prior to endotoxaemia or during the initial pulmonary hypertension following endotoxin, prevented the late phase increase in lung vascular permeability but not the pulmonary hypertension.

McKechnie et al.[165] examined the effects of methylprednisolone on eicosanoid synthesis in the conscious unrestrained rat model following E. coli endotoxin infusion, demonstrating improvement in cardiovascular function as well as several indices of shock severity. This study found that the beneficial effects of methylprednisolone were unrelated to the formation of iTxB$_2$ and i6-keto-PGF$_{1\alpha}$. The effect of methylprednisolone on circulating eicosanoids and on pulmonary and systemic haemodynamics have also been measured in the dog[166]. High-dose methylprednisolone not only failed to inhibit endotoxin stimulation of the arachidonic acid cascade, but enhanced it. This response was observed whether the steroid was administered immediately before endotoxin or whether it was given considerably in advance (2.5 h) to permit synthesis of the factor responsible for suppression of phospholipase A$_2$ activation. They discuss possible differences in pools of arachidonic acid which may not require phospholipase A$_2$ activation, and also the importance of local eicosanoid concentrations rather than circulating levels. However, the mechanisms of the steroid effect on eicosanoid synthesis and on haemodynamic changes in shock remain to be determined.

Almqvist et al.[167] assessed combination therapy with both steroids and NSAIDs. In studies of a canine LD$_{100}$ endotoxin shock model, they reported increased blood pressure as well as survival in shocked animals treated with both methylprednisolone and ibuprofen. Although this group did not investigate the mechanisms responsible, they speculate on inhibition of leukocyte mediation of cardiovascular problems by mechanisms involving both oxygen free radicals and TxA$_2$. In contrast to these results, Elinger et al.[168] found that a combination of methylprednisolone and ibuprofen reduced survival in rats rendered septic by caecal ligation and puncture while neither treatment alone altered mortality. They speculate that the combination therapy impaired host defense mechanisms.

Studies conducted in our laboratories examined the effects of such conjoint therapy with antibiotics on eicosanoid levels and survival in septic shock[139]. In the rat faecal peritonitis model, improved survival time was observed with early treatment with steroids. However, this protection appears to be independent of inhibition of arachidonic acid metabolism. Corticosteroid pretreatment effected no more than a 30 and 40% inhibition of plasma levels of iTxB$_2$ and i6-keto-PGF$_{1\alpha}$ respectively, compared with 100% inhibition with the cyclo-oxygenase inhibitors. Conjoint steroid and NSAID treatment improved survival time compared with each drug employed individually. The combination of steroid, NSAID and gentamicin produced the most significant effect on survival.

Brigham's group also recently examined the effects of conjoint therapy with steroids and NSAIDs in the unanaesthetized sheep model[133]. As noted previously, steroids prevented the late phase increase in lung vascular permeability, but only attenuated the pulmonary hypertension. A combination of methylprednisolone and meclofenamate inhibited the entire pulmonary vascular response to endotoxaemia. They suggest that this beneficial effect was the result of steroid inhibition of granulocyte function and meclofenamate inhibition of cyclo-oxygenase products. In subsequent studies, the accumulation of plasma and lymph iTxB$_2$ and i6-keto-PGF$_{1\alpha}$ was inhibited by the NSAID and steroid but not with the steroid alone[169]. Similar beneficial actions of conjoint steroid and NSAIDs have been observed in endotoxin-induced respiratory failure in pigs[170]. NSAIDs (indomethacin or flunixin meglumine) prevented the phase 1 (0–2 h) endotoxin-induced pulmonary hypertension, increase in pulmonary vascular resistance (PVR), alveolar–arterial O$_2$ gradient,

108

reduction in cardiac index (CI) and lung dynamic compliance (C_{dyn}). During phase 2 (2–4.5 h), the increased PVR and decreased CI and C_{dyn} were not blocked by NSAIDs but were attenuated by dexamethasone. Combination therapy with these agents prevented the respiratory failure in both phase 1 and 2. Hales et al.[166], in studies of a canine endotoxin model, demonstrated that methylprednisolone prevented the fall in systemic blood pressure and vascular resistance. Combined therapy with indomethacin blocked the changes in pulmonary and systemic haemodynamics as well as circulating eicosanoids. Despite the uncertainty of the mechanisms of action, collectively these studies underscore the beneficial actions of conjoint therapy with NSAIDs and steroids.

POTENTIAL ROLE OF LIPOXYGENASE PRODUCTS IN ENDOTOXAEMIA AND ACUTE LUNG INJURY

Evidence for synthesis and metabolism of lipoxygenase products

Lipoxygenase products are potential candidates for a role in endotoxaemia, shock and acute lung injury because of their biological potency as inflammatory mediators, and because they can mimic many pathophysiological features of these conditions[14–21]. As might be predicted for such potent substances, there is rapid elimination from the vascular compartment[171–173]. LTC_4, for example, has a plasma elimination half-life of only 30 seconds[174]. While plasma contains little catabolic activity[175], the cell surface-bound enzymes, γ-glutamyl transferase and dipeptidase (located in kidney, lung and liver), appear to be responsible[24]. Of these organs, the liver exhibits the most rapid uptake with a higher affinity for LTE_4 than LTC_4 and LTD_4[172]. Once in the hepatocyte, there is partial metabolism[172] by acetyl transferase to N-acetyl-LTE_4 which appears as the major metabolite of the leukotrienes in rat bile[176]. Two basic approaches have been used to study leukotriene formation in vivo. The first relies on measurements of leukotriene metabolites in bile or urine[173,176,177]. The second approach is to measure levels by direct sampling of a body compartment, e.g. cannulation of lymph ducts[169] or lung lavage[178].

Evidence for increased leukotriene formation following endotoxin has been found in the bile of rat[176,179,180] and following enterotoxin in the monkey[181] by measurement of metabolites using high-pressure liquid chromatography and radioimmunoassay. Injection of either [^{3}H]LTC_4 or [^{3}H]LTD_4 results in the production of N-acetyl-[^{3}H]LTE_4 as the major metabolite. Endogenous N-acetyl-LTE_4 is, therefore, an index of leukotriene production under pathological conditions, such as endotoxaemia or trauma. In the anaesthetized rat, for example, a leukotriene metabolite (now identified as N-acetyl-LTE_4[174]) was $0.39 \text{ nmol h}^{-1} \text{kg}^{-1}$ immediately following Salmonella minnesota endotoxin compared with a control value of $0.01 \text{ nmol h}^{-1} \text{kg}^{-1}$. These levels returned to control values over 3 h. Measurement of this metabolite after endotoxin probably underestimates endogenous leukotriene production because these rats also showed depressed biliary elimination of N-acetyl-LTE_4 with a concomitant increase in hepatic levels[180]. Indeed, such a mechanism might act

109

synergistically to augment the systemic levels of leukotrienes. Similar increases in biliary N-acetyl-LTE$_4$ occur in rats following thermal injury and trauma[174].

In the monkey (*Macaca fascicularis*), injection of [^{3}H]LTC$_4$ results in the appearance of [^{3}H]LTE$_4$ (rather than [^{3}H]N-acetyl-LTE$_4$) as well as a larger number of polar metabolites of undetermined structure[181]. Within 3–4.5 h of intragastric *Staphylococcal* enterotoxin, bile LTE$_4$ levels increased 45 fold, from 0.2 to 9 nmol l^{-1}. These results demonstrate that enhanced leukotriene production in these conditions is also seen in the primate.

Evidence for increased lipoxygenase metabolism in response to endotoxin has also been shown in the sheep. Ogletree *et al.*[169,182] quantitated arachidonic acid metabolites in the early and late stages of endotoxaemia. As previously noted, iTxB$_2$ increases to peak values in plasma and pulmonary lymph and returns to baseline values within 1 h, while i6-keto-PGF$_{1\alpha}$ levels increase to peak values between 1 and 2 h after endotoxin administration. In the late phase (2.5 h) of endotoxaemia, both 5-hydroxyeicosatetraenoic acid (5-HETE) and 12-HETE[169,182], products of the 5 and 12-lipoxygenase pathway of arachidonic acid, were increased in pulmonary lymph concentrations. The appearance of these lipoxygenase products was coincident with the onset of the late phase increased lung vascular permeability.

Enhanced lipoxygenase metabolism also occurs in a variety of other forms of acute lung injury. Increased 5-HETE concentrations have been measured in the isolated rat lung effluent following oxidant-induced injury with glucose oxidase[183]. Passive Arthus pleurisy in rats, induced by egg albumin and antiserum, is associated with increased concentrations of 5-HETE and leukotrienes LTB$_4$, LTD$_4$, and LTE$_4$ in pulmonary exudate fluid[184]. These metabolites correlate with increased vascular permeability and the migration of inflammatory cells into the pleural cavity. Increased sulphidopeptide leukotriene concentrations have also been measured in bronchoalveolar lavage (BAL) fluid from the following: in isolated rat lungs following acute alveolar hypoxia[185], in BAL fluid of mice after normobaric hyperoxia-induced injury[186], and in BAL fluid from dogs following lung injury with thiourea[187]. Studies conducted in our laboratories have shown enhanced production of iLTC$_4$/D$_4$ and iLTB$_4$ in BAL fluid of rats[178] and dogs[188] following experimental lung injury with oleic acid. Increased levels of these leukotrienes were associated with both increased pulmonary transvascular flux of ^{99}Technetium labelled human serum albumin (^{99}Tc-HSA) and neutropenia[179,188].

The cellular sources of leukotriene production during endotoxaemia and acute lung injury have not yet been elucidated. Leukotriene C$_4$ and D$_4$ are released from human, equine and rat polymorphonuclear granulocytes upon *in vitro* incubation with endotoxin[189–192]. In contrast to granulocytes, macrophages, when stimulated by endotoxin *in vitro*, synthesize cyclo-oxygenase products, iTxB$_2$, i6-keto-PGF$_{1\alpha}$ and iPGE$_2$ but not lipoxygenase products, iLTB$_4$ or iLTC$_4$/D$_4$[87,193]. Possible explanations of this preferential stimulation of cyclo-oxygenase products by endotoxin in these cells have included the existence of separate substrate pools activated by 5-lipoxygenase and fatty acid cyclo-oxygenase[193] and/or a higher intracellular Ca^{2+} requirement for activation of 5-lipoxygenase[194]. Studies by Luderitz *et al.*[195], however, demonstrated endotoxin-stimulated synthesis of leukotrienes by mouse

110

peritoneal macrophages. This study employed measurement of [³H]arachidonic acid products as well as measurement of endogenous LTC_4 and LTE_4 by radioimmunoassay following HPLC. The results of this study, compared with those of Rogers et al.[87] and Humes et al.[193], may reflect differences in length of stimulation with endotoxin, strain of endotoxin or differences in animal species or strain.

Lipoxygenase products are produced by a variety of other inflammatory cells, organ parenchyma and vascular tissue[196–201]. The effect of endotoxin or other noxious stimuli on these tissues and their potential importance as sources of lipoxygenase products in endotoxaemia and sepsis remain to be determined.

Effect of lipoxygenase inhibitors and leukotriene receptor antagonist

Having considered the increased production of lipoxygenase products, the question arises concerning the pathological significance of tissue or circulating levels. Several putative lipoxygenase inhibitors and leukotriene receptor antagonists have been shown to ameliorate the pulmonary vascular permeability changes, histological injury and pulmonary pressor response to various forms of acute lung injury. The lipoxygenase inhibitors tested include diethylcarbamazine[24,174,176,178,179,202,203], AA-861[184,186], nordihydroguaiaretic acid (NDGA)[204], and piriprost, U60,257[204] (a glutathione-S-transferase inhibitor of sulphidopeptide leukotriene synthesis). Dual lipoxygenase and cyclo-oxygenase inhibitors tested include BW755C[165,204] and benoxaprofen[131,132]. These agents have other actions, and caution should therefore be exercised in interpretation of these data. Additionally, in endotoxaemic sheep, the appearance of 12-HETE in lymph in the delayed permeability phase of lung injury is reduced by methylprednisolone[169]. Whether the latter results reflect a direct action of this steroid on the lipoxygenase pathway or reduced 12-HETE as a consequence of less severe vascular injury, is unknown.

Two leukotriene receptor antagonists have been studied: FPL-55712[176,179,205], predominantly a LTC_4 antagonist with lesser antagonism of LTD_4, and the more recently developed compound, LY171883, a selective LTD_4/E_4 antagonist[206]. LY171883 has been used to investigate the involvement of sulphidopeptide leukotrienes in the pathophysiology of oleic acid-induced lung injury in rats[178]. Pretreatment with this compound significantly decreased pulmonary microvascular permeability measured with ^{99}Tc-HSA in oleic acid treated rats, and prevented the oleic acid-induced neutropenia[178]. Despite the reduction in lung oedema, LY171883 did not, however, prevent the hypox-aemia. Previous studies have linked cyclo-oxygenase products rather than leukotrienes to the development of pulmonary hypoxaemia[133,169,207]. These studies have implicated perfusion mismatch as a primary factor in hypoxaemia rather than transvascular protein flux[133,169,207]. The correlation of blood oxygenation of patients with surface area rather than extravascular lung water provides additional evidence for the dissociation between hypoxaemia and oedema[208]. The involvement of arachidonic acid metabolites in oleic acid-induced lung injury is further supported by studies in EFAD rats[209]. The

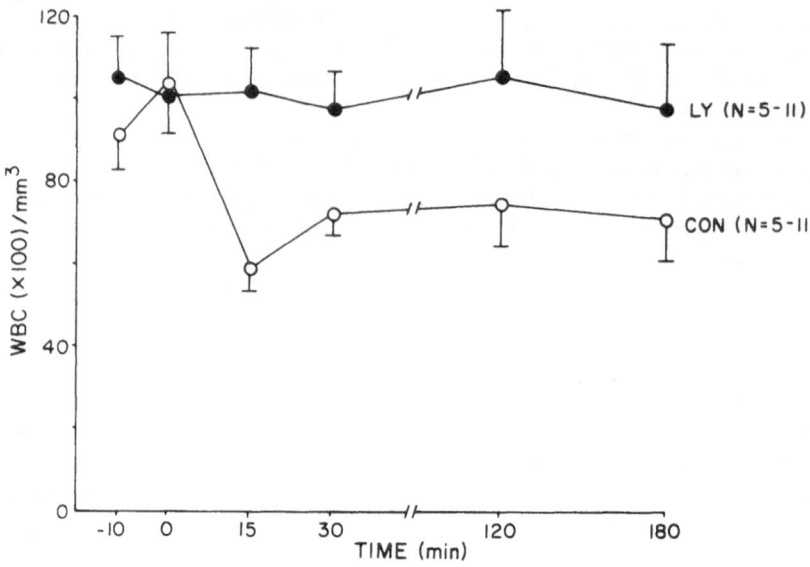

Figure 5.13 Endotoxin-induced leukopenia in rats pretreated with LY171883 (LY), 30 mg kg^{-1}, or isovolumetric vehicle (CON), 10 min before administration of *S. enteritidis* endotoxin (40 mg kg^{-1}). LY or vehicle was started as an infusion 10 mg kg^{-1} h^{-1} at 30 min postendotoxin. The Con group exhibited a significantly more severe leukopenia (0–180) compared with the LY group (analysis of variance, $p < 0.001$). WBC, white blood cells. From Cook *et al.*[211], reprinted with permission of American Society for Pharmacology and Experimental Therapeutics

animals are refractory to lung injury induced by oleic acid, evidencing reduced permeability to ^{99}Tc-HSA as well as the absence of hypoxaemia. In contrast to injured normal rats, bronchoalveolar lavage levels of iLTB$_4$ and i6-keto-PGF$_{1\alpha}$ were not detectable in EFAD rats. Supplementation of these animals with ethyl arachidonic acid increased the permeability index, the hypoxaemia, and the iLTB$_4$ and 6-keto-PGF$_{1\alpha}$ levels in bronchoalveolar lavage fluid[209].

In view of the extensive hepatobiliary elimination of leukotrienes, it is particularly interesting that studies have demonstrated improved liver morphology and reduced damage using both inhibitors and antagonists of leukotrienes. Pretreatment of mice with FPL-55712, Ebselen or diethylcarbamazine reduced the endotoxin-induced hepatic injury and enhanced survival in animals sensitized to endotoxin by D-galactosamine[180,179,202] or amanitin[210]. The dual cyclo-oxygenase–lipoxygenase inhibitor, benoxaprofen, has also been shown to reduce the haemodynamic alterations and improve survival at 24 h in endotoxaemic dogs[131,132]. In contrast, the dual inhibitor, BW755C, failed to improve survival in rats infused with endotoxin[165]. The latter may be explained, in part, by infusion of endotoxin rather than bolus injection.

Support for the involvement of leukotrienes in the pathophysiological sequelae of endotoxaemia also derives from studies with LY171883[211].

112

Pretreatment with LY171883 prevented the endotoxin-induced neutropenia (Figure 5.13), haemoconcentration (Figure 5.14) and acute systemic hypotension observed in rats[211]. The increased haemoconcentration of endotoxic shock, an indirect measure of vascular permeability, suggests enhancement of vascular permeability by endogenous LTD_4/E_4. It is not clear whether the prevention of neutropenia by LY171883 in endotoxaemia is a direct effect of inhibition of the action of sulphidopeptide leukotrienes. For example, these leukotrienes have been shown to stimulate neutrophil adherence to cultured endothelial cells by a platelet activating factor-dependent mechanism[212].

LY171883 prevented the acute haemodynamic alterations of endotoxic shock by significantly improving cardiac output, arterial pressure (Figure 5.15) and blood flow to the heart, kidney and splanchnic regions[213]. Since sulphidopeptide leukotrienes are potent coronary vasoconstrictors[19], the improved cardiac output resulting from LY171883 treatment may, in part, be the result of improved coronary perfusion. Sulphidopeptide leukotrienes are also potent intestinal vasoconstrictors in the rat[214]. Thus, the improvement in splanchnic blood flow[213] and lack of endotoxin-induced small bowel infarction (unpublished observation, Cook) following treatment with LY171883 may be the result of antagonism of the effects of leukotrienes at their receptor. Badr et al.[205] also reported beneficial effects of the antagonist,

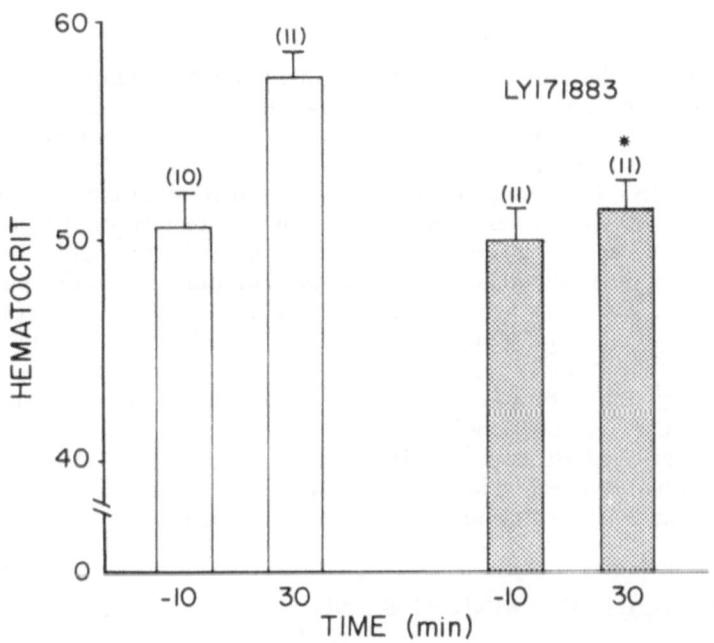

Figure 5.14 Endotoxin-induced haemoconcentration in rats pretreated with LY171883 ($n = 11$) or isovolumetric vehicle ($n = 10-11$). Haematocrit values at 30 min postendotoxin were significantly less ($*p < 0.02$) in the drug-treated group relative to control rats. From Cook et al.[211], reprinted with permission of American Society for Pharmacology and Experimental Therapeutics

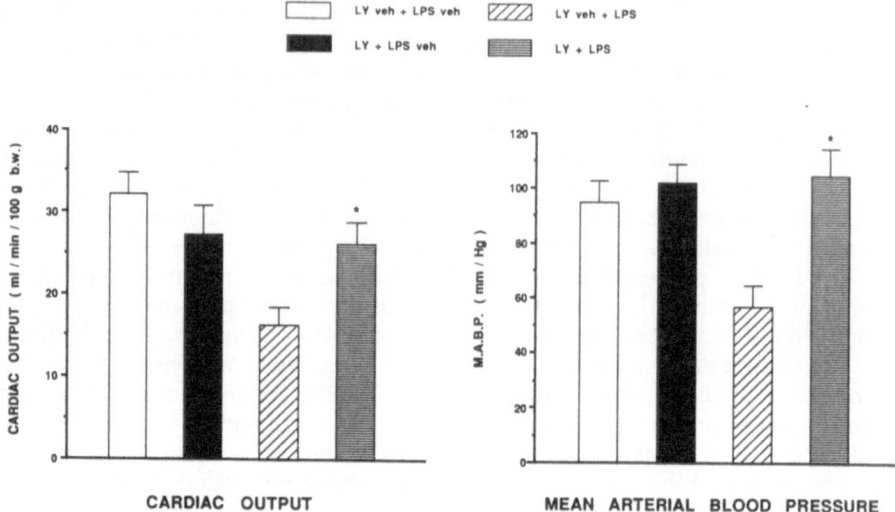

Figure 5.15 Cardiac output and blood pressure measured 30 min postendotoxin (15 mg kg^{-1}). LY171883 (30 mg kg^{-1}) was administered 10 min prior to endotoxin or vehicle. Bars represent mean $\pm$ SEM of 4–6 rats per group. *$p < 0.05$ compared with vehicle + LPS group. From Etemadi et al.[213], reprinted with permission of Alan R. Liss Inc.

FPL55712, in the endotoxaemic rat as measured by improvement in renal blood flow and absence of haemoconcentration. Additionally, pretreatment with LY171883 improved survival and indices of tissue injury in rats subjected to traumatic shock[215].

The relative importance of leukotrienes as pathophysiological mediators may, however, be species dependent. In contrast to rats, pretreatment with this LTD_4/E_4 antagonist in sheep failed to prevent the endotoxin-induced neutropenia, and pulmonary permeability, but did reduce the pulmonary arterial and microvascular pressures[216]. LY171883 failed to prevent the increased rabbit lung permeability induced by oleic acid in the isolated perfused rabbit lung[217].

Although LY171883 is devoid of pharmacological effects on histamine, bradykinin, $PGF_{2\alpha}$ carbachol, serotonin and U46619, this compound is a potent phosphodiesterase inhibitor[206]. This suggests the need for further testing of highly selective leukotriene antagonists and lipoxygenase inhibitors in endotoxaemia, sepsis and forms of acute lung injury.

EICOSANOIDS IN CLINICAL SEPSIS

Meaningful interpretation of eicosanoid levels in plasma or pulmonary oedema fluid during clinical sepsis or ARDS is complicated by the large number of uncontrolled variables compared with experimental sepsis or models of acute lung injury. These include diverse etiological factors precipitating sepsis and ARDS, variation in the stage of severity of these inflammatory conditions and associated renal and hepatic dysfunction which may alter the elimination of eicosanoid products. Nevertheless, several studies suggest that eicosanoid products are increased under these conditions. Reines et al.[218] measured plasma iTxB$_2$ in septic and control patients. The criteria for inclusion in this study were fever, abnormal white blood cell counts, hypotension without pressor drugs and positive blood or peritoneal cultures. In eight patients dying with septic shock, mean central venous plasma iTxB$_2$ was 912 ± 250 pg ml^{-1}. This value was ten times higher than plasma iTxB$_2$ from 4 survivors of septic shock (92 ± 25 pg ml^{-1}) and 6 controls (91 ± 18 pg ml^{-1}). Prothrombin time and partial thromboplastin time were significantly prolonged in non-survivors compared with survivors. Similarly, alveolar–arterial oxygen gradients were significantly raised in non-survivors compared with survivors[218]. Methylprednisolone treatment did not attenuate increases in plasma iTxB$_2$ suggesting that this steroid does not alter conversion of arachidonic metabolites to TxA$_2$ in septic patients[219].

Plasma iTxB$_2$ levels have also been quantitated from burn patients at various times post injury[220] and in patients with ARDS[221]. Levels of iTxB$_2$ were elevated throughout the burn course with a 115 fold increase over control levels occurring in the acute stage of burn injury (within three days post injury) and also in septic burn patients. Increased plasma iTxB$_2$ during ARDS was reported by Deby-Dupont et al.[221]. Of 38 patients studied, plasma levels of greater than 100 pg ml^{-1} at 2–3 days after the appearance of ARDS were observed in 30 patients. iTxB$_2$ levels above 2000 pg ml^{-1} were reported in 7 patients with levels reaching 8000 pg ml^{-1} in one patient. Pretreatment with NSAIDs reduced plasma iTxB$_2$ levels to less than 125 pg ml^{-1} in patients with the highest levels.

Recently, Slotman et al.[222] studied the interaction of iTxB$_2$, i6-keto-PGF$_{1\alpha}$, activated complement and granulocytes in 48 critically ill patients with sepsis and hypotension. Compared with control values of iTxB$_2$ (< 50 pg ml^{-1}) from normal adults, plasma iTxB$_2$ was significantly increased in patients with hypotension, normotensive sepsis or septic shock (approximately 200 pg ml^{-1}). However, there was no significant difference in iTxB$_2$ values among these critically ill patients. Plasma i6-keto-PGF$_{1\alpha}$ levels were greatly increased in septic shock patients (856 ± 439 pg ml^{-1}) compared with other groups. PaO$_2$/FiO$_2$ ratios correlated directly with i6-keto-PGF$_{1\alpha}$ and inversely with C3a and TxB$_2$/6-keto-PGF$_{1\alpha}$ ratios. This strongly suggests the involvement of these mediators in the acute respiratory failure of these patients[213].

In contrast to elevated iTxB$_2$ levels reported by the above studies in sepsis or ARDS, Rie et al.[223] reported that plasma iTxB$_2$ was not significantly increased in 8 patients with positive blood cultures compared with critically ill controls with negative blood cultures. Plasma i6-keto-PGF$_{1\alpha}$ levels were, however, significantly increased from 65 pg ml^{-1} in control patients to 721 ± 411 pg ml^{-1} in septic patients. Studies by Halushka et al.[224] have also shown elevated i6-keto-PGF$_{1\alpha}$ levels in septic patients. Using gas chromatography/mass spectrometry techniques for quantitation of central venous 6-keto-PGF$_{1\alpha}$, median levels of 229 pg ml^{-1} (range 31–21 998) were observed in 8 septic non-survivors compared with 30 pg ml^{-1} (range 22–194) in 6 septic survivors. In control patients without sepsis, 6-keto-PGF$_{1\alpha}$ values were less than $4\,\text{pg ml}^{-1}$. Elevated plasma levels of iPGF$_{2\alpha}$ have been reported in mixed venous and arterial plasma from patients with severe hyperdynamic sepsis[225]. These elevated iPGF$_{2\alpha}$ levels did not, however, correlate individually with respiratory data and pulmonary vascular resistance changes.

Less data are currently available regarding the involvement of lipoxygenase products in clinical pulmonary dysfunction. Stenmark et al.[226] found increased LTC$_4$ and LTD$_4$ in lung lavage fluids of five newborns with a diagnosis of pulmonary hypertension who required ventilatory assistance. In contrast, leukotrienes were non-detectable in a control group of 14 infants requiring ventilatory assistance. Elevated levels of LTD$_4$ in pulmonary oedema fluid in a group of patients with non-cardiogenic pulmonary oedema of various etiologies have been reported by Matthay et al.[227]. Increased iLTD$_4$ was demonstrated in the latter study in the absence of significant increases in iLTB$_4$, iLTC$_4$, iPGE$_2$ and iTxB$_2$,[227]. These investigators also reported elevated iLTD$_4$ and iLTB$_4$ in oedema fluid of a patient with an episode of pulmonary congestion after cardiopulmonary bypass[228].

There have been limited clinical trials assessing the therapeutic efficacy of pharmacological agents which alter eicosanoid metabolism in clinical sepsis and ARDS. Reines et al.[229] studied the effect of the Tx synthetase inhibitor, dazoxiben, in patients with diagnosed septic shock. Dazoxiben significantly lowered elevated central venous plasma levels of iTxB$_2$. However, mean arterial pressure, peripheral vascular resistance, intrapulmonary shunting, extravascular lung water, and haematological parameters were not significantly changed. Dazoxiben treatment has also been studied in ARDS[230]. This compound produced a moderate increase in arterial oxygen pressure and a slight decrease in venous admixture but no effect on pulmonary hypertension[230]. Collectively, these data suggest that Tx synthetase inhibitors will not be beneficial in the management of patients with established septic shock and ARDS. However, the contribution of TxA$_2$ to early pathophysiological sequelae of sepsis, and its value as a marker of the severity of haemodynamic and haemotological dysfunction remain to be determined.

In the absence of published clinical trials with NSAIDs or lipoxygenase inhibitors, the potential pathophysiological importance of other eicosanoids, e.g. PGI$_2$ and leukotrienes, is unknown. The therapeutic efficacy of glucocorticoids, however, in septic shock and ARDS remains controversial[231,232]. In view of the continued high mortality of sepsis and ARDS[2,3], further investigation of therapeutic interventions with pharmacological agents which alter eicosanoid metabolism is warranted.

ACKNOWLEDGEMENTS

This work was supported by NIH GM 27673 and HL 29566. Perry V. Halushka is a Burroughs Wellcome Scholar in Clinical Pharmacology. We appreciate the excellent technical assistance of Mrs Katherine Haines and Ms Sarah Ashton, and the typing of Ms Barbara White and Mrs Leslie Harrelson.

116

REFERENCES

1. Wolff, S.M. and Bennett, J.V. (1974). Gram negative rod bacteremia. *N. Engl. J. Med.*, **291**, 733−734
2. McCabe, W.R. and Jackson, G.G. (1974). Gram-negative bacteremia. *Adv. Intern. Med.*, **19**, 135−158
3. Wardle, N. (1979). Bacteremic and endotoxin shock. *Br. J. Hosp. Med.*, **21**, 223−231
4. National Heart & Lung Institute. (1972). *Respiratory Diseases. Task Force Report on Problems, Research Approaches, Needs.*, p. 167. (DHEW publication no. [NIH] 73−432).
5. Fowler, A.A., Hamman, R.F., Good, J.T., Benson, K.N., Baird, M., Eberle, D.J., Petty, T.L. and Hyers, T.M. (1983). Adult respiratory distress syndrome, risks and common predisposition. *Ann. Int. Med.*, **98**, 593
6. Hasleton, P.S. (1983). Adult respiratory distress syndrome, a review. *Histopathology*, **7**, 307
7. Rinaldo, J.E. and Rogers, R.M. (1982). Medical progress: Adult respiratory distress syndrome: changing concepts of lung injury and repair. *N. Engl. J. Med.*, **306(15)**, 900−909
8. Parratt, J.R. (1983). Neurohumoral agents and their release in shock. In Altura, B.M., Lefer, A.M. and Schumer, W. (eds.) *Handbook of Shock and Trauma.* pp. 311−336 (New York: Raven Press)
9. Bernard, G., Lucht, W., Niedermeyer, M., Snapper, J., Ogletree, M. and Brigham, K. (1984). Effect of *n*-acetylcysteine on the pulmonary response to endotoxin in awake sheep and upon *in vitro* granulocyte function. *J. Clin. Invest.*, **73**, 1772−1782
10. Moncada, S. and Vane, J.R. (1979). Pharmacology and endogenous roles of prostaglandin, endoperoxides, thromboxane A_2 and prostacyclin. *Pharmacol. Rev.*, **30**, 293−331
11. Armstrong, J.M., Lattimer, N., Moncada, S. and Vane, J.R. (1978). Comparison of the vasodepressor effects of prostacyclin and 6-oxo-prostaglandin $F_{1\alpha}$ with those of prostaglandin E_2 in rats and rabbits. *Br. J. Pharmacol.*, **62**, 125−130
12. Weis, H.J. and Turitto, V.T. (1979). Prostacyclin (prostaglandin I_2, PGI_2) inhibits platelet adhesion and thrombus formation on subendothelium. *Blood*, **53**, 244−250
13. Samuelsson, B., Borgeat, P. and Hammarstrom, S. (1979). Introduction of a nomenclature: leukotrienes. *Prostaglandins*, **17**, 785−787
14. Ford-Hutchinson, A.W., Bray, M.A., Doig, M.W., Shiply, M.E. and Smith, M.J.H. (1980). Leukotriene B, a potent chemokinetic and aggregating substance released from polymorphonuclear leukocytes. *Nature (London)*, **286**, 264−265
15. Samuelsson, B. (1983). Leukotrienes: mediators of immediate hypersensitivity reaction and inflammation. *Science*, **220**, 568−575
16. Kreutner, W. and Siegal, M.I. (1984). Biology of leukotrienes. *Annu. Rep. Med. Chem.*, **19**, 241−251
17. Feuerstein, G., Zukowska-Grojec, Z. and Kopin, I.J. (1981). Cardiovascular effects of leukotriene D_4 in SHR and WKY rats. *Eur. J. Pharmacol.*, **76**, 107−110
18. Iacopino, V.J., Fitzpatrick, T.M., Ramwell, R.W., Rose, J.C. and Kot, P.A. (1983). Cardiovascular response to leukotriene C_4 in the rat. *J. Pharmacol. Exp. Ther.*, **227**, 224−247
19. Michalassi, F., Landa, L., Hill, R.D., Lowenstein, E., Watkins, W.D., Petkau, A.J. and Zapol, W.M. (1982). Leukotriene D_4: A potent coronary artery vasoconstrictor associated with impaired ventricular contraction. *Science*, **217**, 841−843
20. Roth, D.M. and Lefer, A.M. (1983). Mechanism of the constrictor action of leukotrienes in cat coronary arteries. *Pharmacologist*, **25**, 142
21. Ford Hutchinson, A.W. and Rackman, A. (1983). Leukotrienes as mediators of skin inflammation. *Br. J. Dermatol.*, **109** (Suppl.), 26−29
22. Ball, H.A., Cook, J.A., Wise, W.C. and Halushka, P.V. (1986). Role of thromboxane, prostaglandins and leukotrienes in endotoxic and septic shock. *Intensive Care Med.*, **12**, 116−126
23. Lefer, A.M. (1986). Leukotrienes as mediators of ischemia and shock. *Biochem. Pharmacol.*, **35**, 123−127
24. Keppler, D., Hagmann, W., Rapp, S., Denzlinger, C. and Koch, H. (1985). The relation of leukotrienes to liver injury. *Hepatology*, **5**, 883−891

25. Hinshaw, L.B. (1985). Cardiovascular dysfunction in shock: An overview with emphasis on septic shock. In: Janssen, H.E. and Barnes, C.A. (eds.) *Circulatory Shock: Basic and Clinical Implications*, pp. 1–19. (New York: Academic Press)
26. Northover, B.J. and Subramanian, G. (1962). Analgesic–antipyretic drugs and antagonists of endotoxic shock in dogs. *J. Pathol. Bacteriol.*, **83**, 463–468
27. Hinshaw, L.B., Solomon, L.A., Erdos, E.G., Reins, D.A. and Gunter, B.J. (1967). Effects of acetylsalicylic acid on the canine response to endotoxin. *J. Pharmacol. Exp. Ther.*, **157**, 665–671
28. Erdos, E.G., Hinshaw, L.B. and Gill, C.C. (1967). Effect of indomethacin in endotoxin shock in the dog. *Proc. Soc. Exp. Biol. Med.*, **157**, 916–919
29. Anderson, F.L., Jubiz, W., Kralios, A.C., Tsagaris, T.J. and Kuida, H. (1972). Plasma prostaglandin levels during endotoxin shock in dogs. *Circulation* (Suppl. III), **46**, 124
30. Anderson, F.L., Jubiz, W., Tsagaris, T.J. and Kuida, H. (1975). Endotoxin-induced prostaglandin E and F release in dogs. *Am. J. Physiol.*, **223**, 410–414
31. Anderson, F.L., Tsagaris, T.J., Jubiz, W. and Kuida, H. (1975). Prostaglandin F and E levels during endotoxin-induced pulmonary hypertension in calves. *Am. J. Physiol.*, **228**, 1479–1482
32. Herman, A.G. and Vane, J.R. (1976). Release of renal prostaglandins during endotoxin-induced hypotension. *Eur. J. Pharmacol.*, **39**, 79–90
33. Fletcher, J.R. and Ramwell, P.W. (1977). Altered lung metabolism of prostaglandins during hemorrhagic and endotoxin shock. *Surg. Forum*, **28**, 184–186
34. Fletcher, J.R. and Ramwell, P.W. (1977). Modification by aspirin and indomethacin of the hemodynamic and prostaglandin releasing effects of E. Coli. endotoxin in the dog. *Br. J. Pharmacol.*, **61**, 174–181
35. Parratt, J.R. and Sturgess, R.M. (1975). E. Coli endotoxin shock in the cat treated with indomethacin. *Br. J. Pharmacol.*, **53**, 485–488
36. Parratt, J.R. and Sturgess, R.M. (1975). The protective effect of sodium meclofenamate in experimental endotoxin shock. *Br. J. Pharmacol.*, **53**, 466
37. Cook, J.A., Wise, W.C. and Halushka, P.V. (1980). Elevated thromboxane levels in the rat during endotoxin shock: Protective effects of imidazole, 13-azaprostanoic acid, or essential fatty acid deficiency. *J. Clin. Invest.*, **65**, 227–230
38. Watkins, W.D., Huttemeier, P.C., Kong, D. and Peterson, M.B. (1982). Thromboxane and pulmonary hypertension following E. coli endotoxin infusion in sheep: Effect of an imidazole derivative. *Prostaglandins*, **23**, 273–285
39. Demling, R.H., Smith, M., Gunther, R., Rlynn, J.T. and Gee, M.H. (1981). Pulmonary injury and prostaglandin production during endotoxemia in conscious sheep. *Am. J. Physiol.*, **240**, H348–H353
40. Casey, L.C., Fletcher, J.R., Zmudka, M.I. and Ramwell, P.W. (1982). Prevention of endotoxin-induced pulmonary hypertension in primates by the use of a selective thromboxane synthetase inhibitor, OKY 1581. *J. Pharmacol. Exp. Ther.*, **222**, 441–446
41. Harris, R.H., Zmudka, M., Maddox, Y., Ramwell, P.W. and Fletcher, J.R. (1980). Relationships of TxB_2 and 6-keto-$PGF_{1\alpha}$ to the hemodynamic changes during baboon endotoxic shock. In Samuelsson, B., Ramwell, R.W. and Paoletti, R. (eds.) *Advances in Prostaglandin Thromboxane Research.* p. 843. (New York: Raven Press)
42. Bottoms, G.D., Templeton, C.B., Fessler, J.F., Johnson, M.A., Roesel, O.F., Ewert, K.M. and Adams, S.B. (1982). Thromboxane, prostacyclin and the hemodynamic changes in equine endotoxin shock. *Am. J. Vet. Res.*, **43**, 999–1002
43. Winn, R., Harlan, J., Nadir, B., Harker, L. and Hildebrandt, J. (1983). Thromboxane A_2 mediates lung vasoconstriction but not permeability after endotoxin. *J. Clin. Invest.*, **72**, 911–918
44. Harlan, J., Winn, R., Hildebrandt, J. and Harkler, L. (1983). Selective inhibition of thromboxane synthesis during experimental endotoxemia in the goat: effects on pulmonary hemodynamics and lung lymph flow. *Br. J. Clin. Pharmacol.*, **15**, 123S–126S
45. Webb, P.J., Westwick, J., Scully, M.F., Zahavi, J. and Kakkar, V.V. (1981). Do prostacyclin and thromboxane play a role in endotoxic shock? *Br. J. Surg.*, **68**, 720–724
46. Coker, S.J., Hughes, B., Parratt, J.R., Rodger, I.W. and Zeitlin, I.J. (1983). The release of prostanoids during the acute pulmonary response to E. coli. endotoxin in anesthetized cats. *Br. J. Pharmacol.*, **78**, 561–570

47. Bult, H., Beetens, J. and Herman, A.G. (1980). Blood levels of 6-oxo-prostaglandin $F_{1\alpha}$ during endotoxin-induced hypotension in rabbits. *Eur. J. Pharmacol.*, **63**, 47–56
48. Furman, B.L., McKechnie, K. and Parratt, J.R. (1984). Failure of drugs that selectively inhibit thromboxane synthesis to modify endotoxin shock in conscious rats. *Br. J. Pharmacol.*, **82**, 289–294
49. Ball, H.A. and Parratt, J.R. (1983). Thromboxane and the pulmonary response to endotoxin in the cat. *Circ. Shock*, **10**, 263
50. Demling, R.H., Winger, H., Hectman, H. and Wong, C. (1985). Role of subcutaneous endotoxin in the production of prostanoid-induced lung injury: Comparison with intravenous endotoxin response. *Circ. Shock*, **17**, 147–161
51. Wise, W.C., Cook, J.A. and Halushka, P.V. (1983). Arachidonic acid metabolism in endotoxin tolerance. *Adv. Shock Res.*, **10**, 131–142
52. Templeton, C.D., Bottoms, G.D., Fessler, J.F., Turek, J.J. and Boon, G.D. (1985). Effects of repeated endotoxin injections on prostanoids, hemodynamics, endothelial cells, and survival in ponies. *Circ. Shock*, **16**, 253–264
53. Ward, D.S., Bottoms, G.D. and Fessler, J.F. (1986). Cardiac function, prostaglandin production and blood chemical alterations in conscious ponies during chronic endotoxemia. *Circ. Shock.*, **18**, 368 (Abstract)
54. Bulter, R.R., Wise, W.C., Halushka, P.V. and Cook, J.A. (1982). Thromboxane and prostacyclin production during septic shock. *Adv. Shock Res.*, **7**, 133–145
55. Fink, M.P., Gardiner, W.M., Roethel, R. and Fletcher, J.R. (1985). Plasma levels of 6-keto-$PGF_{1\alpha}$ but not TxB_2 increase in rats with peritonitis due to cecal ligation. *Circ. Shock*, **16**, 297–305
56. Morgan, D.C., Wise, W.C., Halushka, P.V. and Cook, J.A. (1984). Thromboxane does not play a role in lethality of *E. coli* sepsis. *Physiologist*, **17**(4), 512 (Abstract)
57. Slotman, G.J., Quinn, J.V., Burchard, K.W. and Gann, D.S. (1985). Thromboxane, prostacyclin and the hemodynamic effects of graded bacteremia shock. *Circ. Shock*, **16**, 395–404
58. Casey, L., Bush, D., Roethel, R., Fletcher, J.R., Ramwell, P.W., Chernow, B. and Lake, R. (1983). Plasma prostanoids during live *E. coli* infusion in baboons: The effect of gentamicin in combination with steroids, indomethacin and lidocaine. *Circ. Shock*, **10**, 276 (Abstract)
59. Carmona, R.H., Tsao, T. and Trunkey, D. (1984). The role of prostacyclin and thromboxane in sepsis and septic shock. *Arch. Surg.*, **119**, 189–192
60. Cook, J.A., Halushka, P.V., Tempel, G.E. and Wise, W.C. (1982). Organ sources of arachidonic acid (AA) in endotoxic (LPS) shock in the rat. *Circ. Shock*, **9**, 173
61. Halushka, P.V., Cook, J.A. and Wise, W.C. (1983). Beneficial effects of UK 37,248, a thromboxane synthesis inhibitor, in experimental endotoxic shock in the rat. *Br. J. Clin. Pharmacol.*, **15**, 133s–139s
62. Tempel, G.E., Cook, J.A., Wise, W.C., Halushka, P.V. and Corral, D. (1986). Improvement in organ blood flow by inhibition of thromboxane synthetase during experimental endotoxic shock in the rat. *J. Cardiovasc. Pharm.*, **8**, 514–519
63. Frolich, J.C., Ogletree, M., Peskar, B.A. and Brigham, K.L. (1980). Pulmonary hypertension correlated to pulmonary thromboxane synthesis. In Samuelsson, B., Ramwell, P.W. and Paletti, R. (eds.) *Advances in Prostaglandin and Thromboxane Research*, Vol. 7, pp. 745–750. (New York: Raven Press)
64. Snapper, J.R., Hinson, J.M., Hutchson, A.A., Lefferts, P.L., Ogletree, M.L. and Brigham, K.L. (1984). Effects of platelet depletion on the unanesthetized sheep pulmonary response to endotoxin. *J. Clin. Invest.*, **74**, 1782–1791
65. McDonald, J.W.D., Ali, M., Morgan, E.R., Townsend, E.R. and Cooper, J.D. (1983). Thromboxane synthesis by sources other than platelet in association with complement-induced pulmonary leukostasis and pulmonary hypertension in sheep. *Circ. Res.*, **52**, 1–6
66. Spagnulo, P., Ellner, J. and Hassid, A. (1980). Thromboxane A_2 mediates augmented polymorphonuclear leukocyte adhesiveness. *J. Clin. Invest.*, **66**, 406–414
67. Huttemeier, P.C., Watkin, W.D. and Peterson, M.D. (1982). Acute pulmonary hypertension and lung thromboxane release after endotoxin infusion in normal and leukopenic sheep. *Circ. Res.*, **50**, 688–694
68. Heflin, A.C. and Brigham, K.L. (1981). Prevention by granulocyte depletion of increased vascular permeability of sheep lung following endotoxemia. *J. Clin. Invest.*, **68**, 1253–1260

69. Egan, T.M., Saunders, N.R., Luk, S.C. and Cooper, J.D. (1983). Granulocytes mediate hypoxemia in sheep infused with activated complement. *Physiologist*, **26**, 36
70. Cook, J.A., Wise, W.C., Tempel, G.E. and Halushka, P.V. (1985). Exchange transfusions in rats with a perfluorated blood substitute: Effect on thromboxane B_2 levels during endotoxemia. *Circ. Shock*, **15**, 193–204
71. Morrison, D.C. and Ulevitch, R.J. (1978). The effects of bacterial endotoxins on host mediation system. *Am. J. Pathol.*, **93**, 527–617
72. Mathison, J.C. and Ulevitch, R.J. (1979). The clearance, tissue distribution, and cellular localization of intravenously injected lipopolysaccharide in rabbits. *J. Immunol.*, **123**, 2133–2143
73. Kurland, J.I. and Bockman, R. (1978). Prostaglandin E production by human blood monocytes and mouse peritoneal macrophages. *J. Exp. Med.*, **147**, 952–957
74. Moore, R.N., Urbaschek, R., Wahl, L.M. and Mergenhagen, S.E. (1979). Prostaglandin regulation of colony-stimulating factor production by lipopolysaccharide-stimulated murine leukocytes. *Infect. Immun.*, **26**, 408–414
75. Rietschel, E.T., Schade, U., Luderitz, O., Fischer, H. and Peskar, B.A. (1980). Prostaglandins in endotoxicosis. In Schlessinger, D. (ed.) *Microbiology*, pp. 66–72. (Washington, D.C.: American Society for Microbiology)
76. Cook, J.A., Wise, W.C. and Halushka, P.V. (1981). Thromboxane A_2 and prostacyclin production by lipopolysaccharide stimulated peritoneal macrophages. *J. Reticuloendothel. Soc.*, **30**, 445–450
77. Feuerstein, N., Bash, J.A. Woody, J.N. and Ramwell, P.W. (1981). 3-Deazaadenosine, a transmethylase inhibitor, suppresses the effect of lipopolysaccharide on release of prostacyclin and thromboxane. *J. Pharm. Pharmacol.*, **33**, 401–406
78. Bowers, G.J., MacVittie, T.J., Hirsch, E.F., Conklin, J.C., Nelson, R.D., Roethel, R.J. and Fink, M.P. (1985). Prostanoid production by lipopolysaccharide-stimulated kupffer cells. *J. Surg. Res.*, **38**, 501–508
79. Wahl, L.M. Rosensteich, D.L., Glode, L.M., Sandberg, A.L. and Mergenhangen, S.E. (1979). Defective prostaglandin synthesis by C3H/HeJ mouse macrophages stimulated with endotoxin preparations. *Infect. Immun.*, **23**, 8–13
80. Cook, J.A., Halushka, P.V. and Wise, W.C. (1982). Modulation of macrophage arachidonic acid metabolism: Potential role in the susceptibility of rats to endotoxic shock. *Circ. Shock*, **9**, 605–617
81. Bowers, G.J. Patchen, M.L., MacVittie, T.J., Hirsch, E.F. and Fink, M.P. (1986). A comparative evaluation of particulate and soluble glucan in endotoxin model. *Int. J. Immunopharmacol.*, **8**, 313–321
82. Wise, W.C., Cook, J.A. and Halushka, P.V. (1983). Arachidonic acid metabolism and glucan stimulation of the RES in septic shock. *J. Reticuloendothel. Soc.*, **34**, 190
83. Greisman, S.E. (1983). Induction of endotoxin tolerance. In Nowotny, A. (ed.) *Beneficial Effects of Endotoxin*, pp. 149–178. (New York: Plenum Press)
84. Chedid, L. and Parant, M. (1971). Hypersensitivity and tolerance in reactions to endotoxin. In Kadis', Weinbaum, G. and Ajl, S.J. (eds.) *Microbial Toxins*. Vol. 5: *Bacterial Endotoxins*, pp. 415. (New York–London: Academic Press)
85. Beeson, P.B. (1946). Development of tolerance to bacterial pyrogens and its abolition by reticuloendothelial blockade. *Proc. Soc. Exp. Biol. Med.*, **61**, 248–250
86. Dinarello, C.A., Bodel, P.T. and Atkins, E. (1968). The role of liver in the production of fever and in pyrogenic tolerance. *Trans. Assoc. Am. Physicians*, **81**, 334–344
87. Rogers, T.S., Halushka, P.V., Wise, W.C. and Cook, J.A. (1986). Differential alterations of lipoxygenase and cyclo-oxygenase metabolism by rat peritoneal macrophages induced by endotoxin tolerance. *Prostaglandins*, **31(4)**, 639–650
88. Scott, W.A., Pawlowski, N.A., Murray, H.W., Andreach, M., Srike, S. and Cohn, Z.A. (1982). Regulation of arachidonic acid metabolism by macrophage activation. *J. Exp. Med.*, **155**, 1148–1160
89. Tripp, C.S., Leahy, K.M. and Needleman, P. (1985). Thromboxane is preferentially conserved in active mouse peritoneal macrophages. *J. Clin. Invest.*, **76**, 898–901
90. Brigham, K.L. and Duke, S.S. (1985). Prostaglandins in lung disease: Adult Respiratory Distress Syndrome. *Semin. Respir. Med.*, **7**, 11–16
91. Meyrick, B.O. (1986). Endotoxin mediated pulmonary injury. *Federation Proc.*, **45**, 19–24

92. Harlan, J., Harken, I., Reidy, M., Gaydjusik, C., Schwartz, S. and Striker, G. (1983). Lipopolysaccharide-mediated bovine endothelial cell injury *in vitro*. *Lab. Invest.*, **48**, 269–274

93. Brigham, K.L. and Ogletree, M.L. (1981). Effects of prostaglandins and related compounds on lung vascular permeability. *Bull. Eur. Physiopathol. Respir.*, **17**, 703–722

94. Watkins, W.D., Huttemeier, P.C., Kong, D. and Peteson, M.D. (1982). Thromboxane and pulmonary hypertension following *E. coli* endotoxin infusion in sheep: Effect of an imidazole derivative. *Prostaglandins*, **23**, 273–285

95. Wise, W.C., Cook, J.A., Halushka, P.V. and Knapp, D.R. (1980). Protective effects of thromboxane synthetase inhibitors in rats in endotoxic shock. *Circ. Res.*, **46**, 854–859

96. Smith, E.F., Tabas, J.H. and Lefer, A.M. (1980). Beneficial effects of imidazole in endotoxin shock. *Prostagl. Med.*, **4**, 215–225

97. Ball, H.A., Parratt, J.R. and Zeitlin, I.J. (1983). Effect of dazoxiben, a specific inhibitor of thromboxane synthetase, on acute pulmonary response to *E. coli* endotoxin in anesthetized cat. *Br. J. Clin. Pharmacol.*, **15**, 1275–1315

98. Westwick, J., Fletcher, M.S. and Kakkar, V.V. (1983). Inhibition of thromboxane formation prevents endotoxin-induced renal fibrin deposition in jaundiced rats. In Samuelsson, B., Paoletti, R. and Ramwell, P. (eds.) *Advances in Prostaglandin, Thromboxane and Leukotrienne Research*, Vol. 12, p. 83–91. (New York: Raven Press)

99. Anderegg, K., Anzeveno, P., Cook, J.A., Halushka, P.V., McCarthy, J., Wagner, E. and Wise, W.C. (1983). Effects of a pyridine derivative thromboxane synthetase inhibitor and its inactive isomer in endotoxic shock in the rat. *Br. J. Pharmacol.*, **78**, 725–732

100. Fukumoto, S. and Tanaka, K. (1983). Protective effects of thromboxane A$_2$ synthetase inhibitors on endotoxic shock. *Prosagl. Leuk. Med.* **11**, 179–188

101. Kubo, K. and Kobayashi, T. (1985). Effects of OKY-046, a selective thromboxane synthetase inhibitor, on endotoxin-induced lung injury in unanesthetized sheep. *Am. Rev. Respir. Dis.*, **132**, 494–497

102. Olanoff, L.S., Cook, J.A., Eller, T., Knapp, D.R. and Halushka, P. (1985). Protective effect of *trans*-13-APT, a thromboxane receptor antagonist, in endotoxemia. *J. Cardiovasc. Pharmacol.*, **7**, 114–120

103. Gunther, R.A., Smith, G.J. and Holcroft, J.W. (1984). Pulmonary response to selective inhibition of thromboxane A$_2$ synthesis during endotoxemia utilizing a unique inhibitor. *Surg. Forum*, **35**, 42–44

104. Ball, H.A. and Parratt, J.R. (1983). Thromboxane and the pulmonary response to endotoxin in the cat. *Circ. Shock*, **10**, 263

105. Urbaschek, R., Patscheke, H., Stegmeier, K. and Urbaschek, B. (1985). The effect of a thromboxane receptor blocker in endotoxin shock. *Circ. Shock*, **16**, 71

106. Armstrong, R.A., Jones, R.L. and Wilson, N.H. (1985). Effect of the thromboxane receptor antagonist EP 092 on endotoxin shock in the sheep. *Prostaglandins*, **29**, 703–713

107. Krausz, M.K., Utsumoniya, T., Sunham, B., Valteri, R., Shepro, D. and Hechtman, H.B. (1982). Inhibition of permeability edema with imidazole. *Surgery*, **92**, 299–308

108. Slotman, G.J., Yellin, S.A., Handy, J.R., Hulstyn, M., Husain, S.E. and Gann, D.S. (1986). TxA$_2$ mediates hemodynamic and respiratory dysfunction in graded bacteremia. *Surgery*, **100**, 214–221

109. Bowers, R., Ellis, E., Brigham, K. and Oates, J. (1983). Effects of prostaglandin cyclic endoperoxides on the lung circulation of sheep. *J. Clin. Invest.*, **63**, 131–137

110. Short, B.L., Miller, M.K., Stround, C.Y. and Fletcher, J.R. (1983). Comparison of the thromboxane inhibitors to cyclooxygenase inhibitors on survival in a newborn rat model for group B-streptococcal sepsis. In Samuelsson, B., Paoletti, R. and Ramwell, P. (eds.) *Advances in Prostaglandin, Thromboxane and Leukotriene Research*, Vol. 12, pp. 113–116. (New York: Raven Press)

111. Fletcher, J.R., Short, B.L., Casey, L.C., Walker, R.I., Gardiner, M. and Ramwell, P.W. (1983). Thromboxane inhibition in gram-negative sepsis fails to improve survival. In Samuelsson, B., Paoletti, R. and Ramwell, P. (eds.) *Advances in Prostaglandin, Thromboxane and Leukotriene Research*, Vol. 12, pp. 117–120. (New York: Raven Press)

112. Butler, R.R., Wise, W.C., Halushka, P.V. and Cook, J.A. (1983). Gentamicin and indomethacin in the treatment of septic shock: Effects of prostacyclin and thromboxane A$_2$ production. *J. Pharmacol. Exp. Ther.*, **225**, 94–101

113. Truog, W.C., Soresen, G.K., Standaert, J. and Redding, G.J. (1986). Effect of the thromboxane synthetase inhibitor, Dazmegrel (UK 38,485) on pulmonary gas exchange and hemodynamics in neonatal sepsis. *Pediatr. Res.*, **20**, 481–486

114. Ball, H.A. (1984). Mechanism of the feline cardiopulmonary response to endotoxin. PhD Thesis, University of Strathclyde, Scotland, UK

115. Hassid, A. (1984). Stimulation of prostacyclin synthesis by thromboxane A_2-like prostaglandin endoperoxide analogues in cultured vascular smooth muscle cells. *Biochem. Biophys. Res. Commun.*, **123**, 21–26

116. Rao, P.S., Cavanagh, D. and Gaston, L.W. (1981). Endotoxic shock in the primate, effects of aspirin and dipyridamole administration. *Am. J. Obstet. Gynecol.*, **140**, 914–922

117. Halushka, P.V., Wise, W.C. and Cook, J.A. (1981). Protective effects of aspirin in endotoxic shock. *J. Pharmacol. Exp. Ther.*, **218**, 464–469

118. Halushka, P.V., Wise, W.C. and Cook, J.A. (1983). Studies on the beneficial effects of aspirin in endotoxin shock. Relationship to inhibition of arachidonic acid metabolism. *Am. J. Med.*, **14**, 91–96

119. Parratt, J.R. and Sturgess, R.M. (1976). The effect of a new anti-inflammatory drug, fluribiprofen, on the respiratory, haemodynamic and metabolic response to *E. coli* endotoxin shock in the cat. *Br. J. Pharmacol.*, **58**, 547–551

120. Schrauwen, E., Vandeplassche, G., Laekeman, G. and Houvenaghel, A. (1983). Endotoxin shock in the pig: Release of prostaglandins and beneficial effects of flurobiprofen. *Arch. Int. Pharmacodyn.*, **262**, 332–334

121. Jacobs, E.R., Soulsby, M.E., Bone, R.C., Wilson, F.J. and Hiller, F.C. (1982). Ibuprofen in canine endotoxin shock. *J. Clin. Invest.*, **70**, 536–541

122. Wise, W.C., Cook, J.A., Eller, T. and Halushka, P.V. (1980). Ibuprofen improves survival from endotoxin shock in the rat. *J. Pharmacol. Exp. Ther.*, **215**, 160–164

123. Almqvist, P.M., Kuenzig, M. and Schwartz, S.I. (1984). Treatment of experimental canine endotoxin shock with ibuprofen, a cyclo-oxygenase inhibitor. *Circ. Shock*, **13**, 227–232

124. Gryglewski, R.J. (1978). Screening for inhibitors of prostaglandin and thromboxane biosynthesis. *Adv. Lipid Res.*, **16**, 327–44

125. Ogletree, M.L. and Brigham, K.L. (1982). Effects of cyclo-oxygenase inhibitors on pulmonary vascular responses to endotoxin in unanesthetized sheep. *Prostagl. Leuk. Med.*, **8**, 489–502

126. Fletcher, J.R. and Ramwell, P.W. (1980). Indomethacin improves survival after endotoxin in baboons. In Samuelsson, B., Ramwell, P.W. and Paoletti, R. (eds.) *Advances in Prostaglandin and Thromboxane Research*, Vol. 7, pp. 821–828. (New York: Raven Press)

127. Armstrong, J., Tempel, G.E., Cook, J.A., Wise, W.C. and Halushka, P.V. (1986). The effects of alpha adrenergic blockade on arachidonic acid metabolism and shock sequelae in endotoxemia. *Circ. Shock*, **20**, 151–159

128. Feuerstein, G., Dimicco, J.A., Ramu, A. and Kopin, I.J. (1981). Effect of indomethacin on the blood pressure and plasma catecholamine responses to endotoxemia. *J. Pharm. Pharmacol.*, **33**, 576–579

129. Olson, N.C., Meyer, R.E. and Anderson, D.L. (1985). Effects of flunixin meglumine on cardiopulmonary responses to endotoxin in ponies. *J. Appl. Physiol.*, **59**, 1464–1471

130. Bottoms, G.D., Fessler, J.F., Roesel, O.F., Moore, A.B. and Frauenfelder, H.C. (1981). Endotoxin-induced hemodynamic changes in ponies: Effects of flunixin meglumine. *Am. J. Vet. Res.*, **42**, 1514–1581

131. Toth, P.D., Hamburger, S.A., Hastings, G.H. and Judy, W.V. (1985). Benoxaprofen attenuation of lethal canine endotoxic shock. *Circ. Shock*, **15**, 89–103

132. Toth, P.H., Hamburger, S.A. and Judy, W.V. (1983). Reversal of lethal canine endotoxic shock. *Circ. Shock*, **10**, 233

133. Begley, C., Ogletree, M., Meyrick, B. and Brigham, K. (1984). Modification of pulmonary responses to endotoxemia in awake sheep by steroidal and non-steroidal anti-inflammatory agents. *Am. Rev. Respir. Dis.*, **130**, 1140–64

134. Ogletree, M. and Brigham, K. (1982). Effect of cyclo-oxygenase inhibitors on pulmonary vascular responses to endotoxin in unanesthetized sheep. *Prostagl. Leuk. Med.*, **8**, 489–502

135. Ogletree, M. and Brigham, K.L. (1979). Indomethacin augments endotoxin induced lung vascular permeability in sheep. *Am. Rev. Respir. Dis. (Suppl.)*, **119**, 383

136. Snapper, J., Hutchinson, A., Ogletree, M. and Brigham, K. (1983). Effects of cyclo-oxygenase inhibitors on the alterations in lung mechanics caused by endotoxemia in the unanesthetized sheep. *J. Clin. Invest.*, **72**, 63–76
137. Hanna, C.J., Bach, M.K. and Pare, P.D. (1981). Slow reacting substances (leukotrienes) contract human airway and pulmonary vascular smooth muscle *in vitro*. *Nature (London)*, **290**, 343–344
138. Higgs, G., Eakins, K., Moncada, S. and Vane, J. (1980). The effects of non-steroidal anti-inflammatory drugs on leukocyte migration in carrageenin-induced inflammation. *Eur. J. Pharmacol.*, **68**, 81–86
139. Wise, W.C., Halushka, P.V., Knapp, R.G. and Cook, J.A. (1985). Ibuprofen, methylpred-nisolone and gentamicin as conjoint therapy in septic shock. *Circ. Shock*, **17**, 59–71
140. Kadowitz, P.J., Chapnick, B.M., Feigen, L.P., Hyman, A.L., Nelson, P.K. and Spannhake, E.W. (1978). Pulmonary and systemic vasodilator effects of the newly discovered prostaglandin, PGI_2. *J. Appl. Physiol.*, **45**, 408–413
141. Voelkel, N.F., Gerber, J.G., McMurtry, I.F., Nies, A.S. and Reeves, J.T. (1981). Release of vasodilator prostaglandin, PGI_2, from isolated rat lung during vasoconstriction. *Circ. Res.*, **48**, 207–213
142. Fink, M.P., MacVittie, T.J. and Casey, L.C. (1984). Inhibition of prostaglandin synthesis restores normal hemodynamics in canine hyperdynamic sepsis. *Am. Surg.*, **200**, 619–626
143. Peevy, K.J., Panus, P., Longnecker, L., Chartrand, S.A., Wiseman, H.J., Boerth, R.C. and Olson, R.D. (1986). Prostaglandin synthetase inhibition of Group B streptococcal shock: Hematologic and hemodynamic effects. *Pediatr. Res.*, **20**, 864–866
144. Fink, M.P., Homer, L.D. and Fletcher, J.R. (1985). Diminished pressor response to exogenous norepinephrine and angiotensin II in septic, unanesthetized rats: Evidence for a prostaglandin-mediated effect. *J. Surg. Res.*, **38**, 335–342
145. Hedqvist, P. (1977). Basic mechanisms of prostaglandin action on autonomic neuro-transmission. *Annu. Rev. Pharmacol. Toxicol.*, **17**, 259–279
146. Carmichael, J. and Hankel, S.W. (1985). Effects of non-steroidal anti-inflammatory drugs on prostaglandins and renal function. *Am. J. Med.*, **78**, 992–1000
147. Fink, M.P., MacVittie, T.J. and Casey, L.C. (1984). Effects of non-steroidal anti-inflammatory drugs on renal function in septic dogs. *J. Surg. Res.*, **36**, 516–525
148. Goldberg, A.L., Baracos, V., Rodemann, P., Waxman, L. and Dinarello, C. (1984). Control of protein degradation in muscle by prostaglandins, Ca^{++} and leukocytic pyrogen (interleukin-1). *Fed. Proc.*, **43**, 1301–1306
149. Baracos, V., Rodemann, P., Dinarello, C. and Goldberg, A.L. (1983). Stimulation of muscle protein degradation and prostaglandin E_2 release by leukocytic pyrogen (interleukin-1) (a mechanism for the increased degradation of muscle protein during fever). *N. Engl. J. Med.*, **308**, 553–558
150. Hulton, N.R., Johnson, D.J. and Wilmore, D.W. (1985). Limited effects of prostaglandin inhibitors in *Escherichia coli* sepsis. *Surgery*, **98**, 291–297
151. Cook, J.A., Wise, W.C., Butler, R.R., Reines, H.D., Rambo, W. and Halushka, P.V. (1984). The potential of thromboxane and prostacyclin in endotoxin and septic shock. *Am. J. Emerg. Med.*, **2**, 28–37
152. Ziboh, V.A., Vanderhoek, J.Y. and Lands, W.E.M. (1974). Inhibition of sheep vesicular gland oxygenase by unsaturated fatty acids from skin of essential fatty acid deficient rats. *Prostaglandins*, **5**, 233–240
153. Cook, J.A., Wise, W.C., Knapp, D.R. and Halushka, P.V. (1981). Sensitization of essential fatty acid-deficient rats to endotoxin by arachidonate pretreatment: role of thromboxane A_2. *Circ. Shock*, **8**, 69–76
154. Cook, J.A., Wise, W.C., Knapp, D.R. and Halushka, P.V. (1981). Essential fatty acid deficient rats: A new model for evaluating arachidonate metabolism in shock. *Adv. Shock Res.*, **6**, 93–105
155. Gryglewski, R.J., Panczenko, B., Korbut, R., Grodzinska, L. and Ocetkiewicz, A. (1975). Corticosteroids inhibit prostaglandin release from perfused mesenteric blood vessels of rabbit and from perfused lungs of sensitized guinea pig. *Prostaglandins*, **10**, 343–355
156. Kantrowitz, F., Robinson, D.R. and McGuire, M.B. (1975). Corticosteroids inhibit prostaglandin production by rheumatoid synovia. *Nature (London)*, **258**, 737–738
157. Tashjian, A.H. Jr., Voelkel, N.F. and McDonough, J. (1975). Hydrocortisone inhibits prostaglandin production by mouse fibrosarcoma cells. *Nature (London)*, **258**, 739–741

158. Floman, Y. and Zor, U. (1976). Mechanism of steroid action in inflammation: Inhibition of prostaglandin synthesis and release. *Prostaglandins*, **12**, 403–413
159. Floman, Y., Floman, N. and Zor, U. (1976). Inhibition of prostaglandin E release by anti-inflammatory steroids. *Prostaglandins*, **11**, 591–594
160. Danon, A. and Assouline, G. (1978). Inhibition of prostaglandin biosynthesis by corticosteroid requires RNA and protein synthesis. *Nature (London)*, **273**, 552–554
161. Flower, R.J. and Blackwell, G.J. (1979). Anti-inflammatory steroids induce biosynthesis of a phospholipase A_2 inhibitor which prevents prostaglandin generation. *Nature (London)*, **278**, 456–459
162. Carnuccio, R., DiRosa, M. and Persico, P. (1980). Hydrocortisone-induced inhibitor of prostaglandin biosynthesis in rat leukocytes. *Br. J. Pharmacol.* **68**, 14–16
163. Hinshaw, L.B., Archer, L.T., Beller-Todd, B.K., Coalson, J.J., Flournoy, D.J., Passey, R., Benjamin, B. and White, G.L. (1980). Survival of primates in LD_{100} septic shock following steroid/antibiotic therapy. *J. Surg. Res.*, **28**, 151–170
164. Brigham, K.L., Bowers, R.E. and McKeen, C.R. (1981). Methylprednisolone prevention of increased lung vascular permeability following endotoxemia in sheep. *J. Clin. Invest.*, **67**, 1103–1110
165. McKechnie, K., Furman, B.L. and Parratt, J.R. (1985). Metabolic and cardiovascular effects of endotoxin infusion in conscious unrestrained rats: Effects of Methylprednisolone and BW755C. *Circ. Shock*, **15**, 205–215
166. Hales, C.A., Brandstetter, R.D., Neely, C.F., Peterson, M.B., Kong, D. and Watkins, W.D. (1986). Methylprednisolone on circulating eicosanoids and vasomotor tone after endotoxin. *J. Appl. Physiol.*, **6**, 185–191
167. Almqvist, P.M., Ekstrom, B., Kuenzig, M., Haglund, U. and Schwartz, S.I. (1984). Increased survival of endotoxin-injected dogs treated wth methylprednisolone, naloxone, and ibuprofen. *Circ. Shock*, **14**, 129–136
168. Elinger, J.H., Seyde, W.C. and Longnecker, D.E. (1984). Methylprednisolone plus ibuprofen increase mortality in septic rats. *Circ. Shock*, **14**, 203–208
169. Ogletree, M.L., Begley, C.J., King, G.A. and Brigham, K.L. (1986). Influence of steroidal and nonsteroidal anti-inflammatory agents on the accumulation of arachidonic acid metabolites in plasma and lung lymph after endotoxemia in awake sheep. Measurements of prostacyclin and thromboxane metabolites and 12-HETE. *Am. Rev. Respir. Dis.*, **133**, 55–61
170. Olson, N.C., Brown, T.T. Jr. and Anderson, D.L. (1985). Dexamethasone and indomethacin modify endotoxin-induced respiratory failure in pigs. *J. Appl. Physiol.*, **58**, 274–284
171. Hammarstrom, S. (1983). Leukotrienes. *Ann. Rev. Biochem.*, **52**, 355–377
172. Uehara, N., Ormstad, K., Orning, L. and Hammarstrom, S. (1983). Characteristics of the uptake of cysteine-containing leukotrienes by isolated hepatocytes. *Biochem. Biophys. Acta*, **732**, 69–74
173. Hammarstrom, S., Orning, L., Bernstrom, K., Gustafsson, B., Norin, E. and Kaijser, L. (1985). Metabolism of leukotriene C_4 in rat and man. *Adv. Prostagl. Thrombox. Leuk. Res.*, **15**, 185–188
174. Denzlinger, C., Rapp. S., Hagmann, W. and Keppler, D. (1985). Leukotriene as mediators in tissue trauma. *Science*, **230**, 330–332
175. Koller, M., Schonfeld, W. and Knoller, J. (1985). The metabolism of leukotrienes in blood plasma studied by high-performance liquid chromatography. *Biochim. Biophys. Acta*, **833**, 128–134
176. Hagmann, W., Denzlinger, C. and Keppler, D. (1985). Production of peptide leukotrienes in endotoxin shock. *FEBS Lett.*, **180**, 309–313
177. Craft, D.V., Lefer, D.J., Hock, C.E. and Lefer, A.M. (1986). Significance of production of peptide leukotrienes in murine traumatic shock. *Am. J. Physiol.*, **251**, H80–H85
178. Ball, H.A., Cook, J.A., Spicer, K.M. and Halushka, P.V. (1985). LY171883, a leukotriene D_4/E_4 antagonist, attenuates leak in oleic acid induced pulmonary injury. *Circ. Shock*, **12**, 106
179. Hagmann, W. and Keppler, D. (1982). Leukotriene antagonists prevent endotoxin lethality. *Naturwissenschaffen*, **69**, 594–595
180. Hagmann, W., Denzlinger, C. and Keppler, D. (1984). Role of peptide leukotrienes and their hepatobiliary elimination in endotoxin shock. *Circ. Shock*, **14**, 223–235

181. Denzlinger, C., Guhlmann, A., Scheuber, P.H., Wilker, D., Hammer, D.K. and Keppler, D. (1986). Metabolism and analysis of cysteinyl leukotrienes in the monkey. *J. Biol. Chem.*, **261**, 15601–15606

182. Ogletree, M.L., Oates, J.A., Brigham, K.L. and Hubbard, W.C. (1982). Evidence for pulmonary release of 5-hydroxyeicosatetraenoic acid (5-HETE) during endotoxemia in unanesthetized sheep. *Prostaglandins*, **23**, 459–468

183. Burghuber, O.C., Strife, R.J., Zirrolli, J., Henson, P.M., Henson, J.E., Mathias, M.M., Reeves, J.T., Murphy, R.C. and Voelkel, N.F. (1985). Leukotriene inhibitors attenuate rat lung injury induced by hydrogen peroxide. *Am. Rev. Respir. Dis.*, **131**, 778–785

184. Makino, H., Ashida, Y., Saijo, T. Kuriki, H., Terao, S., and Maki, Y. (1986). Role of leukotrienes in rat reversed passive arthus pleurisy and the effect of AA-861, a 5-lipoxygenase inhibitor. *Int. Arch. Allergy Appl. Immun.*, **79**, 38–44

185. Morganroth, M.L., Stenmark, K.R., Zirrolli, J.A., Mauldin, R., Mathias, M., Reeves, J.T., Murphy, R.C. and Voelkel, N.F. (1984). Leukotriene C_4 production during hypoxic pulmonary vasconstriction in isolated rat lungs. *Prostaglandins*, **28**, 867–875

186. Taniguchi, H., Taki, F., Takagi, K., Satake, T., Sugiyama, S. and Ozawa, T. (1986). The role of leukotriene B_4 in the genesis of oxygen toxicity in the lung. *Am. Rev. Respir. Dis.*, **133**, 805–808

187. Dauber, I., Pluss, W., Stenmark, K., Weil, J. and Voelkel, N. (1983). Leukotrienes in thiourea-induced lung injury edema. *Am. Rev. Respir. Dis.*, **127**, 304

188. Patel, S., Reines, H.D., Spinale, F. and Halushka, P.V. (1986). Leukotrienes are elevated in oleic acid induced lung injury. *Circ. Shock*, **18**, 377

189. Bremm, K.D., Konig, W., Spur, B., Crea, A. and Galanos, C. (1984). Generation of slow-reacting substance (leukotrienes) by endotoxin and lipid from human polymorphonuclear granulocytes. *Immunology*, **53**, 299

190. Konig, W., Scheffer, J., Bremm, K.D., Hacker, J. and Goebel, W. (1985). Role of bacterial adherence and toxin production from *Escherichia coli* on leukotriene generation from human polymorphonuclear granulocytes. *Int. Arch. Allergy Appl. Immun.*, **77**, 118–120

191. Bottoms, G.D., Johnson, M., Ward, D., Fessler, J., Lamar, C. and Turek, J. (1986). Release of eicosanoids from white blood cells, platelets, smooth muscle cells, and endothelial cells in response to endotoxin and A23187. *Circ. Shock*, **20**, 25–34

192. Altavilla, D., Cook, J.A., Halushka, P.V., Chisari, M., Foca, A. and Mastroeni, P. (1985). Determinazione di leucotrieni e trombossano B_2 di leucociti di ratto trattati con LPS batterici. *XXI Congr. Naz. Soc. It. Microbiol*, 4–7 dicembre, Roma

193. Humes, J.L., Sadowski, S., Galavage, M., Goldengerg, M., Subers, E., Bonney, R.J. and Kuehl, F.A. Jr. (1981). Evidence for two sources of arachidonic acid for oxidative metabolism by mouse peritoneal macrophages. *J. Biol. Chem.*, **257**, 1591–1594

194. Tripp, C.S., Mahoney, M. and Needleman, P. (1985). Calcium Ionophore enables soluble agonists to stimulate macrophage 5-lipoxygenase. *J. Biol. Chem.*, **260**, 5895–5898

195. Luderitz, T., Schade, U. and Rietschel, E.T. (1985). Formation and metabolism of leukotriene C_4 in macrophages exposed to bacterial lipopolysaccharide. *Eur. J. Biochem.*, **155**, 377–382

196. Weller, P.F., Lee, C.W., Foster, D.W. *et al.* (1983). Generation and metabolism of 5-lipoxygenase pathway leukotrienes by human eosinophils; predominant production of leukotriene C_4. *Proc. Natl. Acad. Sci. USA*, **80**, 7626–7630

197. Verhagen, J., Bruynzeel, P.L.B. and Koedam, J.A. (1984). Specific leukotriene formation by purified human eosinophils and neutrophils. *FEBS Lett.*, **168**, 23–28

198. Payan, D.G., Goldman, D.W. and Goetzl, E.J. (1984). Biochemical and cellular characteristics of the regulation of human leukocyte function by lipoxygenase products of arachidonic acid. In Chakrin, L.W. and Bailey, D.M. (eds.) *The Leukotrienes, Chemistry and Biology*, pp. 231–245. (Orlando: Academic Press)

199. Perez, H.D., Roll, E.F. and Bissell, D.M. (1984). Production of chemotactic activity for polymorphonuclear leukocytes by cultured rat hepatocytes exposed to ethanol. *J. Clin. Invest.*, **74**, 1350–1357

200. Dembinska-Kiec, A., Simmet, T. and Peskar, B.A. (1984). Formation of leukotriene C_4 like material by rat brain tissue. *Eur. J. Pharmacol.*, **99**, 57–62

201. Dembinska-Kiec, A., Simmet, T. and Peskar, B.A. (1984). Release and vasoconstrictor effect of leukotriene C_4-like immunoreactive material in the guinea pig mesenteric vascular bed. *Eur. J. Pharmacol.*, **101**, 259–262

202. Wendal, A. and Tiegs, G. (1986). A novel biologically seleno-organic compound-VI. Protection by Ebselen (PL51) against galactosamine/endotoxin-induced hepatitis in mice. *Biochem. Pharmacol.*, **35**, 2115–2118
203. Morganroth, M.L., Stenmark, K.R., Morris, K.G., Murphy, R.C., Mathias, M., Reeves, J.T. and Voelkel, N.F. (1985). Diethylcarbamazine inhibits acute and chronic hypoxic pulmonary hypertension in awake rats. *Am. Rev. Respir. Dis.*, **131**, 488–492
204. Burghuber, O., Strife, R., Zirrolli, J., Mathias, M., Henson, J., Henson, P., Reeves, J., Murphy, R. and Voelkel, N. (1984). Leukotriene inhibitors attenuate H_2O_2-induced rat lung injury. *Am. Rev. Respir. Dis.*, **129**, A333
205. Badr, K.F., Kelley, V.E., Rennke, H.G. and Brenner, B.M. (1986). Roles for thromboxane A_2 and leukotrienes in endotoxin-induced acute renal failure. *Kidney Int.*, **30**, 474–480
206. Fleisch, J.H., Rinkema, L.E., Haisch, K.D., Swanson-Bean, D., Goodson, T., Ho, P.K. and Marshall, W.S. (1985). LY171883, 1 < 2 hydroxy-3-propyl-4- < 4(1H-tetrazol-5yl)butoxy > phenyl > ethanone, an orally active leukotriene D_4 antagonist. *J. Pharmacol. Exp. Ther.*, **233**, 148–157
207. Koyama, S., Kiyono, S., Kayaba, K., Kimura, M. and Nishizawa, M. (1985). Cardiovascular and blood gas responses to ketanserin canine pulmonary edema induced by oleic acid. *Anesthesiology*, **62**, 457–461
208. Brigham, K.L., Kariman, K., Harris, T.R., Snapper, J.R., Bernard, G.R. and Young, S.L. (1983). Correlation of oxygenation with vascular permeability-surface area but not with lung water in humans with acute respiratory failure and pulmonary edema. *J. Clin. Invest.*, **72**, 339–349
209. Ball, H.A., Cook, J.A., Spicer, K.M., Wise, W.C. and Halushka, P.V. (1983). Potential role of leukotrienes in oleic acid-induced pulmonary injury: Effects of essential fatty acid deficiency. *Circ. Shock*, **18**, 375
210. Keppler, D., Forsthove, C. and Hagmann, W. (1985). Leukotrienes and liver injury. In Bianchi, L., Gerok, W. and Popper, H. (eds.) *Trends in Hepatology.* pp. 137–145. (Lancaster: MTP Press Limited)
211. Cook, J.A., Wise, W.C. and Halushka, P.V. (1985). Protective effect of a leukotriene antagonist in endotoxic shock. *J. Pharm. Exp. Ther.*, **235**, 470–474
212. McIntyre, T.M., Zimmerman, G.A. and Prescott, S.M. (1986). Leukotrienes C_4 and D_4 stimulate human endothelial cells to synthesize platelet-activating factor and bind neutrophils. *Proc. Natl. Acad. Sci.*, **83**, 2204–2208
213. Etemadi, A.R., Tempel, G.E., Wise, W.C., Halushka, P.V. and Cook, J.A. (1986). The beneficial effects of a leukotriene antagonist on endotoxin induced acute hemodynamic alterations. *Circ. Shock*, (In press)
214. Whittle, B.J.R., Oren-Wolman, N. and Guth, P.H. (1985). Gastric vasoconstrictor actions of leukotriene C_4, $PGF_{2\alpha}$ and thromboxane mimetic U-46619 on rat submucosal microcirculation *in vivo*. *Am. J. Physiol.*, **248**, G580–G586
215. Hock, C.E. and Lefer, A.M. (1985). Protective effects of a new LTD_4 antagonist (LY171883) in traumatic shock. *Circ. Shock*, **17**, 263–272
216. Krausz, M.M., Bendahan, J. and Gross, D. (1986). The effect of the leukotriene antagonist LY171883 in *E. coli* endotoxemia. *Circ. Shock*, **18**, 361
217. Katz, S.A., Etemadi, A.R., Wise, W.C., Halushka, P.V. and Cook, J.A. (1986). Oleic acid-induced lung injury: Effect on vascular permeability and arachidonic acid metabolism. *Fed. Proc.*, **45**, 400
218. Reines, H.D., Halushka, P.V., Cook, J.A., Wise, W.C. and Rambo, W. (1982). Plasma thromboxane concentrations are raised in patients dying with septic shock. *Lancet*, **24**, 174–175
219. Reines, H.D., Halushka, P.V., Cook, J.A. and Loadholt, C.B. (1985). Lack of effect of glucocorticoids upon plasma thromboxane in patients in a state of shock. *Surg. Gynecol. Obstet.*, **160**, 320–322
220. Herndon, D.N., Abston, S. and Stein, M.D. (1984). Increased thromboxane B_2 levels in the plasma of burned and septic burned patients. *Surg. Gynecol. Obstet.*, **159**, 210–213
221. Deby-Dupont, G., Radoux, L., Hass, M., Larbuisson, R., Noel, F.X. and Lamy, M. (1982). Release of thromboxane B_2 during adult respiratory distress syndrome and its inhibition by nonsteroidal anti-inflammatory substance in man. *Arch. Int. Pharmacodyn.*, **259**, 317–319

126

222. Slotman, G.J., Burchard, K.W., Williams, J., D'Arezzo, A. and Yellin, S.A. (1986). Interaction of prostaglandins, activated complement, and granulocytes in clinical sepsis and hypotension. *Surgery*, **99**, 744–750

223. Rie, M., Peteson, M., Kong, D., Quinn, D. and Watkins, D. (1983). Plasma prostacyclin increases during acute human sepsis. *Circ. Shock*, **10**, 232

224. Halushka, P.V., Reines, H.D., Barrow, S.E., Blair, I.A., Dollery, C.T., Rambo, W., Cook, J.A. and Wise, W.C. (1985). Elevated plasma 6-keto-prostaglandin $F_{1\alpha}$ in patients in septic shock. *Crit. Care Med.*, **13**, 451–453

225. Oetinger W.K.E., Walker, G.O., Jensen, U.M., Beyer, A. and Peskar, A. (1983). Endogenous prostaglandin $F_{2\alpha}$ in the hyperdynamic state of severe sepsis in man. *Br. J. Surg.*, **70**, 237–239

226. Stenmark, K.R., James, S.L., Voelkel, N.F., Toews, W.H., Reeves, J.T. and Murphy, R.C. (1983). Leukotriene C_4 and D_4 in neonates with hypoxemia and pulmonary hypertension. *N. Engl. J. Med.*, **309**, 77–80

227. Matthay, M.A., Eschenbacker, W.L. and Goetzl, E.J. (1984). Elevated concentrations of leukotriene D_4 in pulmonary edema fluid of patients with the adult respiratory distress syndrome. *J. Clin. Immunol.*, **4**, 479–483

228. Swerdlow, B.N., Mihm, F.G., Goetzl, E.J. and Matthay, M.A. (1986). Leukotrienes in pulmonary edema fluid after cardiopulmonary bypass. *Anesth. Analog.*, **65**, 306–308

229. Reines, H.D., Halushka, P.V., Olanoff, L.S. and Hunt, P.S. (1985). Dazoxiben in human sepsis and adult respiratory distress syndrome. *Clin. Pharmacol. Ther.*, **37**, 391–395

230. Leeman, M., Boeynaems, J., Degaute, J., Vincent, J. and Kahn, R.J. (1985). Administration of dazoxiben, a selective thromboxane synthetase inhibitor, in the adult respiratory distress syndrome. *Chest*, **87**, 726–730

231. DuToit, H.J., Erasmus, F.R. and Macfarlane, C.M. (1985). Methylprednisolone and the adult respiratory distress syndrome. *S. Afr. Med. J.*, **65**, 1049–1053

232. Sprung, C.L., Caralis, P.V. and Marical, E.H. *et al.* (1984). The effects of high-dose corticosteroids in patients with septic shock: a prospective, controlled study. *N. Engl. J. Med.*, **311**, 1137–1144

6

Eicosanoids in myocardial ischaemia and injury

D. J. Fitzgerald and G. A. FitzGerald

Platelets and smooth muscle cells have been implicated in the development of coronary atherosclerosis and its complications. The potent effects of thromboxane A_2 and other cyclo-oxygenase products of arachidonic acid on these cell types, their production by tissues contiguous with diseased vessels and their local site of action suggest that these eicosanoids may be important in the pathogenesis of ischaemic heart disease. Most attention has focused on their effects on platelets and the development of coronary thrombosis. However, eicosanoids may also be important in the development of athero-sclerosis, in modulating ischaemic and reperfusion-induced myocardial cell death and in arrhythmogenesis. In addition, there is increasing evidence that platelet and vascular smooth muscle cell dysfunction may be important in the development of complications associated with thrombolytic therapy and with transluminal coronary angioplasty, including acute thrombotic occlusion and accelerated restenosis.

METHODOLOGY

A major difficulty in interpreting studies on the role of thromboxane A_2 and prostaglandins in ischaemic heart disease is that the evanescent nature of some of these compounds precludes their direct measurement in biological fluids. Evidence of their role in the pathogenesis of ischaemic heart disease is frequently based, therefore, on measurement of their metabolites. For example, thromboxane A_2 and prostacyclin formation is frequently determined by measurement of their hydrolysis products, and their non-enzymatic conversion to these products thromboxane B_2 and 6-keto-prostaglandin $F_{1\alpha}$ respectively[1–6]. Such measurements are subject to two major sources of error[7]. Firstly, trauma during sampling can result in the *ex vivo* formation of prostaglandins. This is particularly true in the case of thromboxane B_2 which is formed by platelets activated during sampling[8]. Thus, measurements of hydrolysis products in samples obtained using cardiac catheters are highly artifactual[9,10]. Even sampling from a peripheral vein into a syringe containing a cyclo-oxygenase inhibitor results in elevated levels of thromboxane B_2[8,11]. This *ex vivo* artifact can be minimized by measurement of the enzymatic metabolites of thromboxane A_2 in plasma[8]. Secondly, trauma can result in an artifactual increase in prostacyclin and thromboxane A_2 formation *in vivo*, probably reflecting mobilization of precursor arachidonic acid from traumatized tissues. Roy *et al.* have demonstrated increased prostacyclin biosynthesis measured as urinary excretion of its major enzymatic metabolite, 2,3-dinor-6-keto-prostaglandin $F_{1\alpha}$, during cardiac catheterization and pacing[12]. Similarly, in open-chested dogs, a model used frequently in the study of myocardial ischaemia, measurement of eicosanoid biosynthesis is rendered uninterpretable by a massive increase in thromboxane A_2 and prostacyclin formation induced by trauma[13].

Analytical errors also confound measurements of eicosanoids in biological fluids, reflecting poor specificity of the assays[7]. Measurements of plasma thromboxane B_2 and 6-keto-prostaglandin $F_{1\alpha}$ by radioimmunoassay are often orders of magnitude higher than are found by direct physicochemical methods[11,14]. This may, in part, reflect cross-reactivity of the antibody at low levels of plasma metabolites with other eicosanoids which collectively may be present in a high concentration[15]. Indeed, Siess *et al.* have demonstrated plasma levels of 6-keto-prostaglandin $F_{1\alpha}$ in the low $pg\,mg^{-1}$ range by radioimmunoassay[16]. Thus, it is likely that many radioimmunoassays are detecting other products. Both traumatic and analytical errors can be avoided by measurement of the urinary enzymatic metabolites of eicosanoids in non-instrumented subjects by assays utilizing gas chromatography combined with mass spectrometry for quantitation. Such assays have been described for 2,3-dinor-6-keto-prostaglandin $F_{1\alpha}$[17] and for 2,3-dinor-thromboxane B_2[18] and 11-dehydro-thromboxane B_2[8,19], the major enzymatic metabolites of thromboxane A_2. These methods have correctly predicted plasma levels of 6-keto-prostaglandin $F_{1\alpha}$ and thromboxane B_2 in the low $pg\,ml^{-1}$ range[17,20]. In contrast, plasma levels reported using radioimmunoassay[1-6] have frequently been in excess of $100\,pg\,ml^{-1}$.

Evidence that eicosanoids play a pathogenic role in ischaemic heart disease has also been based on the effects of pharmacological inhibitors, particularly of thromboxane A_2, in animal models and in specific clinical conditions. However, interpretation of these studies is confounded by the poor specificity of the compounds used. Cyclo-oxygenase inhibitors, such as aspirin, indomethacin and ibuprofen, decrease thromboxane A_2 formation by preventing conversion of arachidonic acid to prostaglandin endoperoxides[21]. Although relatively selective inhibition of platelet cyclo-oxygenase, and therefore of thromboxane A_2 biosynthesis, can be achieved with low doses of aspirin[22], some inhibition of non-platelet cyclo-oxygenase occurs[23,24] at doses as low as $40\,mg\,day^{-1}$. Thus, inhibition of the proaggregatory and vasoconstrictor effects of thromboxane A_2 by aspirin may theoretically be offset by coincident inhibition of prostacyclin formation *in vivo*[25].

More selective inhibition of thromboxane A_2 biosynthesis can be achieved with thromboxane synthase inhibitors which prevent the conversion[26] of prostaglandin endoperoxides, intermediary products in the cyclo-oxygenase pathway of arachidonic acid metabolism, to thromboxane A_2. However, the platelet-inhibitory effects of these compounds are limited, possibly due to incomplete inhibition of thromboxane A_2 biosynthesis or by accumulation of prostaglandin endoperoxides which are themselves proaggregatory, activating a receptor shared with thromboxane A_2 which mediates platelet aggregation and vascular smooth muscle contraction[27]. In addition, thromboxane synthase inhibition results in increased prostacyclin biosynthesis[28,29], possibly due to shunting of prostaglandin endoperoxides to vascular endothelium and either direct stimulation of prostacyclin formation[30] or their further metabolism by prostacyclin synthase[31,32] (Figure 6.1). Thus, the effects of thromboxane synthase inhibitors *in vivo* may not reflect inhibition of thromboxane A_2 alone. Similarly, the lack of a response to these compounds does not preclude a role for thromboxane A_2. Recently, more selective inhibition of thromboxane A_2 has been achieved with a structurally diverse group of compounds which are antagonists of the shared thromboxane A_2/prostaglandin endoperoxide receptor[33]. While some of these compounds are highly specific, they frequently exhibit other effects including partial agonism at the thromboxane A_2 or other prostaglandin receptors[34,35], antagonism of other eicosanoids, particularly of their constrictor effects on smooth muscle cells[36,37], inhibition of thromboxane synthase at high concentrations and activity against other autocoids[38].

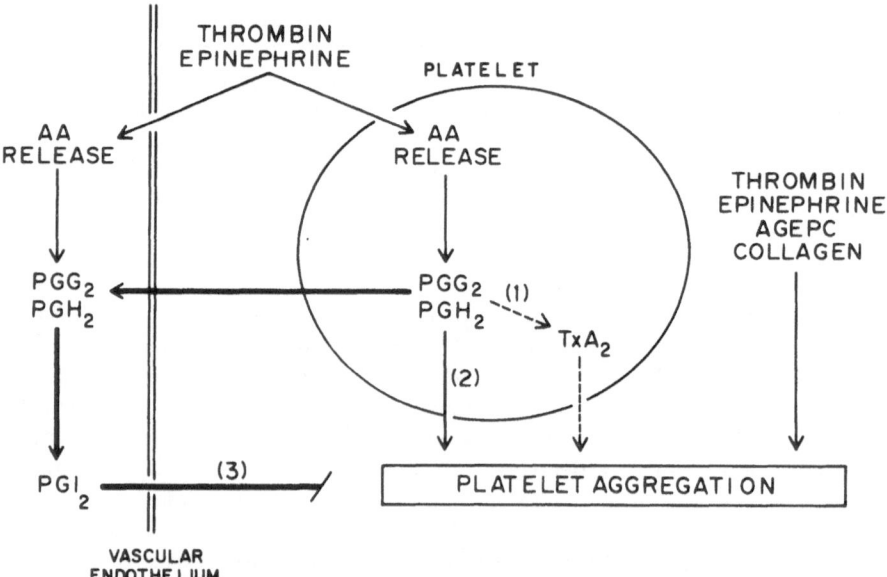

Figure 6.1 Proposed mechanisms of action of thromboxane synthase inhibitors on platelet activity. Thromboxane synthase inhibition prevents the conversion of prostaglandin endoperoxides (PGH$_2$) to thromboxane A_2 (1). Prostaglandin endoperoxides are proaggregatory (2) and are metabolized by endothelium to platelet-inhibitory prostacyclin (3)

In addition, since these compounds are competitive antagonists, the degree of antagonism of the thromboxane A_2/prostaglandin endoperoxide receptor required to achieve a biological response will depend on the amount of agonist formed. Thus, a lack of a response to these compounds would not preclude a role for thromboxane A_2 in a particular clinical setting.

EICOSANOID FORMATION BY CARDIAC TISSUES

The major source of prostaglandins in cardiac tissue is the coronary vasculature[39,40]. Isolated myofibrils exhibit little or no cyclo-oxygenase or thromboxane synthase activity and eicosanoids generated by such preparations probably reflect contamination by vascular elements[39]. The major arachidonic acid product of coronary arteries and veins, as in large vessels from other tissues, is prostacyclin which is largely generated by vascular endothelium[40], although it may also be formed by coronary smooth muscle cells[41]. It has been reported[42] that coronary arteries also generate thromboxane A_2. However, this may reflect contamination by platelets, the major source of thromboxane A_2 in man. No thromboxane synthase activity has been demonstrated in homogenates of bovine coronary arteries or veins[40,43]. Coronary vessels from a number of species also contain prostaglandin H_2–prostaglandin E_2 isomerase activity. This is largely confined to coronary microvessels where prostaglandin E_2 is the major product with little prostacyclin being formed[40,43]. Whether human coronary microvessels also generate prostaglandin E_2 is unknown. However, prostaglandin E_2 is a major product of human foreskin microvessels[44] and is generated from exogenous substrate in the human coronary circulation *in vivo*[45].

In the isolated, perfused heart the major product formed is prostacyclin with lesser amounts of prostaglandin E_2[46,47]. The rate of product formation is increased by a number of stimuli, including vasoactive autocoids, such as adenosine, angiotensin and bradykinin, and by ischaemia[46]. Not surprisingly, the profile of arachidonate products formed also changes following myocardial infarction in which necrotic tissue is initially infiltrated by lymphocytes and fibroblasts and ultimately replaced by scar tissue[48]. Thus, prostacyclin and prostaglandin E_2 production rates in the infarct zone in a canine model increased early following acute myocardial infarction and remained elevated for up to three months. Thromboxane A_2, not present under resting conditions, also increased in the infarcted tissue, probably reflecting deposition of platelet aggregates in the microcirculation[48] although it may also have been generated by other infiltrating inflammatory cells.

There is little information on prostaglandin formation by human cardiac tissue, most of which, based on measurements of thromboxane B_2, prostaglandin E_2 and 6-keto-prostaglandin $F_{1\alpha}$ in aortic and coronary sinus blood, is likely to be highly artifactual. In a recent experiment, Nowak and co-workers[45] infused radiolabelled arachidonic acid into the coronary arteries of male volunteers 3 days following a single dose of aspirin, 600 mg, by which time cyclo-oxygenase activity in endothelial cells, but not in platelets, would have recovered. As in animal models, the major product formed from the radiolabelled substrate was prostacyclin with smaller amounts of prostaglandin E_2 and prostaglandin D_2 also being generated[45].

Physiological effects

Prostaglandins exert marked physiological effects *in vitro* and when administered *in vivo*. Thromboxane A_2 is a potent platelet aggregant in many species, including man[49]. In addition, studies with thromboxane A_2/prostaglandin endoperoxide analogues suggest that thromboxane A_2 is the most potent constrictor of vascular smooth muscle in a variety of human tissues, including the human epicardial artery[50]. Systemic administration of arachidonic acid in a variety of species induces thromboxane A_2-mediated sudden death and platelet consumption[51], demonstrating the potent effect of thromboxane A_2 *in vivo*. Recently, authentic thromboxane A_2 has been synthesized[52] and has been shown to decrease coronary blood flow when administered directly into the coronary artery of dogs[53]. The response was highly variable and thromboxane A_2 was less potent than expected from results with thromboxane A_2/prostaglandin endoperoxide analogues[54], possibly reflecting its chemical lability.

Recent studies suggest that endogenous thromboxane A_2 may also modulate platelet function and vasomotor activity *in vivo*. We have demonstrated inhibition of a canine model of platelet-dependent coronary thrombosis (Figure 6.2) by a thromboxane A_2/prostaglandin endoperoxide receptor antagonist, L636,499 (Figure 6.3). These findings were confirmed with a second, structurally distinct, antagonist, SQ 29,548 (Figure 6.3), suggesting that inhibition of coronary thrombosis reflected thromboxane A_2/prostaglandin endoperoxide receptor antagonism and was not due to a non-specific effect of L 636,499[55]. Consistent with these findings, coronary thrombosis in this model was associated[13] with an increase in thromboxane A_2 biosynthesis, measured as excretion of its urinary metabolite, 2,3-dinor thromboxane B_2. Ashton and co-workers[56] have also demonstrated thromboxane A_2-dependent platelet activation in a canine model of intermittent platelet-thrombosis at a critical coronary stenosis[56]. Partial regulation of platelet activation by endogenous thromboxane A_2 in man is suggested by prolongation of the bleeding time, a platelet-dependent measure of haemostasis, by a variety of thromboxane A_2 inhibitors, including a thromboxane A_2/prostaglandin endoperoxide receptor antagonist[57]. There is little information on the role of endogenous thromboxane A_2 on vascular smooth muscle tone *in vivo*. A recent study in a porcine model of angioplasty in the carotid artery demonstrated a decrease in angiographic luminal diameter distal to the angioplasty site which was prevented by aspirin[58]. This suggests that endogenous thromboxane A_2 released from platelets activated at an angioplasty site may induce local vasoconstriction.

Prostacyclin also exerts potent effects on platelet and vascular smooth muscle function, both *in vitro* and following its administration in a number

132

EICOSANOIDS IN MYOCARDIAL ISCHAEMIA AND INJURY

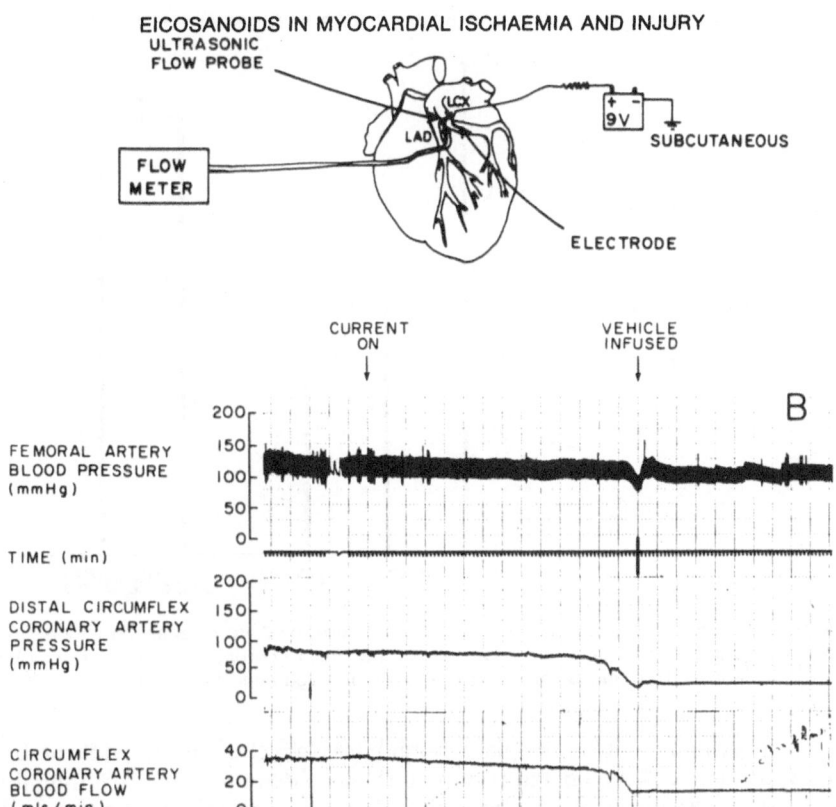

Figure 6.2 Model of platelet-dependent coronary occlusion following electrically-induced endothelial injury in the dog (upper panel). Passage of a 150 μA current results in a fall in coronary artery pressure distal to the electrode and in coronary artery blood flow, with complete occlusion occurring at 70 minutes (lower panel)

of species, including man. *In vitro*, prostacyclin is a potent and non-specific inhibitor of human platelets and vascular smooth muscle, inhibiting aggregation and vasoconstriction induced by a wide range of agonists[59]. Endothelial-derived prostacyclin may play an important role in limiting local thrombosis[60] and the vasoconstrictor response to a number of autocoids, including thromboxane A_2[61]. Systemic administration of prostacyclin in man results[62] in inhibition of platelet aggregation *ex vivo* and a fall in systemic blood pressure at a threshold dose of 4–8 ng kg^{-1} min^{-1}. Prostacyclin induces dilatation of the coronary bed when administered systemically or directly into the coronary artery[63]. In addition, prostacyclin inhibits a number of animal models of platelet-dependent coronary thrombosis[64,65].

Whether endogenous prostacyclin modulates platelet activity *in vivo* is uncertain, but studies using cyclo-oxygenase and thromboxane synthase inhibitors in animal models of thrombosis support this hypothesis. Inhibition of platelet deposition on de-endothelialized rabbit abdominal aorta by aspirin is dose dependent, being less at higher doses at which coincident inhibition

133

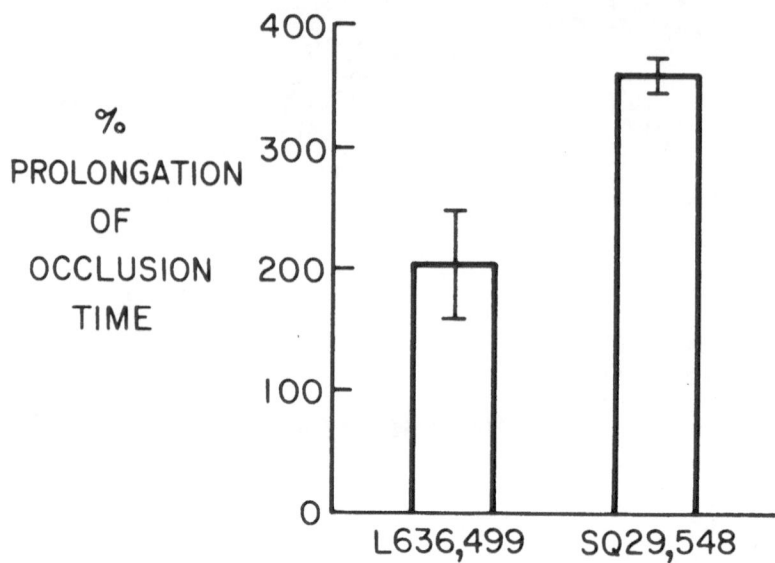

Figure 6.3 Effect of two structurally distinct thromboxane A_2/prostaglandin endoperoxide receptor antagonists, L636,499 and SQ29,548, on the time to coronary occlusion in the canine model of coronary thrombosis following electrically-induced endothelial injury

of prostacyclin may offset the platelet-inhibitory effect of decreased thromboxane A_2 formation[66]. Aiken and co-workers[64] have demonstrated that inhibition of platelet thrombosis at a critical stenosis in the canine coronary artery by a thromboxane synthase inhibitor is reversed by local inhibition of prostacyclin formation[64]. Consistent with these findings, we have demonstrated that addition of a thromboxane synthase inhibitor (U 63,557 A) enhanced the inhibitory effects of a thromboxane A_2/prostaglandin endoperoxide receptor antagonist (L 636,499) in a chronic canine model of coronary thrombosis[67] and that this effect was reversed by aspirin (Figure 6.4). Furthermore, addition of U 63,557 A was associated with an increase in prostacyclin generation during induction of coronary thrombosis coincident with inhibition of thromboxane A_2 biosynthesis[67] (Figure 6.5). This is consistent with the hypothesis that, in the presence of a thromboxane synthase inhibitor, platelet-derived prostaglandin endoperoxides are metabolized by vascular endothelium to prostacyclin, which in turn inhibits platelet aggregation. Thus, even a modest increase in prostacyclin biosynthesis may modulate platelet activity *in vivo*.

A similar interaction between a thromboxane synthase inhibitor and a thromboxane A_2/prostaglandin endoperoxide receptor antagonist on bleeding time suggests that endogenous prostacyclin also plays a platelet regulatory role in man[68]. Consistent with such a role, prostacyclin biosynthesis, measured as excretion of its urinary metabolite, 2,3-dinor-6-keto-prostaglandin $F_{1\alpha}$, is increased in a variety of clinical states associated with platelet activation, including unstable angina[69], atherosclerosis[70] and systemic sclerosis[71], possibly as a compensatory response which limits platelet activation *in vivo*.

134

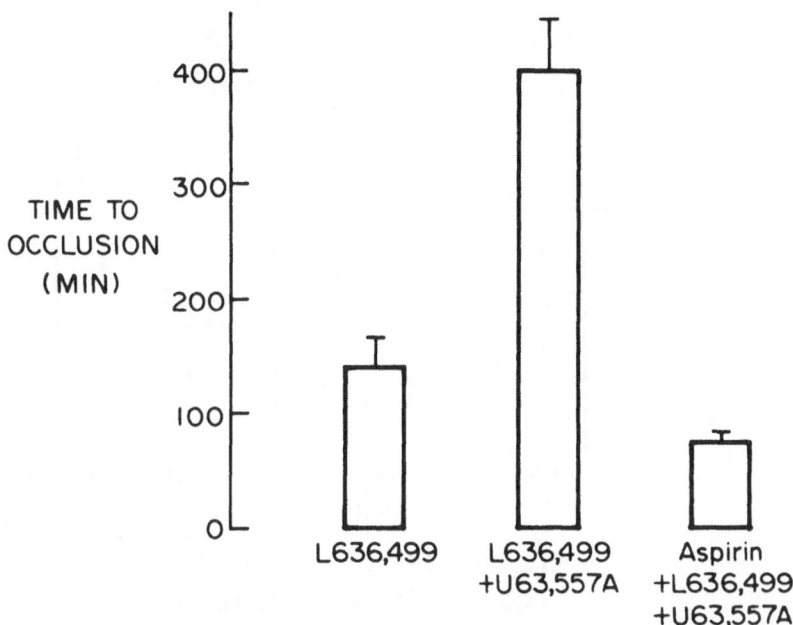

Figure 6.4 Effect of aspirin, 20 mg kg^{-1}, on the response to a combination of a thromboxane A$_2$/prostaglandin endoperoxide receptor antagonist (L 636,499, 20 mg kg^{-1} + 2 mg kg^{-1} min^{-1}) and a thromboxane synthase inhibitor (U63,557 A, 10 mg kg^{-1}) in the chronic canine model of coronary thrombosis. The time to occlusion in controls and in dogs treated with U63,557 A was 81 ± 13 and 112 ± 26 min respectively. The enhanced effect of the combination therapy over the thromboxane A$_2$/prostaglandin endoperoxide receptor antagonist alone was prevented by pretreatment with aspirin

PROSTAGLANDINS IN MYOCARDIAL ISCHAEMIA AND INJURY

Stable angina pectoris

Myocardial ischaemia in patients with stable angina pectoris is thought to reflect inadequate flow through a fixed coronary stenosis. However, variability in the workload required to induce ischaemia suggests that there may also be a dynamic element[72]. In a canine model of a fixed coronary stenosis, spontaneous fluctuations in coronary flow occur and are platelet mediated[73]. These fluctuations can be enhanced by increased heart rate[74] or by infusion of epinephrine[75]. Thus, platelet activation may modulate flow through a severe coronary stenosis. It has also been reported that exercise- and pacing-induced ischaemia in patients with stable coronary artery disease results in platelet activation and an increase in thromboxane B$_2$ concentration in coronary sinus blood[76–78]. Indeed, some studies have shown that the time to exercise- and pacing-induced ischaemia can be increased by cyclo-oxygenase and thromboxane synthase inhibition[79]. These studies suggest, therefore, that platelet activation and increased thromboxane A$_2$ biosynthesis may play a role in mediating stress-related myocardial ischaemia.

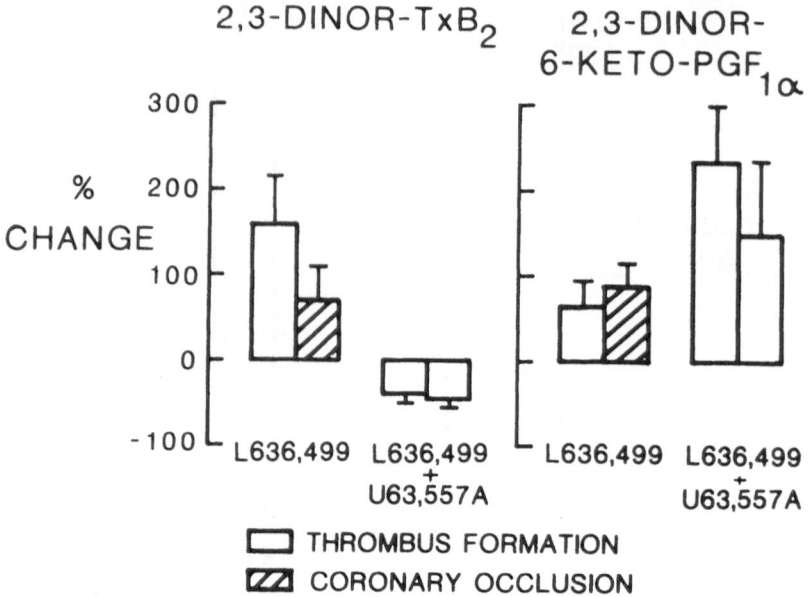

Figure 6.5 Percent change in thromboxane A$_2$ and prostacyclin biosynthesis, measured as excretion of their urinary metabolites, 2,3-dinor-thromboxane (Tx) B$_2$ and 2,3-dinor-6-keto-prostaglandin (PG) F$_{1\alpha}$ respectively, in response to a thromboxane A$_2$/prostaglandin endoperoxide receptor antagonist (L636,499) alone and in combination with a thromboxane synthase inhibitor (U63,557A) in the chronic canine model of coronary thrombosis. (Note that occlusion did not occur in dogs treated with the combination therapy)

Studies in the isolated perfused heart[80] and during pacing[6] and coronary bypass[81] in man suggest that ischaemia also induces an increase in prostacyclin biosynthesis which may, in part, mediate the vasodilator response to this stimulus[82]. It has been further reported that the increase in prostacyclin formation in response to ischaemia is depressed in patients with coronary atherosclerosis and that this may play a role in the pathogenesis of angina pectoris[83]. However, the samples, frequently obtained by cardiac catheters in these studies, are likely to be artifactually elevated, confounding interpretation of the data. In addition, cyclo-oxygenase inhibitors may exert a direct vasoconstrictor effect which may be incorrectly attributed to inhibition of prostaglandin biosynthesis[84]. We have determined thromboxane A$_2$ and prostacyclin biosynthesis during exercise-induced myocardial ischaemia in patients with stable coronary artery disease by measurement of their urinary enzymatic metabolites and by measurement of 11-dehydro-thromboxane B$_2$, the most abundant enzymatic metabolite of thromboxane B$_2$ in plasma[69]. Despite electrocardiographic and clinical evidence of ischaemia, there was no alteration in thromboxane A$_2$ or prostacyclin biosynthesis (Figure 6.6). These findings suggest that prostacyclin and thromboxane A$_2$ do not play a role in the pathogenesis of stable angina pectoris. This is further supported by the failure of a thromboxane A$_2$/prostaglandin endoperoxide receptor antagonist to alter the time to exercise-induced ischaemia in patients with stable angina[85].

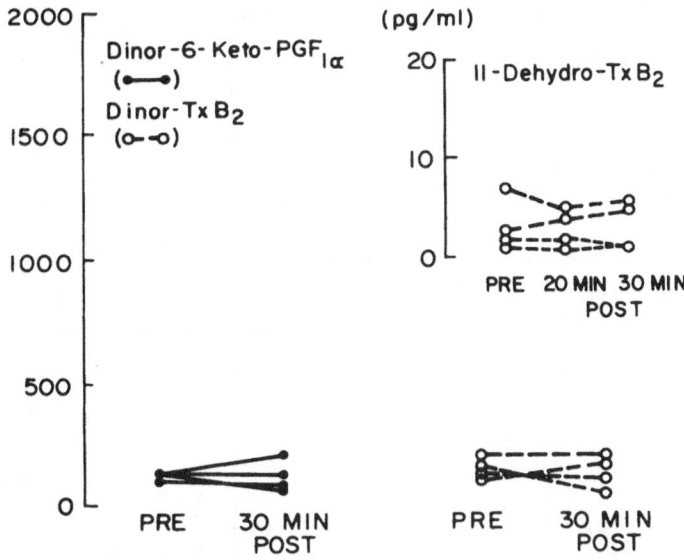

Figure 6.6   Urinary 2,3-dinor-thromboxane (Tx) B_2 and 2,3-dinor-6-keto-prostaglandin (PG) $F_{1\alpha}$ and plasma 11-dehydro-TxB$_2$ (inset) before and following exercise-induced myocardial ischaemia in patients with stable coronary artery disease

Unstable angina

Unstable angina is a condition characterized by spontaneous episodes of myocardial ischaemia in the presence of underlying coronary artery disease and by a high incidence of acute myocardial infarction. Arteriographic and angioscopic evidence suggests that coronary thrombosis is a frequent occurrence in this disease[86–88], as it is in acute myocardial infarction[89]. Indeed, unstable angina and myocardial infarction may represent different clinical presentations of the same underlying pathological process[90]. Detailed histological studies have demonstrated layers of platelet thrombi at the site of active coronary disease in patients with unstable angina preceding death[91]. These studies suggest that periodic platelet activation occurs in unstable angina which, in turn, may result in coronary occlusion, either by formation of an occlusive thrombus or by the release of vasoactive compounds by platelets.

Two clinical studies have demonstrated that aspirin reduces the incidence of myocardial infarction and death by up to 50% in patients with unstable angina, suggesting an important role for thromboxane A_2 in their occurrence[92,93]. Whether platelet activation and thromboxane A_2 also play a role in the episodic ischaemia of unstable angina is unknown. Evidence of platelet activation[94] in patients with unstable angina based on plasma levels of platelet granule proteins, such as β-thromboglobulin and platelet factor 4, is difficult to interpret since such measurements are highly sensitive to *ex vivo* platelet activation[95]. Similarly, studies[1,2] of thromboxane A_2 biosynthesis have been

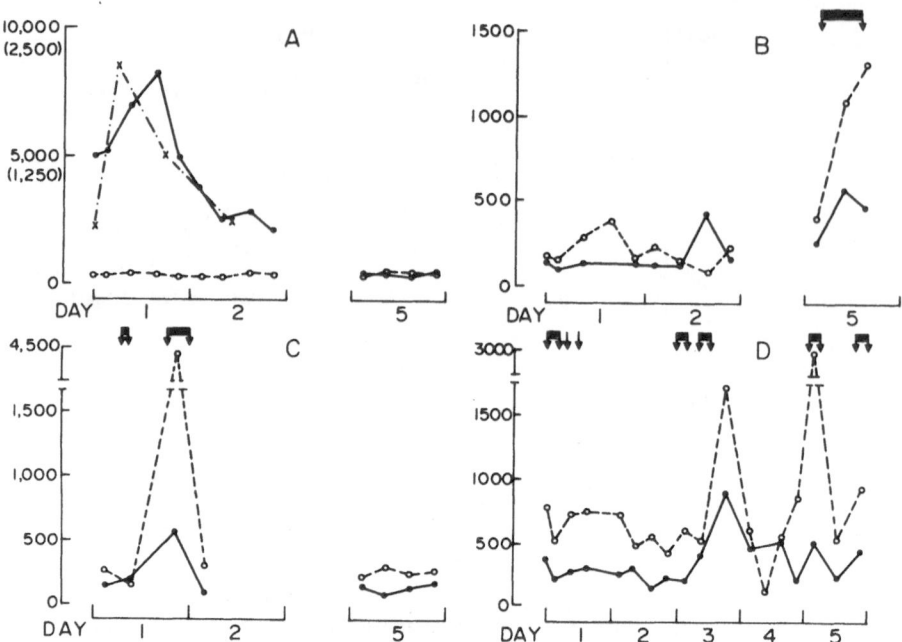

Figure 6.7 Urinary 2,3-dinor-thromboxane (Tx) A_2 (O—O) and 2,3-dinor-6-keto-prosta-glandin (PG) $F_{1\alpha}$ (●—●) in 6 h urine aliquots (expressed in pg/mg creatinine) over 5 days in a patient admitted with acute myocardial infarction (A) and in three patients with unstable angina (B, C and D). Episodes of persistent or recurrent chest pain are indicated by the arrowheads and solid areas above each panel. Total plasma CPK (X—X) is also shown in panel A with the scale (units/ml) shown on the y-axis in parentheses

largely based on measurements of plasma thromboxane B_2 and are confounded by methodological problems and the use of inadequate controls. We have demonstrated episodic increases in thromboxane A_2 and prostacyclin biosynthesis, often coincident with episodes of chest pain, in patients with unstable angina[69] (Figure 6.7). As platelets are the major source of thromboxane A_2 in man, this increase probably reflects episodic platelet activation. Supporting this interpretation, urinary 2,3-dinor-thromboxane B_2 is more frequently increased in cases of unstable angina with angiographic evidence of coronary thrombosis[96]. Interestingly, only 50% of the increases in thromboxane A_2 in patients with unstable angina were associated with chest pain, suggesting that platelet activation did not always induce coronary occlusion[69]. Alternatively, these episodes may have been associated with silent ischaemia, since 50% of ischaemic episodes detected electrocardiographically in patients with unstable angina are not associated with chest pain[97].

Despite the increase in thromboxane A_2 biosynthesis during episodes of ischaemia, aspirin does not appear to alter the frequency of chest pain in patients with unstable angina[92,98]. This might suggest that platelet activation does not play a role in the pathogenesis of these spontaneous ischaemic episodes or that they are not thromboxane A_2 dependent. However, since unstable angina tends to resolve spontaneously[99] and as the use of antianginal therapy was unrestricted in this study, it is difficult to interpret the effect of aspirin on chest pain. Furthermore, prostacyclin biosynthesis increases coincident with an increase in thromboxane A_2 in patients with unstable angina[69,96], suggesting that prostacyclin may also modulate platelet activation in this disease. Thus, failure to alter the frequency of chest pain with aspirin does not exclude a role for thromboxane A_2 since coincident inhibition of prostacyclin biosynthesis would have occurred at the doses used[23]. If prostacyclin does exert a platelet-inhibitory effect, theoretically it should be possible to achieve a greater clinical response with lower, more selective doses of aspirin.

Acute myocardial infarction

Acute myocardial infarction results in nearly all cases from thrombotic occlusion of the coronary artery at a point of atherosclerotic narrowing[89]. Histological studies have demonstrated that the thrombus is largely composed of platelets at its point of attachment to the vessel wall[100], suggesting that platelet activation is the initiating event. In addition, the endothelium is frequently disrupted with haemorrhage from the lumen into the atherosclerotic plaque[101]. Thus, coronary thrombosis may result from platelet activation by exposed subendothelial collagen and subsequent formation of a fibrin clot.

The role of prostaglandins in mediating platelet activation in acute coronary thrombosis is uncertain. Studies in animal models have demonstrated thromboxane A_2/prostaglandin endoperoxide-mediated platelet activation during coronary thrombosis[55,56]. We have demonstrated an increase in thromboxane A_2 biosynthesis in patients admitted with acute myocardial infarction and immediately prior to infarction in a patient with unstable angina[69] (Figure 6.8). A number of clinical studies have examined the effects of aspirin in the prevention of myocardial infarction and death. As discussed above, two studies have demonstrated a marked effect in patients with unstable angina[92,93]. These findings are consistent with a role for thromboxane A_2 in the pathogenesis of acute myocardial infarction. Despite this, studies in patients with a history of prior myocardial infarction and stable coronary artery disease have not demonstrated a significant effect[102-107]. This apparent paradox may be explained in part by the differences in event rates in the two groups. The incidence of myocardial infarction in patients with unstable angina is 10% over the 3–6 months following presentation[92,93]. In contrast, the incidence is considerably lower (about 4% annually), in stable patients so that large numbers of patients are required to demonstrate an effect. Indeed, meta-analysis of the combined data from studies on the secondary prevention of myocardial infarction shows a significant 16% reduction in event rates by aspirin[108].

A second, potentially confounding, factor is that, at the doses of aspirin used, prostacyclin biosynthesis is markedly depressed[23]. Whether prostacyclin limits platelet activation in this disease is not known. However, prostacyclin

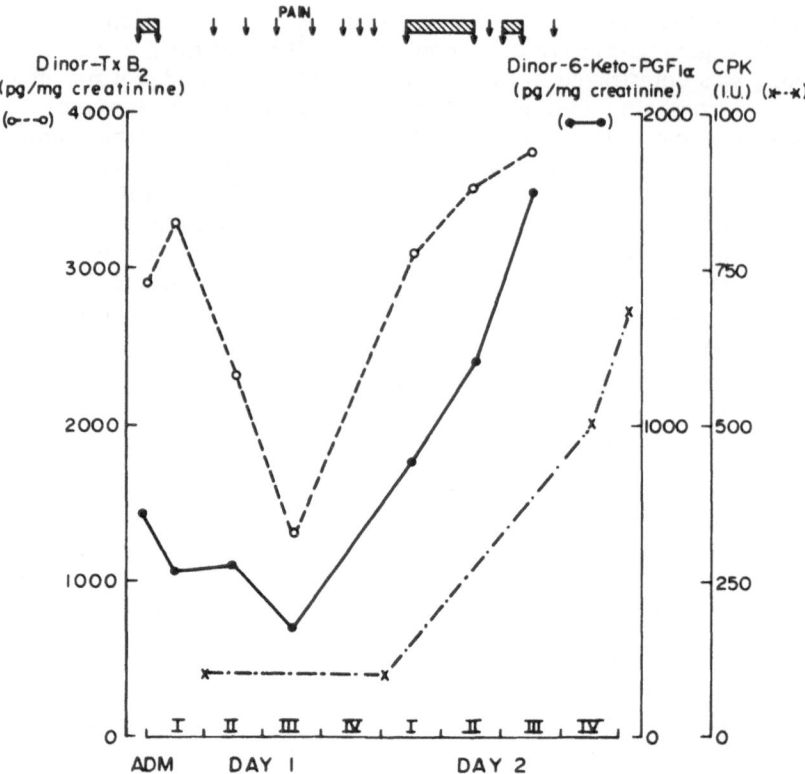

Figure 6.8 Urinary, 2,3-dinor-thromboxane (Tx) B_2 (normal < 350 pg/mg creatinine) and 2,3-dinor-6-keto-prostaglandin (PG) $F_{1\alpha}$ (normal < 220 pg/mg creatinine) in 6 h urine aliquots over 2 days in a patient admitted with unstable angina who subsequently developed an acute myocardial infarction

biosynthesis was found to increase coincident with the rise in thromboxane A_2 formation early in acute myocardial infarction[69] (Figure 6.8) and has been shown to modulate platelet activity in animal models of coronary thrombosis[64,67]. Thus, as discussed for unstable angina, at the doses used, the beneficial effect of aspirin in acute myocardial infarction may have been obscured by a reduction in prostacyclin biosynthesis. Interestingly, a greater reduction in the incidence of myocardial infarction and death with aspirin was seen in the Veterans Administration Co-operative Study in unstable angina, in which the dose used was 325 mg daily[92], than in the Canadian study where the dose of aspirin was three times higher[93].

In addition to their effects on coronary thrombosis, prostaglandins may play a role in modulating the degree of tissue injury in acute myocardial infarction. Infusion of prostacyclin in the isolated perfused heart limits hypoxic injury independent of its effects on tissue perfusion or platelet function, suggesting that prostacyclin exerts a direct myoprotective effect[109]. Prostacyclin biosynthesis increases markedly following acute myocardial infarction in man and remains elevated for 48 h[69]. The increase in prostacyclin biosynthesis correlates with plasma CPK, suggesting that it reflects tissue injury[69]. The source of this increase is uncertain. Arachidonic acid is released from ischaemic myocardial cells both *in vitro* and *in vivo*[110,111]. Although myofibrils contain no prostaglandin synthase activity[40], released arachidonic acid may be metabolized by the cyclo-oxygenase of contiguous vascular tissue which persists in the infarct zone despite marked tissue necrosis. Indeed, cyclo-oxygenase activity increases in infarcted tissue in a canine model of coronary artery ligation[48]. Prostacyclin may also be generated from lymphocytes infiltrating the infarcted tissue, either directly or through release of interleukin-1, a potent stimulus of endothelial prostacyclin formation[112,113]. Whether prostacyclin, or any other prostaglandins generated in the infarct zone, exerts any physiological effects is unknown. Prostaglandin E_2 may be important in mediating the inflammatory response in infarcted tissue, increasing lymphocyte infiltration by increasing vascular permeability and flow in the coronary microcirculation[114]. Consistent with a role for prostaglandins in modulating tissue injury in the infarct zone, indomethacin, a potent cyclo-oxygenase inhibitor, increases infarct size[115,116] at doses which depress tissue cyclo-oxygenase activity, and may decrease scar formation in some animal models of myocardial infarction[117,118].

Thromboxane A_2 has also been shown to modulate myocardial infarct size in animal models independent of its effects on platelets. Thus, infusion of carbocyclic thromboxane A_2, a thromboxane A_2 mimetic with potent vasoconstrictor but little platelet activity, increased infarct size in an isolated perfused heart model[119]. The mechanism of this effect is uncertain, but it may reflect either a reduction in collateral circulation or direct cytotoxicity[119]. Following acute myocardial infarction in man, thromboxane A_2 formation is increased and remains elevated over the first 48 h[69]. The source of this increase is unknown but it may be derived from thrombus in a large epicardial artery or from platelets deposited in the infarct area[120]. Platelet aggregates have been demonstrated in the microcirculation of the infarct zone and this is probably the source of increased thromboxane A_2 formation in tissue homogenates of infarcted tissue[48]. A number of studies have suggested a functional role for thromboxane A_2 generated in the infarct-related circulation. Thus, some studies in animal models suggest that cyclo-oxygenase and thromboxane synthase inhibitors limit infarct size[121,122]. However, the results are variable, and, indeed, indomethacin has been reported to increase the loss of CPK from injured myocardium[115,116]. To some extent, this may reflect simultaneous inhibition of prostacyclin formation. Recent studies demonstrating a reduction in infarct size with specific thromboxane A_2/endoperoxide receptor antagonists in animal models of acute myocardial infarction are consistent with this hypothesis[123,124]. However, these findings need to be confirmed by evidence of long-term improvement in left ventricular function.

Thrombolytic therapy

The clinical response to intravenous thrombolytic therapy in patients with acute myocardial infarction is often limited by failure to reperfuse the occluded coronary artery, despite evidence of a systemic lytic effect[125,126]. Even in

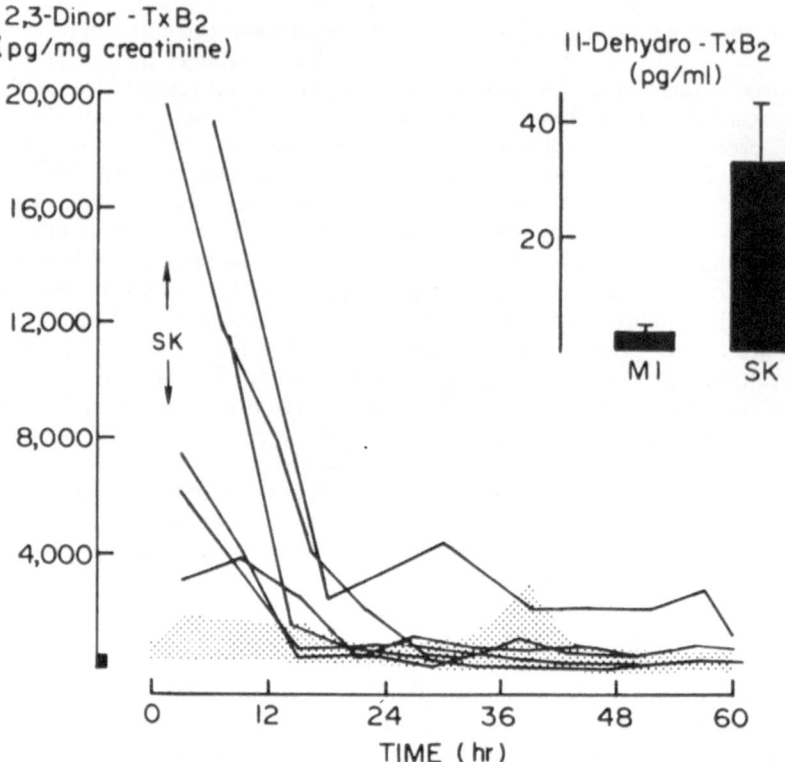

Figure 6.9 Urinary, 2,3-dinor-thromboxane (Tx) B_2 and plasma 11-dehydro-thromboxane B_2 (inset) following administration of streptokinase (SK), 750 000–1 500 000 units intravenously, in patients with acute myocardial infarction. The shaded area represents the range of urinary 2,3-dinor-thromboxane B_2 levels observed in patients with acute myocardial infarction not receiving thrombolytic therapy ($n = 12$). The solid area on the y-axis is the range in healthy volunteers. MI, myocardial infarction not receiving thrombolytic therapy

patients who reperfuse initially, the clinical outcome is often complicated by residual high-grade stenosis[127] and early reocclusion[128]. Evidence from studies in experimental animal models suggest that this may be due, in part, to platelet activation, since interventions which inhibit platelet function enhance the thrombolytic reponse to streptokinase[129] and prevent reocclusion[130]. We have demonstrated a marked increase in thromboxane A_2 metabolites in plasma and urine in patients with acute myocardial infarction who had received intravenous streptokinase[131] (Figure 6.9). This increase was inhibited by aspirin, demonstrating that it reflected de novo thromboxane A_2 biosynthesis and not metabolism of inactive thromboxane B_2 washed out from the coronary circulation. These findings suggest, therefore, that thrombolytic therapy with streptokinase results in marked platelet activation. We have also demonstrated increased thromboxane A_2 biosynthesis following thrombolysis with tissue plasminogen activator in a canine model of coronary thrombosis.

142

In this setting, platelet activation and thromboxane A_2 contribute to early reocclusion[132].

Increased thromboxane biosynthesis following thrombolytic therapy could reflect either a direct effect of the compounds on platelets or platelet activation secondary to thrombolysis and/or coronary reperfusion. Streptokinase enhances the platelet response to a range of platelet agonists *in vitro* at concentrations which are threshold for a fibrinogenolytic effect (Figure 6.10). Platelet activation may therefore occur at the doses used in acute myocardial infarction which are associated with profound systemic fibrinogenolysis[133]. This is further supported by an increase in *ex vivo* platelet activation in patients receiving thrombolytic therapy[134] and in a rabbit model of pulmonary embolism following administration of streptokinase[135]. The mechanism of this proaggregatory effect is unknown. Despite an increase in thromboxane A_2 formation coincident with streptokinase-induced platelet activation, inhibition

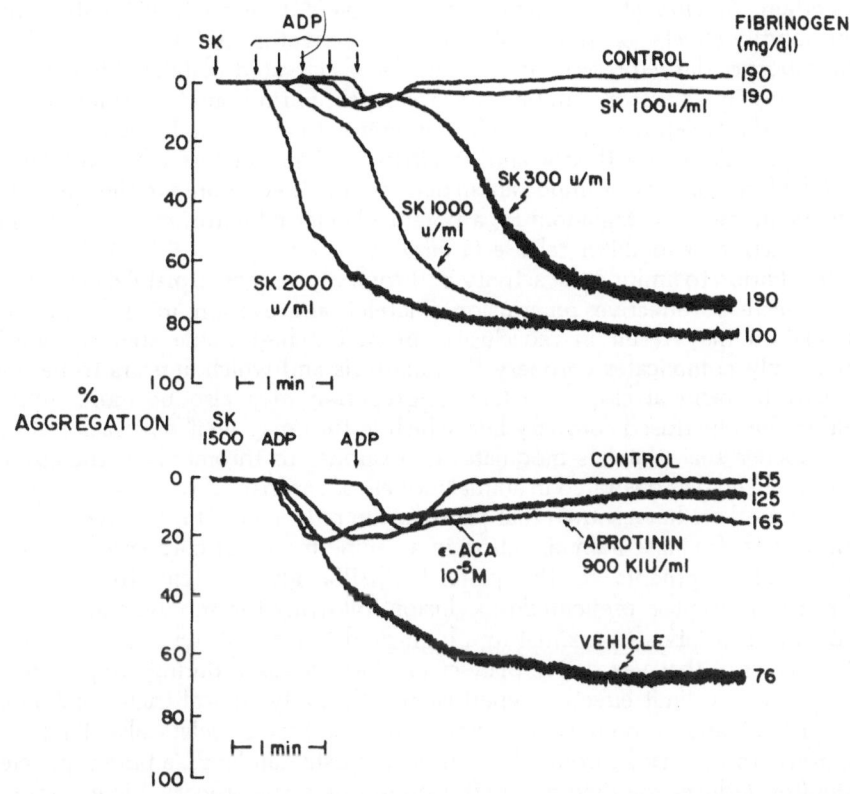

Figure 6.10 Effect of streptokinase (SK) on fibrinogen concentration and platelet aggregation induced by ADP in platelet-rich plasma. Platelets were incubated with streptokinase for 1 minute prior to the addition of ADP, $1 \mu mol\, L^{-1}$, and aggregation monitored by light transmission. Samples for fibrinogen were collected in aprotinin to prevent continued lysis. The fibrinogenolytic and proaggregatory effects of streptokinase were concentration dependent and were inhibited by aprotinin and ε-aminocaproic acid (ε-ACA)

of its formation with aspirin or antagonism of its effect with the thromboxane A_2/prostaglandin endoperoxide receptor antagonist, L 636,499, failed to inhibit platelet aggregation. Thus, release of thromboxane A_2 appears to be a secondary response. It is important to note, however, that such release *in vivo* may exert a physiological effect. Other possible mediators include plasmin, the active fibrinolytic enzyme formed by the action of the streptokinase–plasmin complex on plasminogen[136], and fibrinogen-degradation products, some of which are proaggregatory[137,138]. In addition, it is possible that the increase in platelet activation and thromboxane A_2 biosynthesis *in vivo* following thrombolytic therapy reflects mechanisms other than a direct effect on platelets. Thus, platelets may be activated by exposed subendothelial collagen at the site of the coronary lesion or in the ischaemic coronary bed following reperfusion, or by procoagulant systems on the clot surface[139].

The pathophysiological importance of increased platelet activation following thrombolytic therapy in patients with acute myocardial infarction is uncertain. *In vitro* studies demonstrate a role for platelets in limiting the fibrinolytic effects of tissue plasminogen activator and urokinase. Thus, thrombospondin expressed on the surface of activated platelets binds tissue plasminogen activator, limiting its access to fibrin-bound plasminogen[140]. Activated platelets also release a plasminogen activator inhibitor active against tissue plasminogen activator and urokinase[141]. Thus, factors which modulate platelet function may be important in determining the response to thrombolytic agents. Indeed, prostaglandin E_1, a potent platelet inhibitor, prevents plasminogen activator inhibitor release *in vitro*[141].

In addition to limiting the activity of thrombolytic agents, platelet activation may decrease effective reperfusion. Platelet aggregation in the coronary circulation may result in reocclusion or in the high-grade stenosis which commonly complicates coronary thrombolysis and which appears to be due in part to residual clot[142]. Platelet aggregation may also be more diffuse within the reperfused coronary bed which in turn may limit reperfusion flow.

Evidence that platelets modulate the response to thrombolytic therapy *in vivo* has been demonstrated in animal models of coronary thrombosis. Luchessi and co-workers have shown that prostacyclin reduced the time to reperfusion during streptokinase administration in a canine model of coronary thrombosis[129]. Fab fragments to the platelet IIb/IIIa glycoprotein, the putative fibrinogen receptor, prevented reocclusion following thrombolysis in a canine model of thrombosis proximal to a high-grade coronary stenosis[130]. There is also evidence that vasoactive platelet products released during streptokinase administration limit effective reperfusion[135,143]. Early clinical trials combining antiplatelet and thrombolytic therapy suggest that platelets also limit the response to coronary thrombolysis in man. Prostaglandin E_1, a potent platelet inhibitor, reduces the time to reperfusion during intracoronary administration of streptokinase and decreases the reocclusion rate and degree of residual stenosis in man[144]. Thus, eicosanoids may modulate the response to thrombolytic therapy through their effects on platelets. Prostaglandins may also exert a direct effect on clot lysis as there is evidence that prostacyclin increases endogenous tissue plasminogen activator formation[145].

144

As in acute myocardial infarction, prostaglandins and thromboxane A_2 may also determine the degree of tissue injury following coronary reperfusion, either by a direct effect on myocardial cells or by modulating reperfusion flow. The degree of myocardial damage is inversely related to tissue reflow[146]. Reperfusion flow is limited by platelet-derived vasoactive products, including thromboxane A_2, following thrombolysis in a rabbit model of pulmonary embolism[135] and a similar mechanism may explain the delay in normalization of pulmonary pressures following successful lysis of pulmonary emboli in man[143]. Whether this also occurs in the coronary circulation is unknown. Prostacyclin and prostaglandin E_2 may also play a role in modulating vascular tone, although their effects on vascular resistance in the reperfused coronary bed is uncertain. Studies in animal models and isolated perfused hearts suggest that endogenous prostaglandins may paradoxically enhance reperfusion injury[147]. Thus, cyclo-oxygenase inhibition improved the recovery of contractile function following reperfusion in an isolated rat heart model of ischaemia, an effect reversed by prostacyclin and by prostaglandin E_2[147]. However, contractile function following reperfusion was not correlated with prostacyclin formation, and prostacyclin has been shown to have a protective effect at higher doses in other models[148].

We have demonstrated increased prostacyclin biosynthesis in man following coronary thrombolysis with intravenous streptokinase[131]. This increase was closely related to the increase in thromboxane biosynthesis, consistent with the hypothesis that it reflected platelet activation. In contrast to the findings in acute myocardial infarction, the increase in prostacyclin biosynthesis declined rapidly despite electrocardiographic and biochemical evidence of evolving myocardial infarction. Thus, prostacyclin may not be generated in the reperfused coronary bed. Indeed, it is possible that formation of prostaglandins will be inhibited by reperfusion-induced endothelial injury[149]. Thus, the role of prostaglandins in modulating the degree of myocardial injury during reperfusion is uncertain.

Ventricular arrhythmias

Coronary artery disease is frequently associated with life-threatening ventricular arrhythmias, particularly in the setting of acute myocardial infarction and coronary reperfusion. The mechanism is unknown but prostaglandins have been suggested to play a role in their genesis. Pathological studies[150,151] have demonstrated coronary thrombosis and platelet microaggregates in the coronary circulation of victims of sudden cardiac death which is thought to result from ventricular arrhythmias. Sudden death can also be induced through a thromboxane A_2-dependent mechanism in a number of animal models following systemic administration of arachidonic acid[152] and by inducing platelet aggregate formation in the coronary circulation[153]. In addition, cyclical reductions in coronary blood flow induced by platelet activation at the site of a critical stenosis in the dog are accompanied by reduction in ventricular fibrillation thresholds[154]. These findings suggest a role for platelet activation in the development of ventricular arrhythmias.

145

A number of investigators have demonstrated that ventricular ectopy and fibrillation following coronary occlusion and reperfusion in animal models can be prevented by cyclo-oxygenase and thromboxane synthase inhibitors and by thromboxane A_2/prostaglandin endoperoxide receptor antagonists[155–158]. In addition, Coker and co-workers[159] correlated arrhythmia frequency with thromboxane A_2 biosynthesis during coronary ligation in dogs, suggesting that thromboxane A_2 released during acute myocardial infarction may be arrhythmogenic[159]. However, these measurements were based on radio-immunoassay of plasma thromboxane B_2 in open-chested animals and are therefore likely to be highly artifactual. Kramer et al.[160] failed to demonstrate any alteration, by three different thromboxane synthase inhibitors, in the inducibility of ventricular tachycardia or in regional conduction velocity in either the infarcted or non-infarcted zones. In addition, STA_2, a thromboxane A_2/prostaglandin endoperoxide mimetic had no electrophysiological effects on isolated ventricular tissue[160]. Furthermore, it has been suggested that the antiarrhythmic effect of thromboxane synthase inhibition is not mediated by inhibition of thromboxane A_2 formation but by increased prostacyclin biosynthesis since the antiarrhythmic effect is reversed by cyclo-oxygenase inhibition[161,162]. Therefore, it is uncertain whether thromboxane A_2 plays a role in ischaemia-related arrhythmias.

Prostacyclin has also been reported to exert an effect on ventricular arrhythmias, decreasing their frequency in a number of animal models of myocardial infarction and coronary reperfusion[163–165]. In contrast, PGE_2 has no effect[165]. The antiarrhythmic response to prostacyclin is dose dependent, a proarrhythmic effect occurring at higher doses due to hypotension and a reflex increase in sympathetic activity[166]. The mechanism of the antiarrhythmic activity of prostacyclin is unknown. Prostacyclin has been reported to have a variety of proarrhythmic electrophysiological effects in vitro, including an increase in the maximum rate of depolarization of the transmembrane action potential in isolated Purkinje fibres[167]. In addition, prostacyclin increases, and cyclo-oxygenase inhibitors decrease, the oscillatory afterpotentials induced by acetylstrophanthidin suggesting that prostacyclin mediates the proarrhythmic effects of this cardiac glycoside[168]. In contrast, prostacyclin inhibits digoxin-induced ventricular extrasystoles in the isolated perfused guinea pig heart[169]. Thus, the mechanism of the antiarrhythmic effects of prostacyclin is unclear and may reflect improved myocardial perfusion or a reduction in myocardial injury.

Percutaneous coronary angioplasty

Percutaneous transluminal angioplasty or balloon dilation of the coronary artery results in a dramatic clinical response in many patients. Long-term benefit, however, is dependent on the progression of the disease at the dilated site[170]. The factors which determine the rate of progression of the disease or the development of acute coronary occlusion are not known but pathological evidence of severe trauma with deposition of platelets and endothelial loss at the angioplasty site suggest that eicosanoids may be important[171,172].

Acute coronary occlusion at the time of angioplasty occurs for a number of reasons, including dissection of the vessel and mechanical obstruction by a raised tissue flap[173]. Coronary thrombosis also occurs, as demonstrated by the response to thrombolytic therapy[174] and by pathological studies[171]. Deposition of a layer of platelets at the angioplasty site has been demonstrated in animal models, including a rabbit model of atherosclerosis[175,176]. In addition, studies in man have shown increased uptake of radiolabelled platelets following angioplasty of the femoral artery[177] and multiple myocardial microinfarcts, consistent with platelet embolization, have been reported in a patient following coronary angioplasty[172]. Evidence that platelet activation plays a pathogenic role in acute coronary thrombosis following coronary angioplasty is supported by a preliminary study demonstrating a reduced incidence of acute occlusion in patients receiving intracoronary prostacyclin during the procedure[178]. Furthermore, there is evidence that the risk of coronary thrombosis is not reduced by anticoagulants alone[179]. What determines platelet activation at the angioplasty site is unknown. Experiments in a porcine model of carotid angioplasty failed to demonstrate an alteration in platelet deposition with low- or high-dose aspirin or with the thromboxane A_2/prostaglandin endoperoxide receptor antagonist, SQ 29,548[180]. In contrast, aspirin decreased the uptake of radiolabelled platelets at the angioplasty site in patients with femoral atherosclerosis, suggesting a role for thromboxane A_2 in mediating platelet deposition following angioplasty in man[177].

Coronary angioplasty may also be complicated by coronary vasospasm despite widespread routine pretreatment with calcium channel blockers and nitrates[181,182]. Experiments in animal models suggest an important role for prostacyclin derived from the vessel wall in limiting vasoconstriction of the coronary artery at the angioplasty site[183]. Thus, following angioplasty, the vessel wall demonstrates a decreased contractile response which is reversed by cyclo-oxygenase inhibition. Recent experiments in a porcine model demonstrate thromboxane A_2-mediated vasoconstriction distal to the angioplasty site, suggesting a role for thromboxane A_2 in modulating local vascular tone[58]. Whether the vasospasm which occurs at the time of the procedure[181] or which may supervene during the development of restenosis in man[182] is in part mediated by eicosanoids is unknown.

A more frequent complication is restenosis of the angioplasty site which occurs in 25–30% of patients over 6–9 months[170,184,185]. Pathological studies in patients with recurrence of symptoms are infrequent but demonstrate proliferation of fibroblasts and vascular smooth muscle cells overlying and distinct from the traumatized atherosclerotic plaque[186]. Similar lesions have been described in early atherosclerosis[187] and there is evidence to suggest a role for platelets in the development of such lesions[188], possibly through release of platelet-derived growth factors which stimulate fibroblast and vascular smooth muscle proliferation[189,190]. Thus, depletion or inhibition of platelets prevents the development of atherosclerosis in animal models[191] and aspirin inhibits the accelerated coronary atherosclerosis which occurs in cardiac transplant recipients[192]. Furthermore, restenosis is more frequent when there is evidence of a thrombus at the angioplasty site[193] consistent with previous data suggesting that progression of atherosclerotic lesions involves, at least in part, incorporation of thrombus into the vessel wall[194].

To date, there are no studies directly demonstrating a role for platelets or prostaglandins in the development of restenosis following angioplasty in man. However, King and co-workers demonstrated a trend towards a reduced incidence of restenosis in patients treated with aspirin[195]. There is also preliminary data suggesting that supplementing the diet with eicosapentaenoic acid (EPA), an analogue of arachidonic acid which acts as a substrate for cyclo-oxygenase, may prevent restenosis following angioplasty[196]. This may reflect inhibition of atherogenesis by EPA[197], the mechanism of which is unknown. Incorporation of EPA into the membrane phospholipids of platelets and other tissues and its subsequent release and metabolism during platelet activation may alter thromboxane A_2 and prostacyclin biosynthesis in man. Thus, EPA decreases thromboxane A_2 biosynthesis and is metabolized to thromboxane A_3 which is inactive against platelets. In contrast, prostacyclin biosynthesis is unaltered. Indeed, as the cyclo-oxygenase product of EPA (PGI_3) retains platelet-inhibitory activity and as formation of this eicosanoid is detected during dietary supplementation with EPA, prostacyclin biosynthesis is effectively increased[198]. Whether these changes in eicosanoid biosynthesis mediate the effect of EPA on the rate of restenosis following angioplasty or whether this reflects an independent effect of EPA on the vessel wall in unknown.

SUMMARY

Experimental evidence suggests that eicosanoids play a role in the pathogenesis of ischaemic heart disease through their effects on a variety of cell types. Thromboxane A_2 and prostacyclin exert potent effects on platelets which may initiate coronary thrombosis, an event common to a number of ischaemic heart disease syndromes. Platelets may also be important in atherogenesis, in the restenosis which commonly complicates coronary angioplasty and in limiting the response to thrombolytic therapy. Through their effects on vascular smooth muscle cells, eicosanoids may regulate coronary blood flow which may be an important determinant of myocardial injury. Eicosanoids may also influence myocardial cell survival by a direct effect on myofibrils or by modulating the inflammatory reponse to myocardial infarction. Thromboxane A_2 and prostacyclin have also been reported to play a role in the development of cardiac arrhythmias. The mechanism of this effect is uncertain since neither appear to exert direct electrophysiological effects. Consistent with a role for thromboxane A_2 and prostacyclin in ischaemic heart disease, formation of these eicosanoids is increased in a variety of unstable coronary syndromes in man. Furthermore, clinical trials with aspirin in unstable angina clearly demonstrate a role for thromboxane A_2 in the development of acute myocardial infarction in this disease. Whether eicosanoids exert the same broad spectrum of activity in human ischaemic heart disease as demonstrated in experimental studies is as yet unclear.

ACKNOWLEDGEMENTS

This work was supported by grants HL 40056 and HL 30400 from the National Institutes of Health. Dr D.J. Fitzgerald is a recipient of a Pharmaceutical Manufacturer's Foundation Faculty Development Award. Dr G.A. FitzGerald is an Established Investigator of the American Heart Association.

REFERENCES

1. Neri Serneri, G.G., Gensini, G.F., Abbate, R., Prisco, D., Rogasi, P.G., Laureano, R., Casolo, G.C., Fantini, F., Di Donato, M., Dabizzi, R.P. (1985). Abnormal cardiocoronary thromboxane A_2 production in patients with unstable angina. Am. Heart J., **109**, 732–738
2. Prosdocimi, M., Finesso, M., Gorio, A., Languino, L.R., Maschio, A.D., Castagnoli, M.N., De Gaetano, G. and Dejana, E. (1985). Coronary and systemic 6-ketoprostaglandin-$F_{1\alpha}$ and thromboxane B_2 during myocardial ischemia in the dog. Am. J. Physiol., **248**, H493–H499
3. de Boer, A.C., Turpie, A.G.G., Butt, R.W., Johnston, R.V. and Genton, G. (1982). Platelet release and thromboxane synthesis in symptomatic coronary artery disease. Circulation, **66**, 327–333
4. Walinsky, P., Smith, J.B., Lefer, A.M., Lebenthal, M., Urban, P., Greenspon, A. and Goldberg, S. (1984). Thromboxane A_2 in acute myocardial infarction. Am. Heart J., **108**, 868–872
5. Robertson, R.M., Robertson, D., Roberts, L.J., Maas, R.L., FitzGerald, G.A., Friesinger, G.C. and Oates, J.A. (1981). Thromboxane A_2 in vasotonic angina pectoris. Evidence from direct measurements and inhibitor trials. N. Engl. J. Med., **304**, 998–1003
6. Hirsh, P.D., Hills, L.D., Cambell, W.B., Firth, B.J. and Willerson, J.T. (1981). Release of prostaglandins and thromboxane into the coronary circulation in patients with ischemic heart disease. N. Engl. J. Med., **304**, 685–689
7. FitzGerald, G.A., Pedersen, A.K. and Patrono, C. (1983). Analysis of thromboxane and prostacyclin biosynthesis in cardiovascular disease. Circulation, **67**, 1174–1175
8. Catella, F., Healy, D., Lawson, J.A. and FitzGerald, G.A. (1986). 11-Dehydrothromboxane B_2: a quantitative index of thromboxane A_2 formation in the human circulation. Proc. Natl. Acad. Sci. USA, **83**, 5861–5865
9. Nicholls, A.B., Owen, J., Grossman, B.A., Marcella, J.J., Fleisher, L.N. and Lee, M.M.L. (1984). Effect of heparin bonding on catheter-induced fibrin formation and platelet activation. Circulation, **70**, 843–850
10. Bugiardini, R., Chierchia, S., Crea, F., Gallino, A., Wild, S., Roskovec, A. Lenzi, S. and Maseri, A. (1984). Evaluation of the effects of catheter sampling for the study of platelet behavior in the pulmonary and coronary circulation. Am. Heart J., **108**, 255–260
11. Schweer, H., Kammer, J. and Seyberth, H.W. (1985). Simultaneous determination of prostanoids in plasma by gas chromatography–negative ion chemical ionization–mass spectrometry. J. Chromatogr., **338**, 273–280
12. Roy, L., Knapp, H., Robertson, R.M. and FitzGerald, G.A. (1983). Endogenous biosynthesis of prostacyclin during catheterization and angiography in man. Circulation, **67**, 1174–1177
13. Fitzgerald, D.J., Fragetta, J. and FitzGerald, G.A. (1986). A chronic canine model of coronary thrombosis: minimization of artifactual increases in prostacyclin and thromboxane synthesis in vivo. Clin. Res., **34**, 298A
14. Blair, I.A., Barrow, S.E., Waddell, K.A., Lewis, P.J. and Dollery, C.T. (1982). Prostacyclin is not a circulating hormone in man. Prostaglandins, **23**, 579–589
15. Pederson, A.K., Watson, M. and FitzGerald, G.A. (1983). Inhibition of thromboxane synthase in serum: limitations of the measurement of immunoreactive 6-keto-$PGF_{1\alpha}$. Thrombosis Res., **33**, 99–103
16. Siess, W. and Dray, F. (1982). Very low levels of 6-keto-prostaglandin $F_{1\alpha}$ in human plasma. J. Lab. Clin. Med., **99**, 388–398

149

17. FitzGerald, G.A., Brash, A.R., Falardeau, P. and Oates, J.A. (1981). Estimated rate of prostacyclin secretion into the circulation in normal man. *J. Clin. Invest.*, **68**, 1272–1276
18. Lawson, J.A., Brash, A.R., Doran, J. and FitzGerald, G.A. (1985). Measurement of urinary 2,3-dinor-thromboxane B_2 and thromboxane B_2 using bonded-phase phenylboronic acid columns and capillary gas chromatography–negative-ion chemical ionization mass spectrometry. *Anal. Biochem.*, **150**, 463–470
19. Lawson, J.A., Patrono, C., Ciabottoni, G. and FitzGerald, G.A. (1986). Long lived enzymatic metabolites of thromboxane A_2 in the human circulation. *Anal. Biochem.*, **155**, 195–205
20. Patrono, C., Ciabattoni, G., Pugliese, F., Pierucci, A., Blair, I.A. and FitzGerald, G.A. (1986). Estimated rate of thromboxane secretion into the circulation of normal man. *J. Clin. Invest.*, **77**, 590–593
21. FitzGerald, G.A. and Sherry, S. (1982). The pharmacology and pharmacokinetics of platelet-active drugs under active clinical investigation. *Adv. Prostagl. Thrombox. Leuk. Res.*, **10**, 107–172
22. Patrignani, P., Filabozzi, P. and Patrono, C. (1982). Selective cumulative inhibition of platelet thromboxane production by low-dose aspirin in healthy subjects. *J. Clin. Invest.*, **69**, 1366–1372
23. FitzGerald, G.A., Oates, J.A., Hawiger, J., Maas, R.L., Roberts, L.J. and Brash, A.R. (1983). Endogenous synthesis of prostacyclin and thromboxane and platelet function during chronic aspirin administration in man. *J. Clin. Invest.*, **71**, 676–688
24. Fitzgerald, D.J., Mayo, G., Catella, F., Entman, S.S. and FitzGerald, G.A. (1987). Increased thromboxane biosynthesis in pregnancy largely derives from platelets. *Am. J. Obstet. Gynecol.*, **157**, 325–330
25. Reilly, I.A.G. and FitzGerald, G.A. (1987). Inhibition of thromboxane formation *in vivo* and *ex vivo*: implications for therapy with platelet inhibitor drugs. *Blood*, **69**, 180–187
26. FitzGerald, G.A., Reilly, I.A.G. and Pedersen, A.K. (1985). The biochemical pharmacology of thromboxane synthase inhibition in man. *Circulation*, **72**, 1194–1201
27. Pedersen, A.K. and FitzGerald, G.A. (1985). The human pharmacology of platelet inhibition. *Circulation*, **72**, 1164–1176
28. Reilly, I.A.G., Doran, J.B., Smith, B. and FitzGerald, G.A. (1986). Increased thromboxane biosynthesis in a human model of platelet activation: biochemical and functional consequences of selective inhibition of thromboxane synthase. *Circulation*, **73**, 1300–1309
29. Lorenz, R.L., Fischer, S., Wober, W., Wagner, H.A. and Weber, P.C. (1986). Effects on prostanoid formation and pharmacokinetics of dazmegrel (UK-38,485), a novel thromboxane synthase inhibitor, in man. *Biochem. Pharmacol.*, **35**, 761–766
30. Jeremy, J.Y., Mikhailidis, D.P. and Dandona, P. (1985). Thromboxane A_2 analog (U46619) stimulates vascular PGI_2 synthesis. *Eur. J. Pharmacol.*, **107**, 259–262
31. Schafer, A.I., Crawford, D.D. and Gimbrone, M.M. (1984). Unidirectional transfer of prostaglandin endoperoxides between platelets and endothelial cells. *J. Clin. Invest.*, **73**, 1105–1108
32. Marcus, A.J., Weksler, B.B., Jaffe, E.A. and Brockman, M.J. (1980). Synthesis of prostacyclin from platelet-derived endoperoxides by cultured human endothelial cells. *J. Clin. Invest.*, **66**, 979–986
33. FitzGerald, G.A., Fitzgerald, D.J., Lawson, J.A. and Murray, R. (1987). Thromboxane biosynthesis and antagonism in man. *Adv. Prostagl. Thrombox. Leuk. Res.*, **17**, 199–203
34. Armstrong, R.A., Jones, R.L., Leigh, P.J., MacDermot, J. and Wilson, N.H. (1986). Novel prostaglandin endoperoxide analogues which block thromboxane receptors and mimic prostacyclin. *Br. J. Pharmacol.*, **85**, 643p
35. Armstrong, R.A., Jones, R.L., Peesapati, V., Will, S.G. and Wilson, N.H. (1985). Competitive antagonism at thromboxane receptors in human platelets. *Br. J. Pharmacol.*, **84**, 595–607
36. Ogletree, M.L., Harris, D.N., Greenberg, R., Haslanger, M.F. and Nakane, M. (1985). Pharmacological actions of SQ 29,548, a novel selective thromboxane antagonist. *J. Pharmacol. Exp. Ther.*, **234**, 435–441
37. Carrier, R., Cragoe, E.J., Ethier, D., Ford-Hutchinson, A.W., Girard, Y., Hall, R.A., Hamel, P., Rokach, J., Share, N.N., Stone, C.A. and Yusko, P. (1984). Studies on L-640,035: a novel antagonist of contractile prostanoids in the lung. *Br. J. Pharmacol.* **82**, 389–396

38. Chan, C.C., Nathaniel, D.J., Yusko, P.J., Hall, R.A. and Ford-Hutchinson, A.W. (1984). Inhibition of prostanoid-mediated platelet aggregation *in vivo* and *in vitro* by 3 hydroxymethyl-dibenzo (b,f) thiepin 5,5-dioxide (L-640,035). *J. Pharmacol. Exp. Ther.*, **299**, 276–282

39. Hsueh, W. and Neddleman, P. (1978). Sites of lipase activation and prostaglandin synthesis in isolated and perfused rabbit hearts. *Prostaglandins*, **16**, 661–668

40. Gerristen, M.E. and Printz, M.P. (1981). Sites of prostaglandin synthesis in the bovine heart and isolated bovine coronary microvessels. *Circ. Res.*, **49**, 1152–1163

41. Silberbauer, K., Sinzinger, H. and Winter, M. (1978). Prostaglandin production by vascular smooth muscle cells. *Lancet*, **1**, 1356–1357

42. Ally, A.I. and Horrobin, D.F. (1980). Thromboxane B_2 in blood vessel walls and its physiological significance: relevance to thrombosis and hypertension. *Prostagl. Med.*, **4**, 431–438

43. Gerristen, M.E. and Cheli, C.D. (1983). Arachidonic acid and prostaglandin endoperoxide metabolism in isolated rabbit and coronary microvessels and isolated and cultivated coronary microvessel endothelial cells. *J. Clin. Invest.*, **72**, 1658–1671

44. Charo, I.F., Shak, S., Korasek, M.A., Davison, P.M. and Goldstein, I.M. (1984). Prostaglandin I_2 is not a major metabolite of arachidonic acid in cultured endothelial cells from human foreskin microvessels. *J. Clin. Invest.*, **74**, 914–919

45. Nowak, J., Kaijser, L. and Wennmalm, A. (1980). Cardiac synthesis of prostaglandins from arachidonic acid in man. *Prostagl. Med.*, **4**, 205–214

46. Wennmalm, A. and Ciabattoni, G. (1985). Adenosine-induced coronary release of prostacyclin at normal and low pH in isolated rabbit heart. *Br. J. Pharmacol.*, **85**, 557–563

47. Dedeskere, E.A.M., Nugteren, D.H. and Hoor, T. (1977). Prostacyclin is the major prostaglandin released from the isolated perfused rabbit and rat heart. *Nature (London)*, **268**, 160–163

48. McCluskey, E.R., Corr, P.B., Lee, B.I., Saffitz, J.E. and Needleman, P. (1982). The arachidonic acid metabolic capacity of myocardium is increased during healing of acute myocardial infarction. *Circ. Res.*, **51**, 743–750

49. Granstrom, E., Diczfalusy, U., Hamberg, M., Malmsten, C. and Samuelsson, B. (1982). Thromboxane A_2: biosynthesis and effect on platelets. *Adv. Prostagl. Thrombox. Leuk. Res.*, **10**, 15–57

50. Ginsburg, R., Bristow, M.R. Davis, K., Dibiase, A. and Billingham, M.E. (1984). Quantitative pharmacologic responses of normal and atherosclerotic isolated human epicardial coronary arteries. *Circulation*, **69**, 430–440

51. Silver, M.J., Hock, W., Kocsis, J.J., Ingerman, C.M. and Smith, J.B. (1974). Arachidonic acid causes sudden death in rabbits. *Science*, **138**, 1085–1087

52. Bhagwat, S.S., Hamann, W., Still, W.C., Bunting, S. and Fitzpatrick, F.A. (1985). Synthesis and structure of the platelet aggregation factor thromboxane A_2. *Nature (London)*, **315**, 511–513

53. Bunting, S., Buchanan, L.V. and Holzgrefe, H.H. (1987). The pharmacology of synthetic thromboxane A_2 on the coronary circulation of adult dogs and puppies. *Adv. Prostagl. Leuk. Res.*, **17**, 192–198

54. Hsueh-Hwa. W., Kulkarni, P.S. and Eakins, E.A. (1980). Effects of prostaglandins and thromboxane A_2 on the coronary circulation of adult dogs and puppies. *Eur. J. Pharmacol.*, **66**, 31–41

55. Fitzgerald, D.J., Doran, J., Jackson, E. and FitzGerald, G.A. (1986). Coronary vascular occlusion mediated via thromboxane A_2-prostaglandin endoperoxide receptor activation *in vivo*. *J. Clin. Invest.*, **77**, 496–502

56. Ashton, J.H., Ogletree, M.L., Taylor, A.L., Fitzgerald, C., Rakejo, S., Campbell, W.B., Buja, L.M. and Willerson, J.T. (1985). A thromboxane receptor antagonist, SQ 29,548, abolishes or attenuates cyclic flow variations in severely narrowed canine coronary arteries. *Circulation*, **72**, (Suppl III), III–69

57. Riess, H., Hofling, B., von Arnim, T. and Hiller, E. (1986). Thromboxane receptor blockade versus cyclooxygenase inhibition: antiplatelet effects in patients. *Thrombosis Res.*, **42**, 235–245

58. Lam, J.Y.T., Cheseboro, J.H., Steele, P.M. and Fuster, V. (1987). Is vasospasm related to platelet deposition? *In vivo* relationship in a pig model of arterial injury. *Circulation*, **75**, 342–348

59. Bunting, S., Gryglewski, R., Moncada, S. and Vane, J.R. (1976). Arterial walls generate from prostaglandin endoperoxides a substance (prostaglandin X) which relaxes strips of mesenteric and coeliac arteries and inhibits platelet aggregation. *Prostaglandins*, **12**, 897–913

60. Healy, D., Healy, C., Smith, B., Clanton, J. and FitzGerald, G.A. (1985). High dose aspirin promotes platelet deposition on vascular endotethelium *in vivo. Circulation*, **72**, 773A

61. Miyazaki, M., Yamamoto, M. and Toda, N. (1985). Interaction between non-steroidal antiinflammatory agents and sodium salicylate in the relaxant reponse of dog renal arteries to angiotensin II. *Arch. Int. Pharmacodyn. Ther.*, **274(2)**, 210–222

62. FitzGerald, G.A., Friedman, L.A., Miyamori, I., O'Grady, J. and Lewis, P.J. (1979). A double blind, placebo controlled, cross-over study of prostacyclin in man. *Life Sci.*, **25**, 665–672

63. Ganz, P., Gaspar, J., Colucci, W.S., Barry, W.H., Mudge, G.H. and Alexander, R.W. (1984). Effects of prostacyclin on coronary hemodynamics at rest and in response to cold pressor testing in patients with angina pectoris. *Am. J. Cardiol.*, **53**, 1500–1504

64. Aiken, J.W., Shebuski, R.J., Miller, O.V. and Gorman, R.R. (1981). Endogenous prostacyclin contributes to the efficacy of a thromboxane synthetase inhibitor for preventing coronary artery thrombosis. *J. Pharmacol. Exp. Ther.*, **219**, 299–308

65. Romson, J.L., Hook, B.G. and Luchessi, B.R. (1983). Potentiation of the antithrombotic effect of prostacyclin by simultaneous administration of aminophylline in a canine model of coronary artery thrombosis. *J. Pharmacol. Exp. Ther.*, **227**, 288–294

66. Wu, K.K., Chen, Y.C., Fordham, E., Ts'Ao, C.H., Rayudu, G. and Matayoshi, D. (1981). Differential effects of two doses of aspirin on platelet-vessel wall interaction *in vivo. J. Clin. Invest.* **68**, 382–387

67. Fitzgerald, D.J., Fragetta, J., Fenelon, L.C. and FitzGerald, G.A. (1987). Thromboxane synthase inhibition and thromboxane/endoperoxide receptor antagonism in a chronic canine model of coronary thrombosis. *Adv. Prostagl. Thrombox. Leuk. Res.*, **17**, 496–500

68. Gresele, P., Arnou, J., Deckmyn, H. and Vermylen, J. (1987). Endogenous antiaggregatory prostaglandins can contribute to inhibition of haemostasis: a pharmacological study *in vivo* in man. *Adv. Prostagl. Thrombox. Leuk. Res.* (In press)

69. Fitzgerald, D.J., Roy, L., Catella, F. and FitzGerald, G.A. (1986). Platelet activation in unstable coronary disease. *N. Engl. J. Med.*, **315**, 983–989

70. FitzGerald, G.A., Smith, B., Pedersen, A.K. and Brash, A.R. (1984). Prostacyclin biosynthesis is increased in patients with severe atherosclerosis and platelet activation. *N. Engl. J. Med.*, **310**, 1065–1068

71. Reilly, I.A.G., Roy, L. and FitzGerald, G.A. (1986). Biosynthesis of thromboxane in patients with systemic sclerosis. *Br. Med. J.*, **292**, 1037–1039

72. Hurst, J.W., King, S.B., Friesinger, G.C., Walter, P.F. and Morris, D.C. (1986). Atherosclerotic coronary heart disease: recognition, prognosis and treatment. In Hurst, J.W., Logue, R.B., Rackley, C.E., Schlant, R.C., Sonnenblick, E.H., Wallace, A.G. and Wenger, N.K. (eds.) *The Heart*, pp. 886–1008. (New York: McGraw-Hill Inc.)

73. Folts, J.D., Gallagher, K. and Rowe, G.G. (1982). Blood flow reductions in stenosed canine coronary arteries: vasospasm or platelet aggregation? *Circulation*, **65**, 248–255

74. Bertha, B.G. and Folts, J.D. (1984). Inhibition of epinephrine-exacerbated coronary thrombus formation by prostacyclin in the dog. *J. Lab. Clin. Med.*, **103**, 204–214

75. Walkinsky, P., Lefer, A.M., Frasca, P. and Santamore, W. (1984). Potentiation of coronary vascular platelet adhesion by atrial pacing in the presence of arterial stenosis in dogs. *J. Am. Coll. Cardiol.*, **3**, 1252–1255

76. Laustiola, K., Seppala, E., Nikkari, T. and Vapaatalo, H. (1984). Exercise-induced increase in plasma arachidonic acid and thromboxane B_2 in healthy men: effect of β-adrenergic blockade. *J. Cardiovasc. Pharmacol.*, **6**, 449–454

77. Mehta, J., Mehta, P., Feldman, R.L. and Horalek, C. (1984). Thromboxane release in coronary artery disease: spontaneous versus pacing-induced angina. *Am. Heart J.*, **107**, 286–292

78. Mogensen, K., Knudsen, J.B., Rasmussen, V., Kjoller, E. and Gormsen, J. (1985). Effect of specific thromboxane synthetase inhibition on thromboxane and prostaglandin synthesis in stable angina induced by exercise test. *Thrombosis Res.*, **37**, 259–266

79. Thaulow, E., Dale, J. and Myhre, E. (1984). Effect of a selective thromboxane synthetase inhibitor, dazoxiben, and of acetylsalicylic acid on myocardial ischemia in patients with coronary artery disease. *Am. J. Cardiol.*, **53**, 1255–1258

80. Edlund, A., Fredholm, B.B., Patrignani, P., Patrono, C., Wennmalm, M. and Wennmalm, A. (1983). Release of two vasodilators, adenosine and prostacyclin, from isolated rabbit hearts during controlled hypoxia. *J. Physiol.*, **340**, 487–501
81. Edlund, A., Bomfim, W., Kaijser, L., Olin, C., Patrono, C., Pinca, E. and Wennmalm, A. (1982). Cardiac formation of prostacyclin during cardioplegia in man. *Prostaglandins*, **24**, 5–19
82. Martin, J.L., Fisher, C.A., Untereker, W.J., Laskey, W.K., Hirshfield, J.W., Harken, A.H. and Addonizio, P.V. (1985). Effect of high dose aspirin on coronary hemodynamics during pacing induced myocardial ischemia. *J. Am. Coll. Cardiol.*, **5**, 210–215
83. Neri Serneri, G.G., Gensini, G.F., Abbate, R., Prisco, D., Rogasi, P.G., Castellani, S., Casolo, G.C. Fazi, A., Fantini, F., Di Donato, M. and Dabizzi, R.P. (1986). Impaired cardiac PGI_2 and PGE_2 biosynthesis in patients with angina pectoris. *Am. Heart J.*, **112**, 472–478
84. Edlund, A., Berglund, B. van Dorne, D., Kaijser, L., Nowak, J. Patrono, C., Sollevi, A. and Wennmalm, A. (1985). Coronary flow regulation in patients with ischemic heart disease: release of purines and prostacyclin and the effect of inhibitors of prostaglandin formation. *Circulation*, **71**, 1113–1120
85. Brittain, R.T., Boutal, L., Carter, M.C. *et al.* (1985). AH. 23848: a thromboxane receptor-blocking drug that can clarify the pathophysiological role of thromboxane A_2. *Circulation*, **72**, 1208–1218
86. Vetrovec, G.W., Leinbach, R.C., Gold, H.K. and Cowley, M.J. (1982). Intracoronary thrombolysis in syndromes of unstable ischemia: angiographic and clinical results. *Am. Heart J.*, **104**, 946–952
87. Mandelkorn, J.B., Wolf, N.M., Singh, S., Schecter, J.A., Kersch, R.I., Rodgers, D.M., Workman, M.B., Bentivoglio, L.G., LaPorte, S.M. and Meister, S.G. (1983). Intracoronary thrombus in nontransmural myocardial infarction and in unstable angina pectoris. *Am. J. Cardiol.*, **52**, 1–6
88. Sherman, C.T., Litvack, F., Grundfest, W., Lee, M.E., Chaux, A., Kass, R., Swan, H.J.C., Matloff, J. and Forrester, J.S. (1986). Coronary angioscopy in patients with unstable angina. *N. Engl. J. Med.*, **315**, 913–919
89. DeWood, M.A., Spores, J., Notske, M.D., Mouser, L.T., Burroughs, R., Golden, M.S. and Long, H.T. (1980). Prevalence of total coronary occlusion during the early hours of transmural myocardial infarction. *N. Engl. J. Med.*, **303**, 897–902
90. Ambrose, J.A. Winters, S.L., Arora, R.R., Haft, J.I., Goldstein, J., Rentrop, K.P., Gorlin, R. and Fuster, V. (1985). Coronary angiographic morphology in myocardial infarction: a link between the pathogenesis of unstable angina and myocardial infarction. *J. Am. Coll. Cardiol.*, **6**, 1233–1238
91. Falk, E. (1985). Unstable angina with fatal outcome: dynamic coronary thrombosis leading to infarction and/or sudden death. *Circulation*, **71**, 699–708
92. Lewis, H.D., Davis, J.W., Archibald, D.G., Steinke, W.E., Smitherman, T.C., Doherty, J.E., Schnaper, H.W., LeWinter, M.M., Linares, E., Pouget, J.M. Sabharwal, S.C., Chester, E. and DeMots, H. (1983). Protective effect of aspirin against acute myocardial infarction and death in men with unstable angina. *N. Engl. J. Med.*, **309**, 396–403
93. Carins, J.A., Gent, M., Singer, J., Finnie, K.J., Froggat, C.M., Holder, D.A., Jablonsky, G., Kostuk, W.J., Melendez, L.J., Myers, M.G.G., Sackett, D.L., Sealey, B.J. and Tanswer, P.H. (1985). Aspirin, sulphinpyrazone, or both in unstable angina. *N. Engl. J. Med.*, **313**, 1369–1375
94. Sobel, M., Salzman, E.W. Davies, G.C., Handin, R.I., Sweeney, J., Ploetz, J. and Kurland, G. (1981). Circulating platelet products in unstable angina. *Circulation*, **63**, 300–306
95. Kaplan, K. and Owen, J. (1981). Plasma levels of β-thromboglobulin and platelet factor 4 as indices of platelet activation in vivo. *Blood*, **57**, 199–202
96. Hamm, C.W., Lrenz, R.L., Weber, P.C., Wober, W. and Kupper, W. (1986). Subgroups of patients with unstable angina identified by biochemical evidence of thrombus formation. *Circulation (Suppl. II)*, **74**, II–305
97. Gottlieb, S.O., Weisfeldt, M.L., Ouyang, P., Mellits, E.D. and Lerstenblith, G. (1986). Silent ischemia as a marker for early unfavorable outcomes in patients with unstable angina. *N. Engl. J. Med.*, **31**, 1214–1219
98. Lewis, H.D., Davis, J.W. and Archibald, D.G. (1984). Aspirin and the risk of myocardial infarction. *N. Engl. J. Med.*, **310**, 122–123

99. Mulcahy, R., Daly, L., Graham, I., O'Donoghue, S., Owens, A., Ruane, P. and Tobin, G. (1981). Unstable angina: natural history and determinants of prognosis. *Am. J. Cardiol.*, **48**, 515–530

100. Sandritter, W. and Thomas, C. (1979). *Colour Atlas and Textbook of Histopathology*, pp. 75–76. (Chicago: Year Book Publishers)

101. Constantinides, P. (1970). The role of endothelial injury in arterial thrombosis and atherogenesis. *Adv. Cardiol.*, **4**, 67–71

102. Elwood, P.C., Cochrane, A.L., Burr, M.L., Sweetman, P.M., Williams, G., Welsby, E., Hughes, S.J. and Renton, R. (1974). A randomized controlled trial of acetylsalicylic in the secondary prevention of mortality from myocardial infarction. *Br. Med. J.*, **1**, 436–440

103. The Anturane Reinfarction Trial Research Group (1978). Sulphinpyrazone in the prevention of cardiac death after myocardial infarction. *N. Engl. J. Med.*, **298**, 289–295

104. Aspirin Myocardial Infarction Study Research Group (1980). A randomized controlled trial of aspirin in persons recovering from myocardial infarction. *J. Am. Med. Assoc.*, **243**, 661–665

105. The Persantine-Aspirin Reinfarction Study Group (1980). Persantine and aspirin in coronary heart disease. *Circulation*, **62**, 449–461

106. The EPSIM Research Group (1982). A controlled trial of aspirin or oral anticoagulation in prevention of death after myocardial infarction. *N. Engl. J. Med.*, **307**, 701–708

107. PARIS II Research Study Group (1986). Persantine-aspirin reinfarction study. Part II. Secondary prevention with persantine and aspirin. *J. Am. Coll. Cardiol.*, **7**, 251–269

108. Editorial (1980). Aspirin after myocardial infarction. *Lancet*, **1**, 1172–1173

109. Lefer, A.M., Ogletree, M.L., Smith, J.B., Silver, M.J., Nicolaou, K.C., Barnette, W.E. and Gasic, G. P. (1978). Prostacyclin: a potentially valuable agent for preserving myocardial tissue in acute myocardial ischemia. *Science*, **200**, 52–54

110. Chien, K.R., Sen, A., Reynolds, R., Chang, A., Kim, Y., Gunn, M.D., Buja, M. and Willerson, J.T. (1985). Release of arachidonic acid from membrane phospholipids in cultured neonatal rat myocardial cells during adenosine depletion. Correlation with the progression of cell injury. *J. Clin. Invest.*, **75**, 1770–1178

111. Chien, K.R., Han, A., Sen, A., Buja, M. and Willerson, J.T. (1984). Accumulation of unesterified arachidonic acid in ischemic canine myocardium. Relationship to a phosphatidylcholine deacylation-reacylation cycle and the depletion of membrane phospholipids. *Circ. Res.*, **54**, 313–322

112. Albrighton, C.R., Baenziger, N.L. and Needleman, P. (1985). Exaggerated human vascular cell prostaglandin biosynthesis mediated by monocytes: role of monokines and interleukin 1. *J. Immunol.*, **135**, 1872–1877

113. Montovani, A. and Dejana, E. (1987). Modulation of endothelial function by interleukin-1. A novel target for pharmacological intervention? *Biochem. Pharmacol.*, **36**, 301–305

114. Kaley, G., Hintz, T.H., Panzenbeck, M. and Messina, E.J. (1985). Role of prostaglandins in microcirculatory function. *Adv. Prostagl. Thrombox. Leuk. Res.*, **13**, 27–35

115. Kirmser, R., Berger, J.H., Cohen, L.S. and Wolfson, S. (1976). Effect of indomethacin, a prostaglandin inhibitor on epicardial ST-elevation and myocardial blood flow after coronary occlusion. *Circulation*, **54(Suppl II)**, II–194

116. Ingdott, B.I., Hutching, G.M., Bulkley, B.H. and Becker, L.C. (1979). Effect of indomethacin on collateral blood flow and infarct size in the conscious dog. *Circulation*, **59**, 734–743

117. Hammerman, H., Schoen, F.J. Braunwald, E. and Kloner, R.A. (1984). Drug-induced expansion of infarct: morphologic and functional correlations. *Circulation*, **69**, 611–617

118. Hammerman, H., Kloner, R., Schoen, F.J., Brown, E.J., Hale, S. and Braunwald, E. (1983). Indomethacin-induced scar thinning after experimental myocardial infarction. *Circulation*, **67**, 1290–1295

119. Smith, E.F., Lefer, A.M., Aharony, D., Smith, J.B., Magolda, R.L., Claremon, D. and Nicolaou, K.C. (1981). Carbocyclic thromboxane A$_2$: aggravation of myocardial ischemia by a new synthetic thromboxane A$_2$ analog. *Prostaglandins*, **21**, 443–456

120. Ruf, W., McNamara, J.J., Suehiro, A., Suehiro, G. and Wickline, S.A. (1980). Platelet trapping in myocardial infarct in baboons: therapeutic effect of aspirin. *Am. J. Cardiol.*, **46**, 405–412

121. Jugdutt, B.I., Hutchins, G.M., Bukkley, B.H. and Becker, L.C. (1980). Salvage of ischemic myocardium by ibuprofen during infarction in the conscious dog. *Am. J. Cardiol.*, **46**, 74–82

154

122. Hock, C.E. Phillips, G.R. and Lefer, A.M. (1985). Protective effect of thromboxane synthetase inhibitor in preventing extension of infarct size in acute myocardial infarction. *Prostagl. Leuk. Med.*, **17**, 339–346
123. Hock, C.E. Brezinski, M. and Lefer, A.M. (1986). Anti-ischemic actions of a new thromboxane receptor antagonist, SQ 29,548, in acute myocardial ischemia. *Eur. J. Pharmacol.*, **122**, 213–219
124. Brezinski, M.E., Yanagisawa, A. and Lefer, A.M. (1987). Cardioprotective effects of specific thromboxane receptor antagonist in acute myocardial ischemia. *J. Cardiovasc. Pharmacol.*, **9**, 65–71
125. TIMI Study Group (1985). The thrombolysis in myocardial infarction (TIMI) trial: phase 1 findings. *N. Engl. J. Med.*, **312**, 932–936
126. European Cooperative Study Group (1985). Randomized trial of intravenous recombinant tissue-type plasminogen activator versus intravenous streptokinase in acute myocardial infarction. *Lancet*, **1**, 842–847
127. Sheehan, F.H., Mathey, D.G., Schofer, J., Doge, H.T. and Bolson, E.L. (1985). Factors that determine recovery of left ventricular recovery after thrombolysis in patients with acute myocardial infarction. *Circulation*, **71**, 1121–1128
128. Harrison, D.G., Ferguson, D.W., Collins, S.M., Sherton, D.J., Ericksen, E.E., Kioschar, J.M., Marcus, M.L. and White, C.W. (1984). Rethrombosis after reperfusion with streptokinase: importance of geometry of residual lesions. *Circulation*, **69**, 991–999
129. Schumacher, W.A., Lee, E.C. and Luchessi, B.R. (1985). Augmentation of streptokinase-induced thrombolysis by heparin and prostacyclin. *J. Cardiovasc. Pharmacol.*, **7**, 739–746
130. Yasuda, T., Gold, H.K., Leinbach, R.C., Kanke, M., Fallon, J. Scudder, L.E. and Coller, B.S. (1986). A monoclonal anti-platelet antibody prevents acute coronary reocclusion (RO) following thrombolysis in dogs despite residual high-grade stenosis. *Clin. Res.*, **34**, 634A
131. Fitzgerald, D.J., Roy, L., Catella, F. and FitzGerald, G.A. (1987). Marked platelet activation in vivo after intravenous streptokinase in patients with acute myocardial infarction. *Circulation* (in press)
132. Fitzgerald, D.J., Wright, F. and FitzGerald, G.A. (1987). Platelet dependent reocclusion following coronary thrombolysis with tissue plasminogen activator. *Clin. Res.*, **35**, 278A
133. Mentzer, R.L., Budzynski, A.Z. and Sherry, S. (1986). High-dose, brief duration intravenous doses of streptokinase in acute myocardial infarction: description of effects in the circulation. *Am. J. Cardiol.*, **57**, 1220–1226
134. Griguer, P., Brochier, M., Leroy, J., Leclerc, M., Bertrand, A.H. and Chalons, F. (1980). Platelet aggregation after thrombolytic therapy. *Angiology*, **31**, 91–99
135. Gurewich, V. and Thomas, D.P. (1970). Streptokinase in acute pulmonary embolism. An experimental study. *J. Thorac. Cardiovasc. Surg.*, **59**, 655–661
136. Schafer, A.I., Maas, A.K., Ware, A., Johnson, P.C., Rittenhouse, S. and Salzman, E.W. (1986). Platelet protein phosphorylation, elevation of cytosolic calcium, and inositol phospholipid breakdown in platelet activation induced by plasmin. *J. Clin. Invest.*, **78**, 73–79
137. Larrieu, M.J., Rogollot, C. and Kubisz, P. (1970). Platelet aggregaton induced by soluble fibrin monomers. *Life Sci.*, **9**, 1111–1115
138. Barnhart, M.I., Cress, D.C., Henry, R.I. and Riddle, J.M. (1967). Influence of fibrinogen split products on platelets. *Thrombosis Diathes. Haemorrh.*, **17**, 78–98
139. Eisenberg, P.R., Sherman, L., Rich, M., Schwartz, D., Schecktman, K., Feltman, E.M., Sobel, B.E. and Jaffe, A.S. (1986). Importance of continued activation of thrombin reflected by fibrino-peptide A to the efficacy of thrombolysis. *J. Am. Coll. Cardiol.*, **7**, 1255–1262
140. Silverstein, R.L., Leung, L.K., Harpel, P.C. and Nachman, R.L. (1986). Platelet thrombospondin forms a trimolecular complex with plasminogen and histidine-rich glycoprotein. *J. Clin. Invest.*, **75**, 2065–2073
141. Erickson, L.A., Ginsberg, M.H. and Loskutoff, D.H. (1984). Detection and partial characterization of an inhibitor of plasminogen activator in human platelets. *J. Clin. Invest.*, **74**, 1465–1472
142. Brown, B.G., Gallery, C.A., Badger, R.S., Kennedy, J.W., Mathey, D., Bolson, E.L. and Dodge, H.T. (1986). Incomplete lysis of thrombus in the moderate underlying atherosclerotic lesion during intracoronary infusion of streptokinase for acute myocardial infarction: quantitative angiographic observations. *Circulation*, **73**, 653–661

155

143. Kerstein, M.D. and Adinolfi, M.G. (1986). Pulmonary dysfunction associated with streptokinase therapy. *Arch. Surg.*, **121**, 852–853
144. Sharma, B., Heineman, F., Wyeth, P., Kolath, G. and Gimenez, H. (1987). Alternative intracoronary prostaglandin E_1 and streptokinase infusion in acute myocardial infarction. *Clin. Res.*, **35**, 6A
145. Levin, R.I., Horpel, P.C., Weil, D., Chang, T. and Rifkin, D.B. (1984). Aspirin inhibits vascular plasminogen activator activity *in vivo*. Studies utilizing a new assay to quantify plasminogen activator activity. *J. Clin. Invest.*, **74**, 571–580
146. Buda, A.J., Gallagher, K.P., Wright, L.A. and Krause, L.C. (1986). Effect of critical stenosis on myocardial blood flow, ventricular function and infarct size following coronary reperfusion. *Circulation (Suppl. II)*, **74**, II–18
147. Karmazyn, M. (1986). Contribution of prostaglandins to reperfusion-induced ventricular failure in isolated rat hearts. *Am. J. Physiol.*, **251**, H133–140
148. Nayler, W.G. Purchase, M. and Dusting, G.J. (1984). Effect of prostacyclin infusion during low-flow ischemia in the isolated perfused rat heart. *Basic Res. Cardiol.*, **79**, 125–134
149. Van Bethuysen, K.M., McMurty, I.F. and Horwitz, L.D. (1987). Reperfusion of acute coronary occlusion in dogs impairs endothelium-dependent relaxation to acetylcholine and augments contractile reactivity *in vitro*. *J. Clin. Invest.*, **79**, 257–264
150. Haerem, J.W. (1972). Platelet aggregates in intramyocardial vessels of patients dying suddenly and unexpectedly of coronary artery disease. *Atherosclerosis*, **15**, 199–213
151. Davies, M.J. and Thomas, A. (1984). Thrombosis and acute coronary-artery lesions in sudden cardiac ischemic death. *N. Engl. J. Med.*, **310**, 1137–1140
152. Burke, S.E., Roth, D.M. and Lefer, A.M. (1983). Antagonism of platelet aggregation by 13-azaprostanoic acid in acute myocardial ischemia and sudden death. *Thrombosis Res.*, **29**, 473–488
153. El-Moraghi, N. and Genton, E. (1980). The relevance of platelet and fibrin thromboembolism of the coronary microcirculation, with special reference to sudden cardiac death. *Circulation*, **62**, 936–944
154. Kowey, P.R., Verrier, R.L., Lown, B. and Handin, R.I. (1983). Influence of intracoronary platelet aggregation on ventricular electrical properties during partial coronary artery stenosis. *Am. J. Cardiol.*, **51**, 596–602
155. Coker, S.J. and Parrott, J.R. (1983). Effects of dazoxiben on arrhythmias and ventricular fibrillation induced by coronary occlusion and reperfusion in anesthetized greyhounds. *Br. J. Clin. Pharmacol.*, **15**, 875–955
156. Coker, S.J., Ledingham, I.McA., Parratt, J.R. and Zeitlin, I.J. (1981). Aspirin inhibits the early myocardial release of thromboxane B_2 and ventricular ectopic activity following acute coronary occlusion in dogs. *Br. J. Pharmacol.*, **72**, 593–595
157. O'Conor, K.M., Friehling, T.D., Kelliher, G.J., McNab, M.W., Wetstein, L. and Kowey, P.R. (1986). Effect of thromboxane synthetase inhibition on vulnerability to ventricular arrhythmia following coronary occlusion. *Am. Heart J.*, **111**, 683–688
158. Coker, S.J. and Parratt, J.R. (1985). AH 23848, a thromboxane antagonist, suppresses ischaemia and reperfusion-induced arrhythmias in anaesthetized greyhounds. *Br. J. Pharmacol.*, **86**, 259–264
159. Coker, S.J., Parratt, J.R., Ledingham, I. McA. and Zeitlin, I.J. (1981). Thromboxane and prostacyclin release from ischemic myocardium in relation to arrhythmias. *Nature (London)*, **291**, 323–324
160. Kramer, J.B., Davis, A.G., Dean, R., McCluskey, E.R., Needleman, P. and Corr, P.B. (1985). Thromboxane A_2 does not contribute to arrhythmogenesis during evolving canine myocardial infarction. *J. Cardiovasc. Pharmacol.*, **7**, 1069–1076
161. Wehr, C.J., Hammon, J.W. and Oates, J.A. (1985). Prevention of ventricular fibrillation by thromboxane synthase inhibitors. *Circulation*, **72(Suppl. III)**, III–228
162. Huddleston, C.B., Lupinetti, F.M., Laws, K.M., Collins, J.C., Clanton, J.A., Hawiger, J.J., Oates, J.A. and Hammon, J.W. (1983). The effect of RO-22-4679, a thromboxane synthetase inhibitor, on ventricular fibrillation induced by coronary artery occlusion in conscious dogs. *Circ. Res.*, **52**, 608–613
163. Ribeiro, L.G.T., Brandon, T.A., Hopkins, D.G., Reduto, L.A., Taylor, A.A. and Miller, R.R. (1981). Prostacyclin in experimental myocardial ischemia: effects on hemodynamics, regional myocardial blood flow, infarct size and mortality. *Am. J. Cardiol.*, **47**, 835–840

164. Starnes, V.A., Primm, P.K., Woosley, R.L., Oates, J.A. and Hammon, J.W. (1982). Administration of prostacyclin prevents ventricular fibrillation following coronary occlusion in conscious dogs. *J. Cardiovasc. Pharmacol.*, **4**, 765–769

165. Au, T.L.S., Collins, G.A., Harvie, C.J. and Walker, M.J.A. (1979). The action of prostaglandin I_2 and prostaglandin E_2 on arrhythmias produced by coronary occlusion in the rat and dog. *Prostaglandins*, **18**, 707–720

166. Coker, S.J. and Parratt, J.R. (1983). Prostacyclin – antiarrhythmic or arrhythmogenic? Comparison of the effects of intravenous and intracoronary prostacyclin and ZK 36374 during coronary artery occlusion and reperfusion in anaesthetized greyhounds. *J. Cardiovasc. Pharmacol.*, **5**, 577–567

167. Kecskmeti, V. and Kelemen, K. (1984). Prostaglandins and the cardiac potential. *Prostaglandins*, **27 (Suppl.)**, 107

168. Moffat, M.P. Ferrier, G.R. and Karmazyn, M. (1986). A possible role of endogenous prostaglandins in the electrophysiological effects of acetylstrophanthidin on isolated canine ventricular tissues. *Circ. Res.*, **58**, 486–494

169. Metin, M., Dortlemez, O., Dortlmez, H., Akar, F., Ercan, Z.S. and Turker, R.K. (1984). Prevention by a carbacylin analogue (ZK 36,374) of digoxin-induced ventricular extrasystoles in guinea-pig myocardium. *Eur. J. Pharmacol.*, **98**, 125–128

170. Cowley, M.J. and Block, P.C. (1986). A review of the NHLBI PTCA registry data. In Jang, G.D. *Angioplasty*, pp. 368–378. (New York: McGraw Hill Book Co.)

171. Block, P.C., Myler, R.K., Stertzer, S. and Fallon, J.T. (1981). Morphology after transluminal angioplasty in human beings. *N. Engl. J. Med.*, **305**, 382–385

172. Waller, B., McManus, B.M., Gorfinkel, H.J., Kishel, J.C., Schmidt, E.C.H., Kent, K.M. and Roberts, W.C. (1983). Status of the major epicardial coronary arteries 80–150 days after percutaneous transluminal coronary angioplasty. Analysis of 3 necropsy patients. *Am. J. Cardiol.*, **51**, 82–84

173. Murphy, D.A. and Crover, G.M. (1986). Emergency bypass surgery of patients undergong percutaneous coronary angioplasty. In Jang, G.C. (ed.) *Angioplasty*, pp. 357–367. (New York: McGraw Hill Inc.)

174. Schofer, J., Krebber, H.J., Bleifeld, W. and Mathey, D.G. (1982). Acute coronary occlusion during percutaneous transluminal coronary angioplasty: reopening by intracoronary streptokinase before emergency coronary artery surgery to prevent myocardial infarction. *Circulation*, **66**, 1325–1331

175. Pasternak, R.C., Baughman, K.L., Fallon, J.T. and Block, P.C. (1980). Scanning electron microscopy after coronary transluminal angioplasty of normal canine coronary arteries. *Am. J. Cardiol.*, **45**, 591–597

176. Wilentz, J.R., Sanborn, T.A. Haudenschild, C.C., Valeri, R., Ryan, T.J. and Fanon, D.P. (1987). Platelet accumulation in experimental angioplasty: time course and relation to vascular injury. *Circulation*, **75**, 636–642

177. Cunningham, D.A., Kumar, B., Siegel, B.A., Toty, W.G. and Welch, M.J. (1984). Aspirin inhibition of platelet deposition at angioplasty sites: demonstration by platelet scintigraphy. *Radiology*, **151**, 487–490

178. Knudston, M.L., Dukk, H.J., Flintoft, V.F., Roth, D.L. and Hansen, H.L. (1986). Does short term prostacyclin administration lower the risk of restenosis after PTCA: a prospective randomized trial. *Circulation*, **74 (Suppl II)**, II–282

179. Zeitler, E. (1978). Drug treatment before and after percutaneous transluminal recanalization. In Zeitler, E., Gruentzig, A., Shoop, W. (eds.) *Percutaneous Vascular Recanalization. Technique, Application and Clinical Results*, pp. 120–5. (Berlin–Heidelberg–New York: Springer-Verlag)

180. Chesebro, H.J., Lam, J.Y.T. and Fuster, V. (1986). The pathogenesis and prevention of aortocoronary vein bypass graft occlusion and restenosis after arterial angioplasty: role of vascular injury and platelet thrombus deposition. *J. Am. Coll. Cardiol.*, **8**, 57B–66B

181. Bentivoglio, L.G., Leo, L.R., Wolk, N.M. and Meister, S.G. (1983). Frequency and importance of unprovoked coronary spasm in patients with angina pectoris undergoing percutaneous transluminal coronary angioplasty. *Am. J. Cardiol.*, **51**, 1068–1071

182. Hollman, J., Austin, G.E. Cruentzig, A.R., Douglas, J.S. and King, S.B. (1983). Coronary artery spasm at the site of angioplasty in the first two months after successful percutaneous transluminal coronary angioplasty. *J. Am. Coll. Cardiol.*, 1039–1045

183. Zollikofer, C.L., Cragg, A.H., Einzig, S., Castaneda-Auniga, W., Castaneda, F., Rysavy, J.A., Bruhlmann, W.F., Shebuski, R.J. and Amplatz, K. (1983). Prostaglandins and angioplasty. An experimental study in canine arteries. *Radiology*, **149**, 681–685
184. Holmes, D.R., Vlietstron, R.D., Smith, H.C. *et al.* (1984). Restenosis after percutaneous transluminal coronary angioplasty (PTCA): a report from the PTCA registry of the National Heart, Lung and Blood Institute. *Am. J. Cardiol.*, **53**, 77C–81C
185. Kent, K.M., Borow, R.O., Perins, D.R., Eivels, C.G., Lipson, L.C., McIntosh, C.L., Bacharach, S., Green, M. and Epstein, S.E. (1982). Improved myocardial function during exercise after successful percutaneous transluminal coronary angioplasty. *N. Engl. J. Med.*, **306**, 441–446
186. Austin, G.E., Ratcliff, N.B., Hollman, J., Tobei, S. and Phillipis, D.F. (1985). Intimal proliferation of smooth muscle cells as an explanation for recurrent coronary artery stenosis after percutaneous transluminal coronary angioplasty. *J. Am. Coll. Cardiol.*, **6**, 369–375
187. Thomas, W.A. and Kim, D.N. (1983). Atherosclerosis as a hyperplastic and/or noeplastic process. *Lab. Invest.*, **48**, 245–255
188. Niewiarowski, S. and Rao, A.K. (1983). Contribution of thrombogenic factors to the pathogenesis of atherosclerosis. *Prog. Cardiovasc. Dis.*, **26**, 197–222
189. Nilsson, J. (1986). Growth factors and the pathogenesis of atherosclerosis. *Atherosclerosis*, **62(3)**. 185–189
190. Chesterman, C.N. and Berndt, M.C. (1986). Platelet and vessel wall interaction and the genesis of atherosclerosis. *Clin. Haematol.*, **15(2)**, 323–353
191. Moore, S., Friedman, R.J., Singal, D.P., Souldie, J., Blagchman, M.A. and Roberts, R.S. (1976). Inhibition of injury-induced thromboatherosclerotic lesions by antiplatelet serum in rabbits. *Thrombosis. Diathes. Haemorrh.*, **35**, 70–81
192. Griepp, R.B., Stinson, E.B., Reber, B.A., Copeland, J.G., Oyer, P.E. and Shumway, N.E. (1977). Control of graft atherosclerosis in human heart transplant recipients. *Surgery*, **81**, 262–269
193. Gershony, G., Furman, M., Davis, E., Weintraub, W. and King, S. (1986). Predictors of restenosis after angioplasty in chronic total coronary occlusion. *Circulation*, **74** **(Suppl II)**, II–282
194. Duguid, J.B. (1948). Thrombosis as a factor in the pathogenesis of coronary atherosclerosis. *J. Pathol. Bacteriol.*, **58**, 207
195. Thornton, M.A., Gruentzig, A.R., Hollman, J. King, S.B. and Douglas, J.S. (1984). Coumadin and aspirin in the prevention of recurrence after transluminal coronary angioplasty: a randomized study. *Circulation*, **69**, 721–727
196. Schmitz, J.M., van den Berg, E.K., Prewitt, J.P., Malloy, C.R., Willerson, J.T. and Dehmer, G.J. (1987). Dietary supplementation with n-3 fatty acids may reduce the rate of restenosis after coronary angioplasty. *Clin. Res.*, **35**, 6A
197. Weiner, B.H., Ockene, I.S., Levine, P.H., Cunoud, H.F., Fisher, M., Johnson, B.F., Daoud, A.S., Jarmolych, J., Hosmer, D., Johnson, M.H., Natale, A. Vaudreuil, C. and Hoogasian, J.J. (1986). Inhibition of atherosclerosis by cod-liver oil in hyperlipidemic swine model. *N. Engl. J. Med.*, **315**, 841–846
198. Knapp, H.R., Reilly, I.A.G., Allesandrini, P. and FitzGerald, G.A. (1986). *In vivo* indexes of platelet and vascular function during fish oil administration in patients with atherosclerosis. *N. Engl. J. Med.*, **314**, 937–942

7
Prostanoids in clinical and experimental hypertension

A. Nasjletti and P. G. Baer

In 1965, Lee and co-workers reported the isolation from rabbit renal medulla of two vasodilator and blood pressure-lowering lipids with prostaglandin-like properties[1]. The vasodepressor lipids were subsequently identified as prostaglandins (PG) A_2 and E_2, and a role for prostanoids in blood pressure regulation was suggested[2]. Since that time, the concept that prostanoids contribute to determine the level of arterial blood pressure has gained strength with the demonstration that various prostanoids are capable of affecting the vascular and renal mechanisms involved in blood pressure control, that clinical and experimental hypertension are often accompanied by disturbances in prostanoid levels and/or metabolism by vascular and renal structures, and that treatment with inhibitors of prostanoid synthesis may cause blood pressure to increase or to decrease. It is now known that prostanoids participate in the implementation of both antihypertensive and prohypertensive mechanisms. This review discusses the relationships between prostanoids and blood pressure in normotensive and in hypertensive states.

CONTRIBUTION OF PROSTANOIDS TO THE VASCULAR AND RENAL MECHANISMS OF BLOOD PRESSURE CONTROL

The level of arterial blood pressure is a function of cardiac output and peripheral vascular resistance which, in turn, are determined by many factors working in an interrelated manner. Prostanoids are included among such factors as many members of this class of arachidonic acid metabolites have a demonstrated capacity to influence the vascular and renal mechanisms of blood pressure control.

Contribution of prostanoids to antihypertensive mechanisms

Several renal and vascular actions of PGE_2 and PGI_2 are consistent with their participation in the implementation of antihypertensive mechanisms. For example, PGE_2 and PGI_2 dilate resistance blood vessels[3], reduce the release of norepinephrine from sympathetic nerves[4], attenuate vascular reactivity to pressor hormones[5], and facilitate the excretion of sodium and water[6]. Accordingly, PGE_2 and PGI_2 may subserve antihypertensive processes by counteracting pressor mechanisms that bring about vasoconstriction and conservation of salt and water.

The concept that vasodilatory prostaglandins counteract vasoconstrictor systems was first advanced by McGiff and co-workers[7] who reported release of a prostaglandin-like substance into renal venous blood in response to renal arterial infusion of angiotensin II and noted that the release of prostaglandin was associated with waning of the angiotensin II-induced renal vasoconstriction. It is now known that pressor hormones, including angiotensin II, vasopressin and norepinephrine, stimulate the synthesis of vasodilatory prostanoids, PGE_2 and/or PGI_2, in many tissues[8-12]. It is also known that inhibition of prostaglandin synthesis by indomethacin or similarly acting drugs results in augmentation of the vasoconstrictor effect of angiotensin II in the kidney and heart[11,12], of vasopressin in the kidney[10], and of norepinephrine and/or sympathetic nerve stimulation in the splenic, renal, cutaneous, and mesenteric vasculatures[13-15]. That cyclo-oxygenase inhibitors augment the vasoconstrictor effects of angiotensin II, vasopressin and norepinephrine suggests that endogenous prostaglandins attenuate the vascular actions of such systems. Consistent with this interpretation, a growing body of evidence indicates that prostaglandins play a prominent role in maintenance of renal blood flow in a number of experimental and clinical conditions characterized by increased activity of pressor systems, such as renal ischaemia, hypovolaemia, sodium depletion, chronic liver disease and congestive heart failure[5,16].

Attenuation by endogenous prostaglandins of the vascular actions of pressor systems has a systemic expression, in that treatment with prostaglandin synthesis inhibitors results in magnification of the pressor effect of angiotensin II in animals[17] and normal subjects[18], subjects on a low-sodium diet[19], and patients with Bartter's syndrome[20]. Similarly, inhibition of prostaglandin synthesis increases pressor responsiveness to norepinephrine in patients with Bartter's syndrome[21], and in patients with chronic autonomic failure[22]. That the vasoconstrictor and/or pressor effects of angiotensin II, vasopressin, and norepinephrine are potentiated by inhibitors of prostaglandin synthesis is strong evidence that one or more vasodilatory prostanoids are instrumental in attenuating the vasoconstrictor and pressor effects of such agents. Therefore, vasodilatory prostanoids, such as PGE_2 and PGI_2, may subserve antihypertensive processes by counterbalancing pressor mechanisms that are implemented by the renin–angiotensin system, the sympathetic nervous system and vasopressin.

A role for prostanoids in counteracting salt-and-water conserving systems is suggested by reports that PGE_2 promotes the renal excretion of sodium and water and contributes to the phenomenon of pressure natriuresis. The evidence relating renal prostaglandins to the promotion of salt and water excretion has been reviewed elsewhere[6]. Briefly, PGE$_2$ has been shown to reduce vasopressin-dependent osmotic water permeability of the collecting tubule, enhance medullary blood flow, and inhibit NaCl reabsorption from the thick ascending limb of Henle's loop. These actions of PGE$_2$ have relevance to body fluid homeostasis, since treatment with inhibitors of prostaglandin synthesis results in augmentation of the antidiuretic effect of vasopressin[23] and in elevation of chloride reabsorption in the ascending limb of Henle's loop and/or the cortical and outer medullary collecting tubule[24]. From these observations, it is apparent that renal PGE$_2$ may subserve mechanisms that promote diuresis and natriuresis. One of these mechanisms is the pressure natriuresis mechanism(s) which brings about marked augmentation of sodium excretion in response to slight increases in renal perfusion pressure. This view is supported by a recent study demonstrating that inhibition of prostaglandin synthesis with indomethacin attenuates the pressure natriuresis response[25].

Contribution of prostanoids to prohypertensive mechanisms

Several prostanoids possess actions that are conducive to their participation in prohypertensive mechanisms. For example, TxA$_2$ causes vasoconstriction[3], PGF$_{2\alpha}$ reduces venous compliance leading to elevation of cardiac output[26], and both PGE$_2$ and PGI$_2$ stimulate renin secretion[27,28]. The involvement of prostanoids in the control of renin secretion has been investigated extensively. Renal prostanoids appear to contribute to both the renal baroreceptor-mediated and the macula densa-mediated release of renin[27,28]. The extent of their contribution appears to be substantial since treatment with prostaglandin synthesis inhibitors results in lowering of plasma renin activity in both normotensive and hypertensive conditions[29–32]. Treatment with prostaglandin synthesis inhibitors was shown to produce correlated decrements of plasma renin activity and blood pressure in renin-dependent hypertension, which is consistent with the concept that prostanoids can contribute to prohypertensive mechanisms by promoting renin release[31,32]. In relation to this point, it has been shown that chronic renal arterial infusion of PGE$_2$ in conscious dogs causes elevation of plasma renin activity and hypertension[33].

In summary, a substantial body of evidence indicates the participation of various prostanoids in the vascular and renal mechanisms controlling blood pressure. Reports that PGE$_2$ and PGI$_2$ dilate resistance blood vessels, reduce the release of norepinephrine from sympathetic nerves, attenuate vascular reactivity to pressor hormones, and facilitate the renal excretion of sodium and water are all supportive of the notion that PGE$_2$ and PGI$_2$ subserve antihypertensive processes by opposing pressor mechanisms that bring about vasoconstriction and conservation of salt and water. On the other hand, reports that TxA$_2$ causes vasoconstriction, that PGF$_{2\alpha}$ reduces venous compliance, and that PGE$_2$ and PGI$_2$ stimulate renin secretion are supportive of the concept that these prostanoids subserve mechanisms that cause blood pressure to increase. Inasmuch as prostanoids participate in the implementation of both prohypertensive and antihypertensive mechanisms, hypertension may be caused by an uncompensated excess in prostanoids subserving prohypertensive functions, or by a deficit in prostanoids subserving antihypertensive functions.

PROSTANOID LEVELS IN HYPERTENSION

Studies constrasting normotensive and hypertensive subjects in terms of renal prostanoid excretion and prostanoid production by vascular and renal structures are abundant and provide compelling evidence that hypertension, both clinical and experimental, is commonly associated with disturbances in the arachidonic acid–prostanoid system.

Experimental hypertension

Rioux and co-workers[34] reported augmentation of *in vitro* prostanoid release by strips of aorta from spontaneously hypertensive rats, DOCA-salt hypertensive rats, and two kidney–one clip hypertensive rats. These early findings are in general agreement with the results of later studies demonstrating enhanced formation of PGI_2 by aortic rings from spontaneously hypertensive rats[35], one kidney–one clip hypertensive rats[36], and rats made hypertensive by chronic angiotensin II infusion[37]. Increased production of PGI_2 by aortas from spontaneously hypertensive rats has been attributed to an increase in vascular cyclo-oxygenase activity[38,39] associated with enhancement of phospholipase A_2 activity[40]. In general, the level of arterial blood pressure *in vivo* appears to correlate positively with indices of aortic PGI_2 production *in vitro*. Furthermore, in spontaneously hypertensive rats, the overproduction of aortic PGI_2 *in vitro* does not precede the development of hypertension, supporting the notion that the increased vascular PGI_2 production is secondary to the hypertension[41]. However, proportionality between the level of blood pressure and aortic prostaglandin synthesis is not always apparent. For example, the reversal of hypertension following unclipping in one kidney–one clip hypertensive rats is associated with an increase rather than a decrease in aortic PGI_2 synthesis[42]. Be that as it may, the alterations in aortic PGI_2 production *in vitro* are difficult to interpret as they may not be indicative of a general alteration in arterial and arteriolar PGI_2 synthesis. Pertaining to this point, it was recently reported that the urinary excretion of 2,3-dinor-6-keto-$PGF_{1\alpha}$, an index of total PGI_2 production, is diminished rather than increased in the spontaneously hypertensive rat[43].

Many studies indicate an association between high blood pressure in experimental animals and abnormalities in urinary prostanoid excretion, a presumed index of the balance between renal prostanoid production and catabolism *in vivo*, and in rates of prostanoid synthesis and catabolism by renal structures and subcellular fractions *in vitro*. The urinary excretion of PGE_2 is unchanged[44] or decreased[43] in spontaneously hypertensive rats, decreased in genetically hypertensive mice[45], in female genetically hypertensive rats (New Zealand strain)[46], and in hypertensive Dahl salt-sensitive rats[47], and either unchanged[48] or increased[49] in rats with two kidney–one clip

162

hypertension. Renal $PGF_{2\alpha}$ excretion is unaffected[44] or increased[50] in spontaneously hypertensive rats. Urinary excretion of 6-keto-$PGF_{1\alpha}$ is increased in genetically hypertensive rats of the Lyon strain[51] and in rats with angiotensin II-induced hypertension[37], but is unchanged in rats with two kidney–one clip hypertension[48,49]. Urinary TxB_2 excretion is increased in spontaneously hypertensive rats[52,53]. The concentration in renal venous plasma of PGE_2 and $PGF_{2\alpha}$ is unchanged in spontaneously hypertensive rats[44] but is increased transiently in dogs with two kidney–one clip hypertension[54]. The renal venous output of 6-keto-$PGF_{1\alpha}$ is increased within the first 10 min after the onset of unilateral renal artery constriction in conscious dogs[55].

The release of prostaglandins elicited by arachidonic acid infusion in isolated perfused kidneys does not change in rats with two kidney–one clip hypertension but increases in spontaneously hypertensive rats and in rats with deoxycorticosterone-salt hypertension[56]. In rats with two kidney–one clip hypertension, the release of PGE_2 by the renal medulla *in vitro* is diminished[57,58], as is the prostaglandin release elicited by norepinephrine in the perfused kidney of one kidney–one clip hypertensive rats[59]. The release of prostaglandins and TxB_2 by isolated glomeruli is increased in spontaneously hypertensive rats[60]. Prostanoid release by glomeruli from clipped kidneys exceeds the release of glomeruli from untouched kidneys in two kidney–one clip hypertensive rats but is not different from the corresponding values in normotensive controls[61].

The biochemical mechanisms underlying the abnormalities in renal prostanoids featured by hypertensive animals are incompletely understood. Quite often, efforts to relate an abnormality of renal prostanoids *in vivo* to alteration in *in vitro* indices of renal prostanoid synthesis and catabolism have yielded quite confusing results. For example, in spontaneously hypertensive rats, the activity of renal 15-hydroxyprostaglandin dehydrogenase is decreased[62,63], whereas the activity of renomedullary cyclo-oxygenase is increased[64] as is the basal and/or the hormone-induced release of arachidonic acid[65] and prostanoids[65,66] from renal medulla slices or perfused kidney. These are intriguing findings as, in spontaneously hypertensive rats, the renal excretion of PGE_2 is unchanged or reduced rather than increased[43,44]. In hypertensive Dahl salt-sensitive rats, having reduced renal PGE_2 excretion[47], the metabolism of arachidonic acid to prostaglandins by renal medulla microsomes is reduced and the activity of renal 15-hydroxyprostaglandin dehydrogenase is enhanced[67], suggesting that the deficit in renal PGE_2 excretion is the manifestation of both reduced production and increased catabolism of renal prostaglandins. However, in New Zealand strain genetically hypertensive rats, renal 15-hydroxyprostaglandin dehydrogenase activity is reduced in males but not females, yet urinary PGE_2 excretion by females is reduced while that by males is unaltered[46].

Clinical hypertension

Abnormalities in renal prostanoids have been detected in several forms of clinical hypertension, including essential hypertension, renovascular hypertension and eclampsia.

According to reports by several investigators over the past decade, the urinary excretion of PGE_2 is depressed in patients with essential hypertension[68-71]. However, there is substantial overlap in the urinary PGE_2 excretion values of normotensive and essential hypertensive subjects, so that not all patients with hypertension exhibit reduction of urinary PGE_2 excretion[72-74]. Apparently, diminished PGE_2 excretion is prevalent in subsets of essential hypertensive patients over the age of forty[72], patients having low plasma renin activity[73], or patients maintained on a low-sodium intake[74]. The urinary excretion of 6-keto-$PGF_{1\alpha}$, the product of non-enzymatic breakdown of PGI_2, was also reported as diminished in a small group of patients with essential hypertension[75]. The renal excretion of TxB_2 in essential hypertensive subjects was found to be increased in one study[76] and unchanged in another[74]; the excretion of $PGE_{2\alpha}$ is comparable in normotensive and essential hypertensive subjects[74]. Little information is available on circulating prostanoids in essential hypertension; PGE_2 was reported to be increased in the central venous blood[77], whereas the concentration of 6-keto-$PGF_{1\alpha}$ in peripheral venous blood was increased in one study[78] and decreased in another[79].

The urinary excretion of PGE_2 is normal in patients with primary aldosteronism[69] and in patients with hypertension secondary to chronic renal disease[80]. In renovascular hypertension, renal PGE_2 excretion is either normal[69] or increased[81], and the concentration of PGE_2 in renal venous plasma is higher on the stenotic than on the non-stenotic side[82,83]. In pre-eclampsia, the urinary excretion rates of PGE_2, 6-keto-$PGF_{1\alpha}$, 2,3-dinor-6-keto-$PGF_{1\alpha}$ and 15-keto-13,14-dihydro-2,3-dinor-6-keto-$PGF_{1\alpha}$ are reduced relative to corresponding values in normotensive pregnant women[84-86]. That pre-eclampsia is a state of PGI_2 deficiency is also suggested by reports that the *in vitro* release of 6-keto-$PGF_{1\alpha}$ by placental tissue from pre-eclampsia patients is reduced relative to release values for tissue from normotensive pregnant subjects[87].

In summary, hypertension in both humans and experimental animals is commonly associated with disturbances in the arachidonic acid–prostanoid system as revealed by abnormalities in urinary excretion of prostanoids and/or in various indices of prostanoid production and catabolism by renal and vascular structures *in vitro*. The significance of abnormalities in prostanoid levels and/or metabolism in relation to the pathophysiology of hypertension is yet to be resolved. Conceivably, both a deficit in prostanoids subserving antihypertensive functions and an excess in prostanoids subserving prohypertensive functions may contribute to produce hypertension. For example, hypertension may be the expression of a deficit in antihypertensive functions mediated by PGE_2 and/or PGI_2 in subsets of patients with essential hypertension having reduced urinary PGE_2 excretion[69-74], and in pre-eclampsia patients and hypertensive Dahl salt-sensitive rats having diminished urinary excretion of PGE_2 and 2,3-dinor-6-keto-$PGF_{1\alpha}$[43,85]. Also, in models of renal hypertension having increased plasma renin activity and renal venous blood concentration of PGE_2 and 6-keto-$PGF_{1\alpha}$[54,55,82,83], the hypertension may be the manifestation of prohypertensive mechanisms involving excessive stimulation of renin secretion by PGE_2 and/or PGI_2. Additionally, abnormalities in prostanoids may be the consequence rather than the cause of hypertension. For example, the finding of increased *in vitro* aortic PGI_2

production in several models of experimental hypertension raises the possibility that the abnormality in vascular prostanoid synthesis is a secondary event, perhaps reflecting activation of a blood pressure lowering mechanism. Clearly, however, it is difficult to interpret the significance of disturbances in prostanoid levels and/or metabolism in relation to the pathophysiology of hypertension since there are prostanoids, viz. PGE_2 and PGI_2, that can participate in the implementation of both prohypertensive and antihypertensive mechanisms.

BLOOD PRESSURE AS AFFECTED BY INHIBITORS OF PROSTANOID SYNTHESIS

Blood pressure has been reported to increase, decrease, or remain unaffected during treatment with inhibitors of prostanoid synthesis. This variability in response is not unexpected. Since prostanoids participate in the implementation of both antihypertensive and prohypertensive mechanisms, the blood pressure response to treatment with inhibitors of prostanoid synthesis may reflect the relative contribution of such prostanoid-mediated mechanisms to setting the level of arterial blood pressure. For example, augmentation of blood pressure in response to treatment with an inhibitor of prostanoid synthesis may be the manifestation of a deficit in prostanoid-mediated antihypertensive mechanisms. Conversely, lowering of blood pressure in reponse to prostanoid synthesis inhibition may be the expression of a deficit in prostanoid-mediated prohypertensive mechanisms. The effect on blood pressure of treatment with cyclo-oxygenase inhibitors to reduce prostanoid synthesis has been investigated in both normotensive and hypertensive animals and man. Treatment with inhibitors of cyclo-oxygenase bring about reduction in the synthesis of all prostaglandins and of TxA_2.

Effect of inhibitors of prostanoid synthesis on blood pressure in normotensive animals and man

In conscious rabbits, blood pressure was reported to be unchanged[88,89] or slightly increased[90] within one hour of the onset of treatment with an inhibitor of cyclo-oxygenase, indomethacin or meclofenamate. The blood pressure increase elicited in rabbits by short-term treatment with cyclo-oxygenase inhibitors is associated with elevation of total peripheral vascular resistance and reduction of cardiac output[90]. Also, in sheep, short-term treatment with indomethacin causes augmentation of blood pressure and total peripheral vascular resistance and lowering of cardiac output[91]. Blood pressure is unchanged during acute treatment with indomethacin in sodium-replete dogs and rats but falls substantially in sodium-depleted animals[92,93]. The indomethacin-induced lowering of blood pressure in sodium-depleted dogs and rats is associated with reduction of plasma renin activity[92,93]. Short-term infusion of indomethacin in normotensive, healthy humans causes augmentation of blood pressure and total peripheral vascular resistance associated with lowering of cardiac output[94]. Indomethacin also increases blood pressure acutely in normotensive patients with coronary artery disease[95] and in patients with severe congestive heart failure and hyponatraemia[96].

Chronic treatment with sodium meclofenamate in normotensive rats was reported to have no effect on blood pressure[97]. Similarly, blood pressure did not change in rabbits receiving indomethacin at 3 or $10 \, mg \, kg^{-1} day^{-1}$ for 10 days[98,99]. However, blood pressure was reported[100] to increase substantially in rabbits treated for 14 days with indomethacin at $15 \, mg \, kg^{-1} day^{-1}$. For healthy humans, most investigators agree that the administration of indomethacin at $1–2 \, mg \, kg^{-1} \, day^{-1}$ for 3–7 days is without effect on blood pressure, although it causes reduced plasma renin activity, reduced plasma norepinephrine concentration and increased pressor responsiveness to angiotensin II[101–103]. In one study, however, treatment with indomethacin for 5 days in normotensive subjects resulted in a small, but significant, pressure elevation[104]. In the same study, blood pressure did not increase during treatment with aspirin[104]. In patients with autonomic failure, treatment with indomethacin for 7 days caused elevation of the reclining but not of the standing blood pressure[103].

Effect of inhibitors of prostanoid synthesis on blood pressure in hypertensive animals and man

In two kidney–one clip hypertensive rabbits without significant impairment of renal function, treatment with indomethacin for 10 days is without effect on blood pressure although it reduces plasma renin activity[98]. In contrast, in two kidney–one clip hypertensive rabbits having high plasma renin activity and depressed renal haemodynamics, chronic treatment with indomethacin aggravates both the hypertension and the renal function impairment[98]. In the latter study, plasma renin activity, which initially was reduced by indomethacin, returned on subsequent days to pretreatment levels *pari passu* with the increase in blood pressure and the deterioration of renal function[98]. Chronic indomethacin treatment also exacerbates the hypertension, and depresses renal excretory function, in rats with two kidney–one clip hypertension[57]. However, short-term treatment with indomethacin lowers blood pressure, associated with reduction of plasma renin activity, in rats with two clip–one kidney hypertension[93]. Indomethacin also produces correlated decrements of blood pressure and plasma renin activity in rats made hypertensive by complete ligation of the aorta between the renal arteries[32]. In contrast, short-term treatment with indomethacin or meclofenamate is without effect on blood pressure in dogs with two kidney–one clip hypertension[105].

In rabbits with one kidney–one clip hypertension, treatment with indomethacin for 10 days aggravates the hypertension and causes deterioration of renal haemodynamic and excretory functions, while reducing plasma renin activity[98]. In contrast, short-term treatment with indomethacin was reported to reduce both blood pressure and plasma renin activity in dogs with one kidney–one clip hypertension[106]. Treatment with meclofenamate prior to and following bilateral renal artery constriction markedly attenuates, in the acute phase, the development of hypertension in rats[97]. However, once the hypertension is established, chronic treatment with meclofenamate does not affect blood pressure in rats with two kidney—one clip hypertension[97].

Chronic treatment with indomethacin results in aggravation of hypertension in rats with DOCA-salt hypertension[107] and in rats with adrenal enucleation hypertension[108]. Similarly, in adult spontaneously hypertensive rats maintained on a high salt intake, chronic treatment with meclofenamate causes aggravation of hypertension associated with reduction of renal blood flow and glomerular filtration rate[109]. Blood pressure in adult spontaneously hypertensive rats also increases following short-term treatment with indomethacin, meclofenamate or other inhibitors of prostanoid synthesis[110]. However, chronic treatment with aspirin, commencing at 3 weeks of age, was reported to arrest the development of hypertension in spontaneously hypertensive rats[111]. Chronic treatment with CV-4151, an inhibitor of thromboxane synthesis, also was found to attenuate the development of hypertension in 4-week-old spontaneously hypertensive rats, associated with diuresis and natriuresis[52]. In contrast, 6 weeks of treatment with UK-38485, another inhibitor of thromboxane synthesis, does not affect the development of hypertension, or renal haemodynamic and excretory functions, in 3.5-week-old spontaneously hypertensive rats[112]. Yet, in another study, chronic treatment with UK-38485 caused lowering of blood pressure in 16-week-old spontaneously hypertensive rats[53]. Similarly, 14 weeks of treatment with the thromboxane synthesis inhibitor, OKY-046, commencing at 8 weeks of age, clearly attenuated the hypertension and improved renal function in spontaneously hypertensive rats[113].

In patients with essential hypertension, indomethacin, given by in intramuscular injection at $1 \, mg \, kg^{-1}$, increases blood pressure and total peripheral vascular resistance associated with diminution of cardiac output[114]. However, reports that indomethacin, given orally at $75-200 \, mg \, day^{-1}$ for 4–7 days, increases blood pressure in patients with untreated, uncomplicated, essential hypertension contrasts with reports that it does not[115-117]. Cyclo-oxygenase inhibitors, indomethacin and ibuprofen, were also without effect on blood pressure in patients with renovascular hypertension[30]. Yet, in two siblings with renin-dependent hypertension and aldosteronism, the administration of indomethacin at $250 \, mg \, day^{-1}$ for 16 days was found to lower blood pressure and plasma renin activity, despite promoting slight retention of salt and water[31].

Mechanism(s) of the blood pressure disturbances elicited by prostanoid synthesis inhibitors

The net blood pressure response to treatment with inhibitors of prostanoid synthesis is determined by the sum of the alterations in cardiovascular and renal functions resulting from the deficit in prostanoid-mediated prohypertensive and antihypertensive mechanisms. In general, augmentation of blood pressure during chronic treatment with inhibitors of prostanoid synthesis is a response more frequent in hypertensive than in normotensive states and is usually accompanied by deterioration of renal haemodynamic and excretory functions[31,57,98]. Since vasodilatory prostanoids, such as PGE_2 and PGI_2, contribute to maintenance of renal blood flow and glomerular filtration when pressor systems are overactive[5,16], promote diuresis and natriuresis[6], and attenuate the renal and extrarenal vasoconstrictor actions of pressor hormones[5], the rise in pressure elicited by prostanoid synthesis inhibitors is probably the manifestation of a deficit in prostanoids which oppose the renal and extrarenal vascular actions of pressor systems and contribute to maintenance of body fluids homeostasis.

Reduction of blood pressure during the administration of inhibitors of prostanoid synthesis is noted in both normotensive and hypertensive conditions characterized by elevated plasma renin activity and is accompanied by marked lowering of plasma renin[29-32]. Since renal prostanoids promote renin secretion[27,28], the reduction in blood pressure elicited by prostanoids synthesis inhibitors is probably the manifestation of a deficit in prostanoid-mediated renin release. Reduced synthesis of thromboxane also may contribute to lowering of blood pressure during treatment with inhibitors of prostanoid synthesis. This possibility is supported by the demonstration that specific inhibitors of thromboxane synthetase can lower blood pressure in spontaneously hypertensive rats[52,53,113].

INTERACTION OF PROSTANOIDS AND ANTIHYPERTENSIVE DRUGS

Reports that antihypertensive drugs increase prostanoid levels in blood and urine and that their blood pressure lowering effect is diminished during treatment with cyclo-oxygenase inhibitors suggest interactions among antihypertensive drugs and prostanoids. Prostanoid levels in human blood or urine have been shown to increase during treatment with a variety of antihypertensive agents, including captopril, furosemide and thiazide diuretics. Captopril increases the urinary excretion of PGE_2 and the plasma levels of 6-keto-$PGF_{1\alpha}$ and of 13,14-dihydro-15-keto-PGE_2, a metabolite of PGE_2[118-120]; the action of captopril in increasing prostanoid levels in blood and urine is thought to be the result of prostanoid synthesis stimulation by the drug itself or by kinins[120]. Furosemide increases the urinary excretion of PGE_2 and 6-keto-$PGF_{1\alpha}$, effects which have been attributed to augmentation of renal prostanoid synthesis due to increased availability of free arachidonic acid to cyclo-oxygenase[115,121-123]. The urinary excretion of PGE_2 also increased during repeated administration of hydrochlorothiazide[124] and triamterene[125], and the plasma level of 6-keto-$PGF_{1\alpha}$ is increased during therapy with bendrofluazide[126]. Plasma PGE_2 levels were shown to increase in response to treatment with hydralazine in dogs[127] and with propranolol in rats[128].

That therapy with various types of antihypertensive agents causes prostanoid levels to increase, raises the possibility that the accompanying blood pressure lowering effect is related to the increase in prostanoids. Pertaining to this point, several studies have demonstrated that indomethacin treatment at $75-200\,mg\,day^{-1}$ consistently raises blood pressure, sometimes by as much as 30 mmHg, in hypertensive patients undergoing therapy with a variety of antihypertensive drugs. Specifically, indomethacin has been shown to counteract the antihypertensive effect of captopril[118,120], furosemide[115], thiazides[117,129], propranolol and other blockers of β-adrenoreceptors[117,129,130], dihydralazine[131] and verapamil[132]. This effect of indomethacin, particularly as it relates to the antihypertensive effect of furosemide and other diurectics, is manifested despite reduction of plasma renin activity, an action of indomethacin which is conducive to lowering of blood pressure.

The mechanism(s) underlying the rise in blood pressure caused by indomethacin in hypertensive patients undergoing antihypertensive therapy with a wide spectrum of drugs is not defined as yet. Prostaglandins are proposed to contribute to the blood pressure lowering effect of kinins, which increase with captopril[120], to the renal vasodilatory and natriuretic actions of furosemide[121], to the vasodilatory effect of hydralazine[127], and to the effect of propranolol in antagonizing the facilitation of sympathetic transmission elicited by angiotensin II[128]. Therefore, the rise in blood pressure elicited by indomethacin in patients undergoing antihypertensive treatment with the aforementioned drugs may be the consequence of diminished synthesis of prostaglandins acting as mediators of antihypertensive drug actions. It is also possible that the pressor effect of indomethacin in such patients is the expression of diminished prostanoid synthesis in a setting in which the effectiveness of prostanoid-mediated antihypertensive mechanisms is amplified. Finally, the possibility must be considered that indomethacin increases blood pressure in subjects receiving antihypertensive drug treatment via a mechanism(s) unrelated to prostanoid synthesis inhibition. Relative to this point, inhibitors of cyclo-oxygenase other than indomethacin were either ineffective or less effective than indomethacin in raising blood pressure in patients undergoing antihypertensive treatment[133].

REFERENCES

1. Lee, J.B., Corvino, B.G., Rakman, B.H. and Smith, E.R. (1965). Renomedullary vasodepressor substance. Medullin: isolation, chemical characterization and physical properties. *Circ. Res.*, **7**, 57–77
2. Lee, J.B., Crowshaw, K., Takman, B.H., Attrep, K.A. and Gougoutas, J.Z. (1967). Identification of prostaglandins E_2, $F_{2\alpha}$ and A_2 from rabbit kidney medulla. *Biochem. J.*, **105**, 1251–1260
3. Moncada, S. and Vane, J.R. (1978). Pharmacology and endogenous roles of prostaglandin endoperoxides, thromboxane A_2 and prostacyclin. *Pharmacol. Rev.*, **30**, 293–331
4. Hedqvist, P. (1979). Actions of prostacyclin (PGI_2) on adrenergic neuroeffector transmission in the rabbit kidney. *Prostaglandins*, **17**, 249–258
5. Nasjletti, A. and Malik, K.U. (1981). Interrelationships among prostaglandins and vasoactive substances. *Med. Clin. N. Am.*, **65**, 881–889
6. Stokes, J.B. (1981). Integrated actions of renal medullary prostaglandins in the control of water excretion. *Am. J. Physiol.*, **240**, F471–F480
7. McGiff, J.C., Crowshaw, K., Terragno, N. and Lonigro, A.J. (1970). Release of a prostaglandin-like substance into the renal venous blood in response to angiotensin II. *Circ. Res.*, **26**, and **27** (Suppl. I), I-121–I-130
8. Dunn, M.J., Greely, H.P., Valtin, H., Kinter, L.B. and Beeuwkes, R. (1978). Renal excretion of prostaglandins E_2 and $F_{2\alpha}$ in diabetes insipidus rats. *Am. J. Physiol.*, **235**, E624–E627

9. Nadler, J., Zipser, R.D., Coleman, R. and Horton, R. (1983). Stimulation of renal prostaglandins by pressor hormones in man: Comparison of prostaglandins E_2 and prostacyclin (6-keto-$PGF_{1\alpha}$). *J. Clin. Endocrinol. Metab.*, **56**, 1260–1265

10. Oliver, J.A. Sciacca, R.R., Le Gren, G. and Cannon, P.J. (1982). Modulation by prostaglandins of the renal vascular action of arginine vasopressin. *Prostaglandins*, **24**, 641–656

11. Aiken, J.W. and Vane, J.R. (1973). Intrarenal prostaglandin release attenuates the renal vasoconstrictor activity of angiotensin. *J. Pharmacol. Exp. Ther.*, **184**, 678–687

12. Gunther, S. and Cannon, P.J. (1980). Modulation of angiotensin II coronary vasoconstriction by cardiac prostaglandin synthesis. *Am. J. Physiol.*, **238**, 895–901

13. Malik, K.U. and McGiff, J.C. (1975). Modulation by prostaglandins of adrenergic transmission in the isolated perfused rabbit and rat kidney. *Circ. Res.*, **36**, 599–609

14. Malik, K.U., Ryan, P. and McGiff, J.C. (1976). Modification by prostaglandin E_1 and E_2, indomethacin, and arachidonic acid of the vasoconstrictor responses of the isolated perfused rabbit and rat mesenteric arteries to adrenergic stimuli. *Circ. Res.*, **39**, 163–168

15. Zimmerman, B.G., Ryan, M.J., Gomer, S. and Kraft, E. (1973). Effect of prostaglandin synthesis inhibitors indomethacin and eicosa-5,8,11,14-tetraynoic acid on adrenergic responses in dog cutaneous vasculature. *J. Pharmacol. Exp. Ther.*, **187**, 315–323

16. DiBona, G.F. (1986). Prostaglandins and nonsteroidal anti-inflammatory drugs. Effects on renal hemodynamics. *Am. J. Med.*, **80** (Suppl. 1A), 12–21

17. Rowe, B.P. and Nasjletti, A. (1983). Biphasic blood pressure response to angiotensin II in the conscious rabbit: Relation to prostaglandins. *J. Pharmacol. Exp. Ther.*, **225**, 559–563

18. Negus, P., Tannen, R.L. and Dunn, M.J. (1976). Indomethacin potentiates the vasoconstrictor actions of angiotensin II in normal man. *Prostaglandins*, **12**, 175–180

19. Speckart, P., Zia, P., Zipser, R. and Horton, R. (1977). The effect of sodium restriction and prostaglandin inhibition on the renin–angiotensin system in man. *Clin. Endocrinol. Metab.*, **44**, 832–837

20. Gill, J.R., Frohlich, J.C., Bowden, R.E., Taylor, A.A., Keiser, H.R., Seyberth, H.W., Oates, J.A. and Bartter, F.C. (1976). Bartter's syndrome: a disorder characterized by high urinary prostaglandins and a dependence of hypereninemia on prostaglandin synthesis. *Am. J. Med.*, **61**, 43–61

21. Silverberg, A.B., Mennes, P.A. and Cryer, P.E. (1978). Resistance to endogenous norepinephrine in Bartter's syndrome. Reversion during indomethacin administration. *Am. J. Med.*, **64**, 231–235

22. Davies, I.B., Bannister, R., Hensby, C. and Sever, P.S. (1980). The pressor actions of noradrenaline and angiotensin II in chronic autonomic failure treated with indomethacin. *Br. J. Clin. Pharmacol.*, **10**, 223–229

23. Anderson, R.J., Berl, T., McDonald, K.M. and Schrier, R.W. (1975). Evidence for an in vivo antagonism between vasopressin and prostaglandin in the mammalian kidney. *J. Clin. Invest.*, **56**, 420–426

24. Higashihara, E., Stokes, J.B., Kokko, J.P., Campbell, W.B. and DuBose, T.D. (1979). Cortical and papillary micropuncture examination of chloride transport in segments of the rat kidney during inhibition of prostaglandin production: a possible role for prostaglandins in the chloruresis of acute volume expansion. *J. Clin. Invest.*, **64**, 1277–1287

25. Carmines, P.K., Bell, P.D., Roman, R.J., Work, J. and Navar, L.G. (1985). Prostaglandins in the sodium excretory response to altered renal artery pressure in dogs. *Am. J. Physiol.*, **248**, F8–F14

26. Ducharme, D.W., Weeks, J.R. and Montgomery, R.G. (1968). Studies on the hypertensive effect of prostaglandin $F_{2\alpha}$. *J. Pharmacol. Exp. Ther.*, **160**, 1–10

27. Henrich, W.L. (1981). Role of the prostaglandins in renin secretion. *Kidney Int.*, **19**, 822–828

28. Gerber, J.G., Olson, R.D. and Nies, A.S. (1981). Interrelationship between prostaglandins and renin release. *Kidney Int.*, **19**, 16–21

29. Frohlich, J.C., Hollifield, J.W., Dormois, J.C., Frolich, B.L., Seyberth, H., Michelakis, A.M. and Oates, J.A. (1976). Suppression of plasma renin activity by indomethacin in man. *Circ. Res.*, **39**, 447–452

30. Speckart, P., Zia, P., Zipser, R., Croxson, C., Mayeda, S. and Horton, R. (1978). Effect of prostaglandin inhibition on the renin and aldosterone response to posture in normal and hypertensive man. *Mineral Electrolyte Metab.*, **1**, 208–215
31. de Jong, P.E., Donker, A.J.M., Van der Wall, E., Erkelens, D.W., Van der Hem, G.K. and Doorenbos, H. (1980). Effect of indomethacin in two siblings with a renin-dependent hypertension, hyperaldosteronism and hypokalemia. *Nephron*, **25**, 47–52
32. Jackson, E.K., Oates, J.A. and Branch, R.A. (1981). Indomethacin decreases arterial blood pressure and plasma renin activity in rats with aorta ligation. *Circ. Res.*, **49**, 180–185
33. Hockel, G. and Cowley, A.W. (1979). Prostaglandin E$_2$-induced hypertension in conscious dogs. *Am. J. Physiol.*, **237**, H449–H454
34. Rioux, F., Quirion, R. and Regoli, D. (1977). The role of prostaglandins in hypertension. I. The release of prostaglandins by aorta strips of renal, DOCA-salt, and spontaneously hypertensive rats. *Can. J. Physiol. Pharmacol.*, **55**, 1330–1338
35. Pace-Asciak, C.R., Carrara, M.C., Rangaraj, G. and Nicolaou, K.C. (1978). Enhanced formation of PGI$_2$, a potent hypotensive substance, by aortic rings and homogenates of the spontaneously hypertensive rat. *Prostaglandins*, **15**, 1005–1012
36. Dusting, G.J., Dickens, P.A., DiNicolantonio, R. and Doyle, A.E. (1984). Vascular prostacyclin and Goldblatt Hypertensive rats. *J. Hypertens.*, **2**, 31–36
37. Diz, D.I., Baer, P.G. and Nasjletti, A. (1983). Angiotensin II-induced hypertension in the rat. Effects on the plasma concentration, renal excretion, and tissue release of prostaglandins. *J. Clin. Invest.*, **72**, 466–477
38. Limas, C.J. and Limas, C. (1977). Vascular prostaglandin synthesis in the spontaneously hypertensive rat. *Am. J. Physiol.*, **233**, H493–H499
39. Skidgel, R. and Printz, M.P. (1980). Vascular PG synthesis in hypertensive and normotensive rats. *Adv. Prostagl. Thrombox. Res.*, **7**, 803–805
40. Limas, C., Goldman, P. and Limas, C.J. (1981). Aortic phospholipid deacylation-reacylation cycle in spontaneously hypertensive rats. *Am. J. Physiol.*, **240**, H33–H38
41. Pace-Asciak, C.R. and Carrara, M.C. (1979). Age-dependent increase in the formation of prostaglandin I$_2$ by the intact and homogenised aortae from the developing spontaneously hypertensive rat. *Biochim. Biophys. Acta*, **574**, 177–181
42. McGowan, H.M., Vandongen, R., Codde, J.P. and Croft, K.D. (1986). Increased aortic PGI$_2$ and plasma lyso-PAF in the unclipped one-kidney hypertensive rat. *Am. J. Physiol.*, **251**, H1361–H1364
43. Martineau, A., Robillard, M. and Falardeau, P. (1984). Defective synthesis of vasodilator prostaglandins in the spontaneously hypertensive rat. *Hypertension*, **6**, (Suppl I), I-161–I-165
44. Dunn, M.J. (1978). Renal prostaglandin production in the japanese (Kyoto) spontaneously hypertensive rat. *Clin. Sci. Mol. Med.*, **55**, 191s–193s
45. Sustarsic, D.L., McPartland, R.P., Rapp, J.P., Schlager, G.S. and Tan, S.Y. (1980). Urinary kallikrein and urinary prostaglandin E$_2$ in genetically hypertensive mice. *Proc. Soc. Exp. Biol. Med.*, **163**, 193–199
46. Baer, P.G. and Cagen, L.M. (1981). Renal prostaglandin excretion and metabolism in male and female New Zealand normotensive and genetically hypertensive rats. *Hypertension*, **3**, 257–261
47. Sustarsic, D.L., McPartland, R.P. and Rapp, J.P. (1981). Developmental patterns of blood pressure and urinary protein, kallikrein, and prostaglandin E$_2$ in Dahl salt-hypertension susceptible rats. *J. Lab. Clin. Med.*, **98**, 599–606
48. Vandongen, R. and O'Dwyer, J. (1984). Urinary 6-keto-PGF$_{1\alpha}$ and PGE$_2$ in two kidney–one clip hypertension in the rat. *Prostgl. Leuk. Med.*, **13**, 289–293
49. Lahera, V., Duran, F., Cachofeiro, V., Canizo, F.J., Tresguerres, J.A.F. and Rodriguez, F.J. (1986). Different excretion pattern of urinary PGE$_2$ and 6-keto-PGF$_{1\alpha}$ in two kidney–one clip goldblatt rats. *Prostagl. Leuk. Med.*, **24**, 35–41
50. Ahnfelt-Ronne, I. and Arrigoni-Marterlli, E. (1978). Increased PGF$_{2\alpha}$ synthesis in renal papilla of spontaneously hypertensive rats. *Biochem. Pharmacol.*, **27**, 2363–2367
51. Benzoni, D., Vincent, M. and Sassard, J. (1984). Urinary 6-ketoprostaglandin F$_{1\alpha}$ in genetically hypertensive rats of the Lyon Strain. *Clin. Sci.*, **66**, 453–457
52. Shibouta, Y., Terashita, Z., Inada, Y. and Nishikawa, K. (1985). Delay of the initiation of hypertension in spontaneously hypertensive rats by CV-4151, a specific thromboxane A$_2$ synthetase inhibitor. *Eur. J. Pharmacol.*, **109**, 135–144

171

53. Purkerson, M.L., Martin, K.J., Yates, J., Kissane, J.M. and Klahr, S. (1986). Thromboxane synthesis and blood pressure in spontaneously hypertensive rats. *Hypertension*, **8**, 1113–1120

54. Dighe, K.K., Smith, G.W., Ungar, A. and Whelpdale, P.H. (1978). Renal prostaglandins in renal hypertensive dogs. *Clin. Sci. Mol. Med.*, **54**, 561–566

55. Jackson, E.K., Gerkens, J.F., Brash, A.R. and Branch, R.A. (1982). Acute renal artery constriction increases renal prostaglandin I_2 biosynthesis and renin release in the conscious dog. *J. Pharmacol. Exp. Ther.*, **222**, 410–413

56. Shibouta, Y., Terashita, Z., Inada, Y., Nishikawa, K. and Kikuchi, S. (1981). Enhanced thromboxane A_2 biosynthesis in the kidney of spontaneously hypertensive rats during development of hypertension. *Eur. J. Pharmacol.*, **70**, 247–256

57. Pugsley, D.J., Beilin, L.J. and Peto, R. (1975). Renal prostaglandin synthesis in the Goldblatt hypertensive rat. *Circ. Res.*, **36** and **37** (Suppl. I), 81–88

58. Sirois, P. and Gagnon, D.J. (1974). Release of renomedullary prostaglandins in normal and hypertensive rats. *Experientia*, **30**, 1418–1419

59. Leary, W.P., Ledingham, J.G. and Vane, J.R. (1974). Impaired prostaglandin release from the kidneys of salt-loaded and hypertensive rats. *Prostaglandins*, **7**, 425–432

60. Konieczkowski, M., Dunn, M.J., Stork, J.E. and Hassid, A. (1983). Glomerular synthesis of prostaglandins and thromboxane in spontaneously hypertensive rats. *Hypertension*, **5**, 446–452

61. Stahl, R.A.K., Helmchen, U., Paravicini, M., Ritter, L.J. and Schollmeyer, P. (1984). Glomerular prostaglandin formation in two-kidney, one-clip hypertensive rats. *Am. J. Physiol.*, **247**, F975–F981

62. Pace-Asciak, C.R. (1976). Decreased renal prostaglandin catabolism precedes the onset of hypertension in the developing spontaneously hypertensive rat. *Nature (London)*, **263**, 510–512

63. Limas, C.J. and Limas, C. (1977). Prostaglandin metabolism in the kidneys of spontaneously hypertensive rats. *Am. J. Physiol.*, **233**, H87–H92

64. Dunn, M.J. (1976). Renal prostaglandin synthesis in the spontaneously hypertensive rat. *J. Clin. Invest.*, **58**, 862–870

65. Limas, C. and Limas, C.J. (1979). Enhanced renomedullary prostaglandin synthesis in spontaneously hypertensive rats: Role of phospholipase A_2. *Am. J. Physiol.*, **236**, H65–H72

66. Shibouta, Y., Inada, Y., Terashita, Z., Nishikawa, K., Kikuchi, S. and Shimamoto, K. (1979). Angiotensin II-stimulated release of thromboxane A_2 and prostacyclin (PGI_2) in isolated, perfused kidneys of spontaneously hypertensive rats. *Biochem. Pharmacol.*, **28**, 3601–3609

67. Limas, C., Goldman, P., Limas, C.J. and Iwai, J. (1981). Effect of salt on prostaglandin metabolism in hypertension-prone and resistant Dahl rats. *Hypertension*, **3**, 219–224

68. Abe, K., Yasujima, M., Irokawa, N., Seino, M., Chiba, S., Sakurei, Y., Sato, M., Imai, Y., Saito, K., Ito, T., Haruyama, T., Otsuka, Y. and Yoshinaga, K. (1978). The role of intrarenal vasoactive substances in the pathogenesis of essential hypertension. *Clin. Sci. Mol. Med.*, **55**, 363s–366s

69. Tan, S.Y., Bravo, E. and Mulrow, P.J. (1978). Impaired renal prostaglandin E_2 biosynthesis in human hypertensive states. *Prostagl. Med.*, **1**, 76–85

70. Weber, P.C., Scherer, B., Held, E., Siess, W. and Stoffel, H. (1979). Urinary prostaglandins and kallikrein in essential hypertension. *Clin. Sci.*, **57**, 259s–261s

71. Level, M. and Grose, J.H. (1982). Renal prostaglandins in borderline and sustained essential hypertension. *Prostagl. Leuk. Med.*, **8**, 409–418

72. MacKenzie, T., Zawada, E.T., Johnson, M.D. and Green, S. (1984). The importance of age on prostaglandin E_2 excretion in normal and hypertensive men. *Nephron*, **38**, 178–182

73. Rathaus, M., Korzets, Z. and Bernheim, J. (1983). The urinary excretion of prostaglandins E_2 and $F_{2\alpha}$ in essential hypertension. *Eur. J. Clin. Invest.*, **13**, 13–17

74. Campbell, W.B., Holland, O.H., Adams, B.V. and Gomez-Sanchez, C.E. (1982). Urinary excretion of prostaglandin E_2, prostaglandin $F_{2\alpha}$, and thromboxane B_2 in normotensive and hypertensive subjects on varying sodium intakes. *Hypertension*, **4**, 735–741

75. Grose, J.H., Lebel, M. and Gbeassor, F.M. (1980). Diminished urinary prostacyclin metabolite in essential hypertension. *Clin. Sci.*, **59**, 121s–123s

76. Hornych, A., Safar, M., Bariety, J. and Milliez, P. (1983). Thromboxane B_2 in borderline and essential hypertensive patients. *Prostagl. Leuk. Med.*, **10**, 145–155
77. London, G.M., Hornych, A., Safar, M.E., Levenson, J.A. and Simon, A.C. (1982). Plasma prostaglandins PGE_2 and $PGF_{2\alpha}$, total effective vascular compliance and renal plasma flow in essential hypertension. *Nephron*, **32**, 118–124
78. Roy, L., Mehta, J. and Mehta, P. (1983). Increased plasma concentrations of prostacylin metabolite 6-keto-$PGF_{1\alpha}$ in essential hypertension. *Am. J. Cardiol.*, **51**, 464–467
79. Chen, L.S., Ito, T., Ogawa, K., Shikano, M. and Satake, T. (1984). Plasma concentrations of 6-keto-prostaglandin $F_{1\alpha}$, thromboxane B_2 and platelet aggregation in patients with essential hypertension. *Jpn. Heart J.*, **25**, 1001–1009
80. Ruilope, L., Garcia, Robles, C., Bernis, C., Barrientos, A., Alcazar, J., Tresguerres, J.A.F., Sancho, J. and Rodicio, J.L. (1982). Role of renal prostaglandins E_2 in chronic renal disease hypertension. *Nephron*, **32**, 202–206
81. Zia, P., Zipser, R., Speckart, P. and Horton, R. (1978). The measurement of urinary prostaglandin E in normal subjects and in high renin states. *J. Lab. Clin. Med.*, **92**, 415–422
82. Zipser, R.D., Speckart, P.F., Zia, P.K., Hahn, J.A., Boswell, W.P. and Horton, R. (1978). Release of immunoassayable prostaglandin E by the human ischemic kidney. *J. Clin. Endocrinol. Metab.*, **47**, 914–917
83. Tabuchi, Y., Ogihara, T. and Kumahara, Y. (1985). Renal vein prostaglandins in renovascular hypertensive patients. *Prostagl. Leuk. Med.*, **19**, 219–226
84. Pedersen, E.B., Christensen, N.J., Christensen, P., Johannesen, P., Kornerup, H.J., Kristensen, S., Lauritsen, J.G., Leyssac, P.P., Rasmussen, A. and Wohlert, M. (1983). Preeclamsia–A state of prostaglandin deficiency? Urinary prostaglandin excretion, the renin–aldosterone system, and circulating catecholamines in preeclamsia. *Hypertension*, **5**, 105–111
85. Goodman, R.P., Killam, A.P., Brash, A.R. and Branch, R.A. (1982). Prostacyclin production during pregnancy: Comparison of production during normal pregnancy and pregnancy complicated by hypertension. *Am. J. Obstet. Gynecol.*, **142**, 817–822
86. Ylikorkala, O., Pekonen, F. and Viinikka, L. (1986). Renal prostacyclin and thromboxane in normotensive and preeclamptic women and their infants. *J. Clin. Endocrinol. Metab.*, **63**, 1307–1312
87. Walsh, S.W. (1985). Preeclamsia: An imbalance in placental prostacyclin and thromboxane production. *Am. J. Obstet. Gynecol.*, **152**, 335–340
88. Rowe, B.P. (1986). The influence of indomethacin on blood pressure during infusion of vasopressors. *Hypertension*, **8**, 772–778
89. Banks, R.A., Beilin, L.J. and Soltys, J. (1983). Dose-dependent effects of meclofenamate on peripheral vasculature of conscious rabbits. *Clin. Sci.*, **64**, 471–474
90. Beilin, L.J. and Bhattacharya, J. (1977). The effect of prostaglandin synthesis inhibitors on renal blood flow distribution in conscious rabbits. *J. Physiol.*, **269**, 395–405
91. Mason, R.T., Coghlan, J.P., Denton, D.A., Graham, W.F., Humphery, T.J., Scoggins, B.A. and Whitworth, J.A. (1984). Prostaglandin synthesis inhibition with indomethacin in ACTH-induced hypertension. *J. Cardiovasc. Pharmacol.*, **6**, 288–292
92. DeForrest, J.M., Davis, J.O., Freeman, R.H., Seymour, A.A., Rowe, B.P., Williams, G.M. and Davis, T.P. (1980). Effects of indomethacin and meclofenamate on renin release and renal hemodynamic function during chronic sodium depletion in conscious dogs. *Circ. Res.*, **47**, 99–107
93. Stahl, R., Dienemann, H., Besserer, K., Kneissler, U. and Helmchen, U. (1981). Effect of indomethacin on blood pressure in rats with renovascular hypertension: Dependence on plasma renin activity. *Klin. Wochenschr.*, **59**, 245–246
94. Wennmalm, A. (1978). Influence of indomethacin on the systemic and pulmonary vascular resistance in man. *Clin. Sci. Mol. Med.*, **54**, 141–145
95. Friedman, P.L., Brown, E.J., Gunther, S., Alexander, R.W., Barry, W.H., Mudge, G.H. and Grossman, W. (1981). Coronary vasoconstrictor effect of indomethacin in patients with coronary-artery disease. *N. Engl. J. Med.*, **305**, 1171–1175
96. Dzau, V.J., Packer, M., Lilly, L.S., Swartz, S.L., Hollenberg, N.K. and Williams, G.H. (1984). Prostaglandins in severe congestive heart failure. Relation to activation of the renin–angiotensin system and hyponatremia. *N. Engl. J. Med.*, **310**, 347–352
97. McQueen, D. and Bell, K. (1976). The effects of prostaglandin E_1 and sodium meclofenamate on blood pressure in renal hypertensive rats. *Eur. J. Pharmacol.*, **37**, 223–235

98. Romero, J.C. and Strong, C.G. (1977). The effect of indomethacin blockade of prostaglandin synthesis on blood pressure of normal rabbits and rabbits with renovascular hypertension. *Circ. Res.*, **40**, 35–40
99. Muirhead, E.E., Brooks, B. and Brosius, W.L. (1976). Indomethacin and blood pressure control. *J. Lab. Clin. Med.*, **88**, 578–583
100. Colina-Chourio, J., McGiff, J.C. and Nasjletti, A. (1979). Effect of indomethacin on blood pressure in the normotensive unanesthetized rabbit: Possible relation to prostaglandin synthesis inhibition. *Clin. Sci.*, **57**, 359–365
101. Vierhapper, H., Waldhausl, W. and Nowotny, I. (1981). Effect of indomethacin upon angiotensin-induced changes in blood pressure and plasma aldosterone in man. *Eur. J. Clin. Invest.*, **11**, 85–89
102. Gullner, H.G., Gill, J.R., Bartter, F.C. and Dusing, R. (1980). The role of the prostaglandin system in the regulation of renal function in normal women. *Am. J. Med.*, **69**, 718–724
103. Gullner, H.G., Lake, C.R., Bartter, F.C. and Kafka, M.S. (1979). Effect of inhibition of prostaglandin synthesis on sympathetic nervous system function in man. *J. Clin. Endocrinol. Metab.*, **49**, 552–556
104. Mills, E.H., Whitworth, J.A., Andrews, J. and Kincaid-Smith, P. (1982). Non-steroidal anti-inflammatory drugs and blood pressure. *Aust. NZ J. Med.*, **12**, 478–482
105. Zimmermann, B.G. (1978). Effect of meclofenamate on renal vascular resistance in early Goldblatt hypertension in conscious and anesthetized dogs. *Prostaglandins*, **15**, 1027–1033
106. Dietz, J.R., Davis, J.O., DeForrest, J.M., Freeman, R.H., Echtenkamp, S.F. and Seymour, A.A. (1981). Effects of indomethacin in dogs with acute and chronic renovascular hypertension. *Am. J. Physiol.*, **240**, H533–H538
107. Pugsley, D.J., Mullins, R. and Beilin, L.J. (1976). Renal prostaglandin synthesis in hypertension induced by deoxycorticosterone and sodium chloride in the rat. *Clin. Sci. Mol. Med.*, **51**, 253s–256s
108. Paulson, D.J. and Eversole, W.J. (1977). Effects of prostaglandin E$_2$ and prostaglandin inhibitors on adrenal regeneration hypertension. *Am. J. Physiol.*, **232**, E95–E99
109. Chrysant, S.G., Townsend, S.M. and Morgan, P.R. (1978). The effects of salt and meclofenamate administration on the hypertension of spontaneously hypertensive rats. *Clin. Exp. Hypertens.*, **1**, 381–391
110. Levy, J.V. (1977). Changes in systolic arterial blood pressure in normal and spontaneously hypertensive rats produced by acute administration of inhibitors of prostaglandin biosynthesis. *Prostaglandins*, **13**, 153–160
111. Tuttle, R.S., Banziger, V., Patel, S. and Northrup, N. (1985). Inhibition by metroprolol of the antihypertensive effect of aspirin in young rats. *J. Pharmacol. Exp. Ther.*, **234**, 166–171
112. Grone, H.J., Grippo, R.S., Arendhorst, W.J. and Dunn, M.J. (1986). Role of thromboxane in control of arterial pressure and renal function in young spontaneously hypertensive rats. *Am. J. Physiol.*, **250**, F488–F496
113. Uderman, H.D., Jackson, E.K., Puett, D. and Workman, R.J. (1984). Thromboxane synthetase inhibitor UK 38,485 lowers blood pressure in the adult spontaneously hypertensive rat. *J. Cardiovasc. Pharmacol.*, **6**, 969–972
114. Safar, M.E., Hornych, A.F., Levenson, J.A., Simon, A.C., London, G.M., Bariety, J.L. and Milliez, P.L. (1981). Central haemodynamics and plasma prostaglandin E$_2$ in borderline and sustained hypertensive patients before and after indomethacin. *Clin. Sci.*, **61**, 323s–325s
115. Patak, R.V., Mookerjee, B.K., Bentzel, C.J., Hysert, P.E., Babej, M. and Lee, J.B. (1975). Antagonism of the effects of furosemide by indomethacin in normal and hypertensive man. *Prostaglandins*, **10**, 649–658
116. Ylitalo, P., Pitkajarvi, T., Metsa-Ketela, T. and Vapaatalo, H. (1978). The effect of inhibition of prostaglandin synthesis on plasma renin activity and blood pressure in essential hypertension. *Prostagl. Med.*, **1**, 479–488
117. Lopez-Ovejero, J.A., Weber, M.A., Drayer, J.I.M., Sealey, J.E. and Laragh, J.H. (1978). Effects of indomethacin alone and during diuretic or β-adrenoreceptor-blockade therapy on blood pressure and the renin system in essential hypertension. *Clin. Sci. Mol. Med.*, **55**, 203s–205s

174

118. Abe, K., Ito, T., Sato, M., Harayuma, T., Sato, K., Omata, K., Hiwatari, M., Sakurai, Y., Imai, Y. and Yoshinaga, K. (1980). Role of prostaglandin in the antihypertensive mechanism of captopril in low renin hypertension. *Clin. Sci.*, **59**, 141s–144s
119. Someya, N., Kodama, K. and Tanaka, K. (1985). Effect of captopril on plasma prostacyclin concentration in essential hypertensive patients. *Prostgl. Leuk. Med.*, **20**, 187–195
120. Swartz, S.L. and Williams, G.H. (1982). Angiotensin-converting enzyme inhibition and prostaglandins. *Am. J. Cardiol.*, **49**, 1405–1409
121. Ciabattoni, G., Pugliese, F., Cinotti, G.A., Stirati, G., Ronci, R., Castrucci, G., Peirucci, A. and Patrono, C. (1979). Characterization of furosemide-induced activation of the renal prostaglandin system. *Eur. J. Pharmacol.*, **60**, 181–187
122. Patrono, C.F., Pugliese, F., Ciabattoni, G., Patrignani, P., Maseri, A., Chierchia, S., Peskar, B.A., Cinotti, G.A., Simonetti, B.M. and Pierucci, A. (1982). Evidence for a direct stimulatory effect of prostacyclin on renin release in man. *J. Clin. Invest.*, **69**, 231–239
123. Weber, P.C., Scherer, B. and Larsson, C. (1977). Increase of free arachidonic acid by furosemide in man as the cause of prostaglandin and renin release. *Eur. J. Pharmacol.*, **41**, 329–332
124. Kramer, H.J., Dusing, R., Stinnesbeck, B., Prior, W., Backer, A., Eden, J., Kipnowski, J., Glanzer, K. and Kruck, F. (1980). Interaction of conventional and antikaliuretic diuretics with the renal prostaglandin system. *Clin. Sci.*, **59**, 67–70
125. Chiba, S., Abe, K., Yasujima, M., Irokawa, N., Saito, K., Sakurai, Y., Ito, T., Sato, M. Otsuka, Y. and Yoshinaga, K. (1979). Effect of triamterene on urinary excretion of immunoreactive prostaglandin E in essential hypertension. *Tohoku J. Exp. Med.*, **129**, 249–256
126. Webster, J., Dollery, C.T. and Hensby, C.N. (1980). Circulating prostacyclin concentrations may be increased by bendrofluazide in patients with essential hypertension. *Clin. Sci.*, **59**, 125s–128s
127. Haeusler, G. and Gerold, M. (1979). Increased levels of prostaglandin-like material in the canine blood during arterial hypotension produced by hydralazine, dihydralazine and minoxidil. *Naunyn-Schmiedebergs Arch. Pharmacol.*, **310**, 155–167
128. Jackson, E.K., and Campbell, W.D. (1981). A possible antihypertensive mechanism of propranolol: Antagonism of angiotensin II enhancement of sympathetic nerve transmission through prostaglandins. *Hypertension*, **3**, 23–33
129. Watkins, J., Abbott, E.C., Hensby, C.N., Webster, J. and Dollery, C.T. (1980). Attenuation of hypotensive effect of propranolol and thiazide diuretics by indomethacin. *Br. Med. J.*, **281**, 702–705
130. Ylitalo, P., Pitkajarvi, T., Pyykonen, M.L., Nurmi, A.K., Sappala, E. and Vapaatalo, H. (1985). Inhibition of prostaglandin synthesis by indomethacin interacts with the antihypertensive effect of atenolol. *Clin. Pharmacol. Ther.*, **38**, 443–449
131. Reimann, I.W., Ratge, D., Wisser, H. and Frolich, J.C. (1981). Are prostaglandins involved in the antihypertensive effect of dihydralazine? *Clin. Sci.*, **61**, 319s–321s
132. Das, U.N. (1982). Modification of anti-hypertensive action of verapamil by inhibition of endogenous prostaglandin synthesis. *Prostgl. Leuk. Med.*, **9**, 167–169
133. Chalmers, J.P., West, M.J., Wing, L.M.H., Bune, A.J.C. and Graham, J.R. (1984). Effects of indomethacin, sulindac, naproxen, aspirin, and paracetamol in treated hypertensive patients. *Clin. Exp. Hypertens.* **A6(6)**, 1077–1093

8
Prostacyclin receptors

J. MacDermot

Prostacyclin (epoprostenol, PGI_2) was discovered a little over 10 years ago by Vane and his colleagues[1] when they were examining the products of vascular cyclo-oxygenase metabolism. They remarked on its chemical instability, and much of the information regarding the detailed pharmacological properties of this molecule has been obtained with potent and stable structural analogues. The biological activities of PGI_2 are described in more detail in other chapters of this book, and, in each case, the response at a cellular level is mediated by activation of adenylate cyclase (ATP pyrophosphate-lyase(cyclizing): EC 4.6.1.1). There is compelling evidence, which is reviewed in more detail below, that PGI_2 mediates its effects by interaction with high-affinity cell-surface receptors which are distributed widely in mammalian tissues. Detailed knowledge of PGI_2 receptors is confined largely to platelets[2-5], blood vessels[6,7] and a number of cell culture systems (both primary cell cultures and established cell lines)[5], although PGI_2 receptors have been identified and partially characterized in other tissues[8,9].

ADENYLATE CYCLASE ACTIVATION (NCB-20 CELLS)

Adenylate cyclase is bound to the inner aspect of the plasma membrane. Its catalytic activity mediates hydrolysis of ATP to form cyclic AMP, and may be measured in fractured membranes *in vitro* by the conversion of radiolabelled ATP to cyclic AMP[10]. The activity of the enzyme may also be measured by following changes in intracellular cyclic AMP in whole cells in the absence or presence of a phosphodiesterase inhibitor[11,12]. A full discussion of the relative merits of the two assay systems lies beyond the scope of the present review, but most information on the detailed biochemistry of receptor-mediated responses has been obtained by direct measurement of the enzymatic activity (i.e. conversion of labelled substrate to labelled product) in washed membrane preparations.

The ready availability of transformed cell lines, and the capacity to manipulate with great precision the growth environment of cultured cells, have made possible a large number of experiments directed to an examination of PGI_2 receptors that would not be possible in whole animals or tissues, and certainly not in man. PGI_2 receptors have been identified on a number of cell lines, but have been most profitably exploited to date in the NCB-20 neuronal somatic hybrid[13]. These cells were 'made' some years ago by Minna and his colleagues, and have been made available generously since then. NCB-20 cells are the product of Sendai virus-induced fusion of an HGPRT⁻ mutant mouse neuroblastoma (N18TG2)[14] and embryonic brain cells of Chinese hamster (18 days *in utero*). This cell was derived as part of an extensive programme of research to examine differentiated neuronal function *in vitro*, especially cell–cell recognition and synapse formation. NCB-20 cells are cholinergic, they are electrically excitable, and are competent to form synapses with cultured myotubes *in vitro*[15]. These cells express numerous cell surface receptors for hormones and neurotransmitters, including muscarinic cholinergic, serotonergic, α-adrenergic, opiate, adenosine (A_2) and, of interest to the present discussion, PGI_2[16].

A comparison of the capacity of three PGI_2 structural analogues (PGI_2, PGE_1 and 6β-PGI_1) to activate adenylate cyclase is shown in Figure 8.1. It will be immediately apparent that each compound is a 'full agonist', increasing

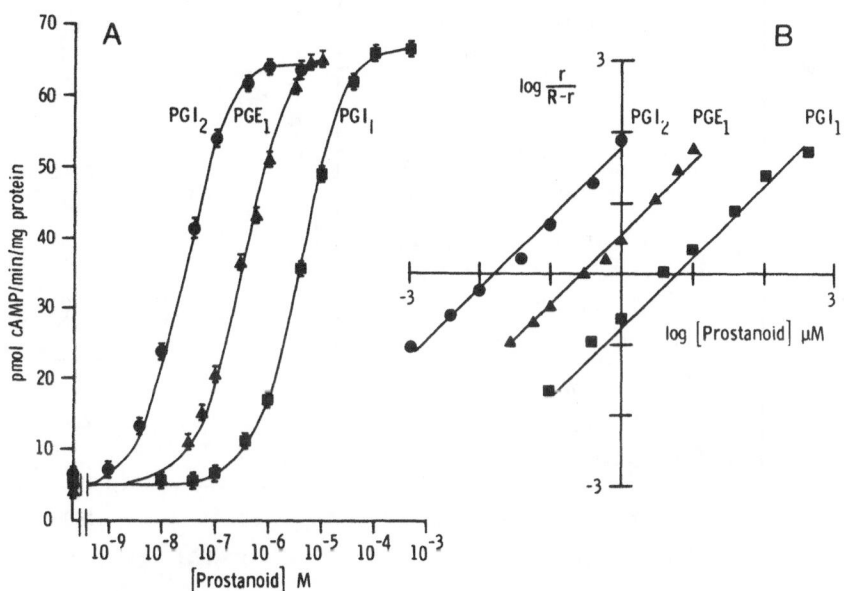

Figure 8.1 Prostanoid-dependent activation of adenylate cyclase in whole homogenates of NCB-20 cells. Results in (A) show means ± SEM of triplicate determinations of adenylate cyclase activity in the presence of increasing concentrations of prostacyclin (●), PGE_1 (▲) and 6β-PGI_1 (■). The same data are presented in (B) as Hill plots, where r is the increase in enzyme activity above basal levels at each concentration of prostanoid, and R is the maximum activation produced by each prostanoid. (Reproduced from reference 16 with permission)

basal enzyme activity more than 10-fold (Figure 8.1a). The corresponding Hill transformations of the same concentration curves (Figure 8.1b) show straight lines with values of the slopes (n) approximating closely to 1.0. This suggests a simple 1:1 stoichiometric relationship in each ligand-receptor interaction, with little likelihood of multiple functional receptors, and no evidence of co-operativity. 6β-PGI$_1$ is the most stable of the three eicosanoids shown in Figure 8.1, and was selected therefore for further analysis of receptor-mediated adenylate cyclase activation[16]. In individual incubations of NCB-20 homogenates, the accumulation of cyclic AMP was linear in the absence or presence of 6β-PGI$_1$ (at 2 concentrations) for times up to 20 min (Figure 8.2a). This observation is a prerequisite for the Eadie–Hofstee transformation of a concentration curve. The increase in enzyme activity as a function of 6β-PGI$_1$ concentration is shown in Figure 8.2b, and the inset shows the corresponding Eadie–Hofstee plot. The linear relationship between the two co-ordinate scales provides compelling evidence for a single biologically active PGI$_2$ receptor species in the plasma membrane of NCB-20 cells. This point has been addressed in some detail here, as there is some

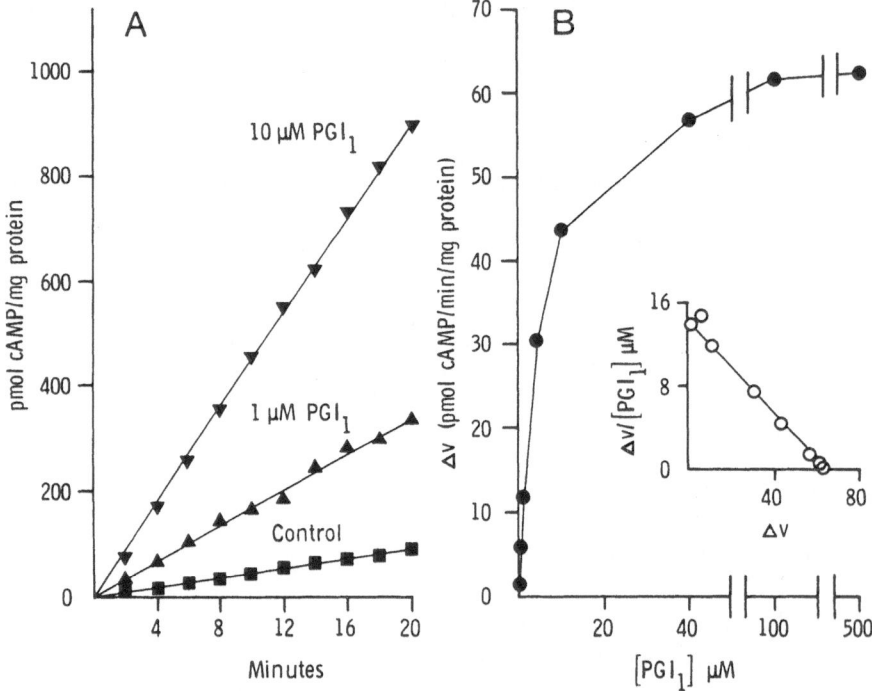

Figure 8.2 Activation of adenylate cyclase by 6β-PGI$_1$ in a whole homogenate of NCB-20 cells. Results in (A) show the cyclic AMP formed/mg protein as a function of time in the absence (■) or presence of 1.0 μmol L^{-1} (▲) or 10 μmol L^{-1} (▼) 6β-PGI$_1$. The results in (B) show the increase in adenylate cyclase activity above the basal level (5.2 pmol cyclic AMP min^{-1} (mg protein)$^{-1}$ at selected concentrations of 6β-PGI$_1$. The inset shows an Eadie–Hofstee plot of the same data, where Δv is the increase in enzyme activity at any particular 6β-PGI$_1$ concentration. (Reproduced from reference 16 with permission)

uncertainty on this point in similar responses measured in platelet membranes (see below).

The receptor-mediated activation of adenylate cyclase in all neurotransmitter or hormonal systems that have been studied to date requires the presence of GTP[17,18]. Within the plasma membrane of most cells, there are numerous guanyl nucleotide-binding regulatory proteins (variously called N- or G-proteins) that are responsible for receptor-mediated stimulation (G_s) or inhibition (G_i) of the catalytic subunit of adenylate cyclase (for reviews, see references 19, 20). The G-proteins have subunit structure, and are constituted as heterotrimers with α, β and γ subunits. G_s and G_i share the same β and γ subunits, but have unique α subunits that determine stimulatory or inhibitory effects on the catalytic adenylate cyclase subunit. Further details of this complex system are described later. The activation of adenylate cyclase by PGI_2 analogues is dependent on the presence of GTP[16], and this provides the most compelling evidence for a functional membrane receptor for PGI_2, as distinct from a non-specific membrane or other effect of PGI_2 in cell homogenates *in vitro*. Figure 8.3 shows the 6β-PGI_1-dependent accumulation of cyclic AMP with time, and the requirement for GTP in this reponse. Measurement of the 6β-PGI_1-dependent increase in adenylate cyclase activity at selected GTP concentrations (Figure 8.4) shows that the concentration of GTP producing half-maximum enzyme activation was about 0.3 μmol L^{-1} and was within the range observed in other systems.

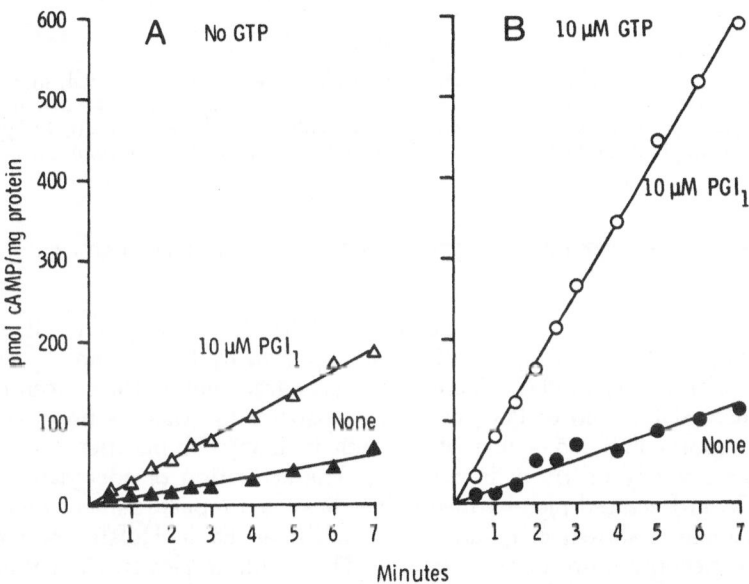

Figure 8.3 GTP requirement for activation of adenylate cyclase by 6β-PGI_1 in a washed particulate preparation of NCB-20 cells. Results show the accumulation of cyclic AMP/mg protein with time in the absence (A) or presence (B) of 10 μmol L^{-1} GTP. Assays were performed in each case in the absence (▲●) or presence (△○) of 10 μmol L^{-1} 6β-PGI_1. (Reproduced from reference 16 with permission)

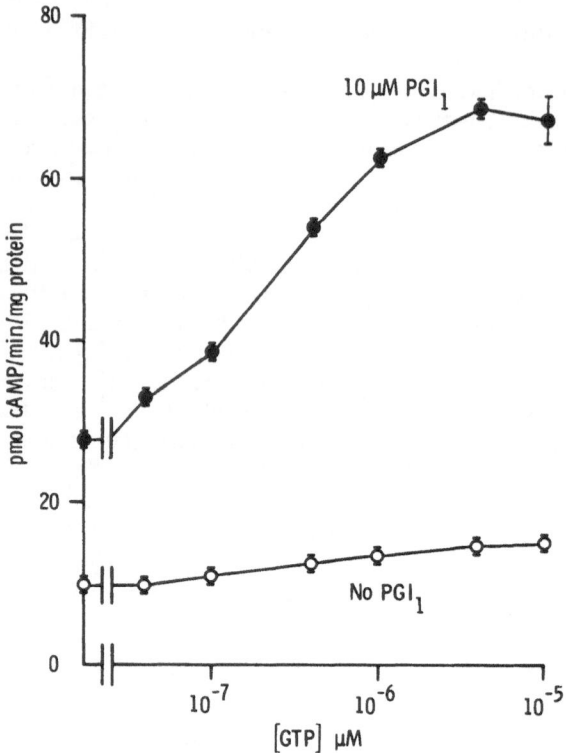

Figure 8.4 GTP requirement for activation of adenylate cyclase by 6β-PGI₁ in a washed particulate fraction of NCB-20 cells. Results show the means ± SEM of triplicate determinations of adenylate cyclase activity at increasing GTP concentrations, in the absence (○) or presence (●) of 10 μmol L⁻¹ 6β-PGI₁. (Reproduced from reference 16 with permission)

ADENYLATE CYCLASE ACTIVATION (PLATELETS AND BLOOD VESSELS)

The first demonstration of the molecular mechanism(s) by which PGI₂ acts as an inhibitor of platelet aggregation was reported by two groups[11,12] shortly after the discovery of PGI₂. There was broad agreement on the concentration-response relationship of PGI₂ in the two papers, and there is no doubt that these reports initiated a line of research in many laboratories that is still pursued actively nearly a decade later. The activation of adenylate cyclase by PGI₂ in fractured platelet membranes has been repeated many times, and an example is shown in Figure 8.5, which is an Eadie–Hofstee plot of the PGI₂ concentration-response curve[21]. The result is clearly similar to that obtained in NCB-20 homogenates, but it must be emphasized that, in at least one report[3], there is a suggestion of a second biologically active receptor type. This conclusion is dependent on a non-linear relationship between the co-ordinate values which may be resolved into two straight lines, each one of which, it is proposed, corresponds to a specific, biologically active receptor

180

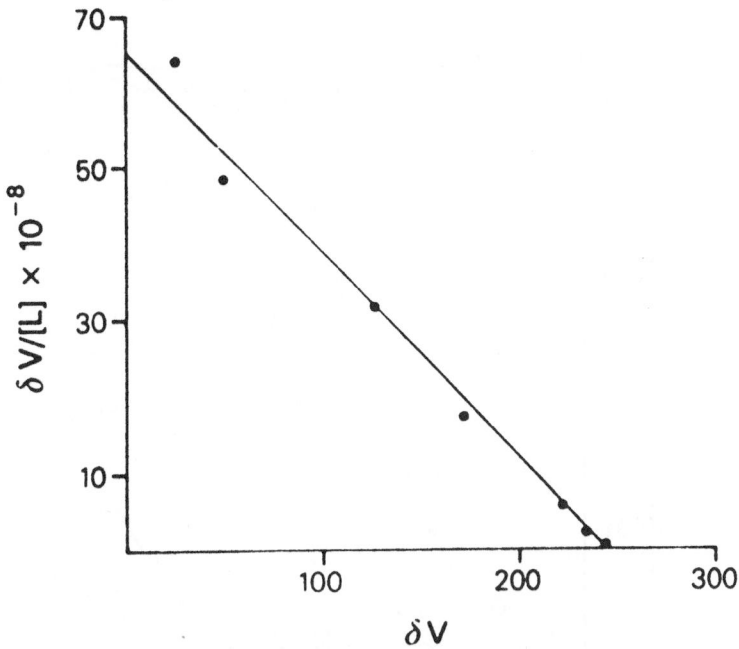

Figure 8.5 PGI$_2$-dependent activation of platelet adenylate cyclase. The data are presented as an Eadie–Hofstee plot. δv is the increase in adenylate cyclase activity above basal enzyme activity, and [L] the PGI$_2$ concentration (nmol L^{-1}). (Reproduced from reference 21 with permission)

site. This discrepancy in the published data can be of little general interest, and, for the time being, remains unresolved.

A more intriguing anomaly relates, however, to the interaction between PGE$_1$ and the PGI$_2$ receptor. The I-series prostaglandins make up a vanishingly small proportion of the total complement of eicosanoids in mammalian systems, and are certainly present at concentrations far too low to have any biological effect. However, *in vitro* experiments reveal that PGE$_1$ is a full agonist at PGI$_2$ receptors[16], provided measurements are made of adenylate cyclase activity in incubations containing fractured platelet or other membranes (e.g see Figure 8.1). However, if PGE$_1$-dependent increases in intracellular cyclic AMP concentrations are compared in whole platelets with those mediated by PGI$_2$, the results suggest a partial agonist activity for PGE$_1$[11,12]. There is, at present, no explanation for these results, although (somewhat unsatisfactorily) possible explanations have included PGI$_2$ receptor sub-types that are revealed or lost during cell fracture, or even PGE$_1$-dependent activation of phosphodiesterase in the intact cell.

PGI$_2$-dependent activation of adenylate cyclase has been demonstrated[22] in homogenates of guinea-pig lung (Figure 8.6). A more detailed analysis of the concentration curves revealed linear Eadie–Hofstee plots, and Hill interaction coefficients approximating closely to 1.0, suggesting once again

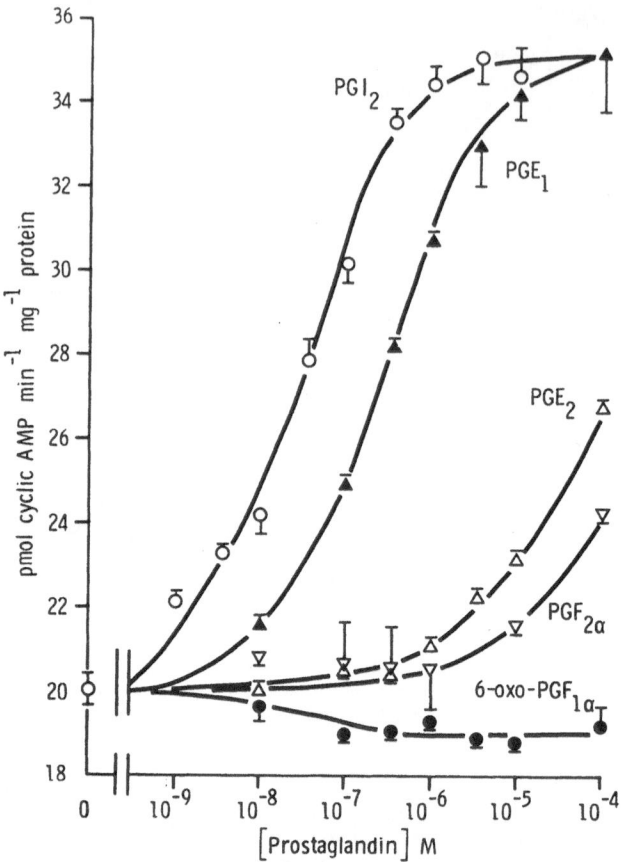

Figure 8.6 PGI$_2$-dependent activation of adenylate cyclase of a guinea-pig lung homogenate. Results show the means $\pm$ SEM of adenylate cyclase activity measured in the presence of increasing concentrations of PGI$_2$ (○), PGE$_1$ (▲), PGE$_2$ (△), PGF$_{2\alpha}$ (▽) and 6-oxo-PGF$_{1\alpha}$ (●). (Reproduced from reference 22 with permission)

that there is a single functional PGI$_2$ receptor with no evidence of co-operativity. Comparison of the densities of PGI$_2$ receptors in different lung tissues has shown the greatest number of receptors to be located peripherally in small blood vessels[23]. Contraction or relaxation of these vessels regulates pulmonary artery pressure, and it is proposed that the vasodilator effects of PGI$_2$ in both the systemic and pulmonary arterial beds is mediated by a direct effect of PGI$_2$ on vascular smooth muscle[24].

LIGAND BINDING TO PGI$_2$ RECEPTORS

There have been several reports in the last few years of [³H]PGI$_2$ binding to platelet[2], vascular[25] or cultured cell membranes[26]. Many of these studies[2] have used 9β-[³H]PGI$_2$, which was available previously from New England Nuclear

182

as the tetramethylammonium salt and, more recently, as the methyl ester which is readily hydrolysed to yield the free acid under alkaline conditions. We reported from this laboratory[27] a synthesis of 11β-[^{3}H]PGI$_2$, which has also been used in similar studies to identify membrane PGI$_2$ receptors. Both of these tritiated materials, whether labelled in the 11β- or 9β-positions, are, however, very far from ideal radioligands. The major problem is that of instability, which necessitates measurement of ligand binding under alkaline conditions (usually pH 8.5) to minimize the spontaneous hydrolysis of PGI$_2$ to 6-oxo-PGF$_{1\alpha}$.

There are numerous carbacyclic (and other) chemically stable structural analogues of PGI$_2$, and one of these, [^{3}H]iloprost, is now available from Amersham International. Similar compounds may well become available from other commercial sources in the near future. In the experience of this laboratory at least, [^{3}H]iloprost is the best of the available radioligands at present, on the basis of substantially greater chemical stability than PGI$_2$, a lower proportion of 'non-specific' binding, and a higher binding affinity. PGE$_1$ binds to PGI$_2$ receptors[26], but, in spite of moderate chemical stability, it is unsuitable as a radioligand. The problem here is one of affinity, which for PGE$_1$ is of the order[26] of 50–220 nmol L^{-1}.

The binding of [^{3}H]iloprost to NCB-20 membranes is representative of the binding to other PGI$_2$-sensitive tissues that have been examined in this laboratory, namely human platelets and lung membranes. In these experiments[28], 'specific binding' was defined as that displaced by 10 μmol L^{-1} carbacyclin (6α-carbaprostaglandin I$_2$) in parallel tubes. The association of 15 nmol L^{-1} [^{3}H]iloprost to the PGI$_2$ receptor of NCB-20 membranes is shown in Figure 8.7. At this ligand concentration, the non-specific binding represented about 15% of the total. This compares very favourably with [^{3}H]PGI$_2$, for which the proportion of non-specific binding (at least in our experience) is often in excess of 40–50%. A pseudo-1st-order rate plot of these data had a slope (observed rate constant, k_{obs}) of 4.2 × 10^{-3} s^{-1}. The forward rate constant (k_{+1}) was 2.01 × 10^{-5} (mol L^{-1})$^{-1}$ s^{-1} determined from the relationship $k_{+1} = (k_{obs} - k_{-1})/$[ligand], where k_{-1} is the 1st-order rate constant for the dissociation of the ligand–receptor complex. The numerical value of k_{-1} was determined by measurement of the rate of dissociation of the ligand and receptor, after addition of an excess of unlabelled iloprost (final concentration, = 4 μmol L^{-1}). The results are shown in Figure 8.8. A semilogarithmic plot of the data (Figure 8.8b) revealed a half-time for dissociation ($t_{1/2}$) of 584.5s, whence k_{-1} was calculated to be 1.19 × 10^{-3} s^{-1}. The value of the dissociation constant (K_d) was determined from the ratio k_{-1}/k_{+1}, and was 5.9 nmol L^{-1}.

Iloprost binding was also measured at equilibrium at selected concentrations of [^{3}H]iloprost up to 100 nmol L^{-1}. The result is shown in Figure 8.9, and, from the corresponding Scatchard plot (Figure 8.9b), the values were obtained for the equilibrium dissociation constant (K_d = 29.9 nmol L^{-1}) and the maximum binding capacity of the membranes (B_{max} = 347 fmol mg^{-1} protein). An important point needs to be made here relating to the linearity of the Scatchard plot in Figure 8.9b which suggests a single receptor type. If the concentration curve includes free ligand concentrations in excess of this value

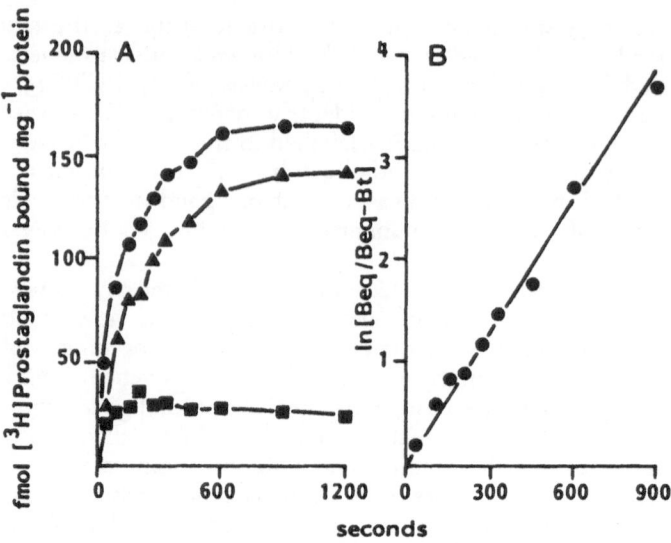

Figure 8.7 Association of [³H]iloprost with the membrane receptor of NCB-20 cells. Total (●), non-specific (■), and specific binding (▲) of 15 nmol L⁻¹ [³H]iloprost at 20°C are shown in A. A pseudo first-order rate plot of the data up to 900 s is shown in B. Beq is the specific [³H]iloprost binding at equilibrium, and Bt is the specific binding at each time, t. (Reproduced from reference 28 with permission)

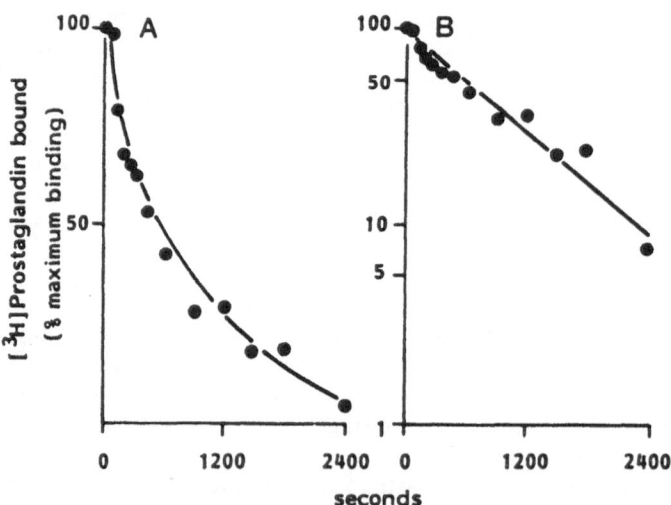

Figure 8.8 Dissociation of [³H]iloprost from the receptor of NCB-20 membranes. An equilibrium was established at 20°C for 20 min with 15 nmol L⁻¹ [³H]iloprost. At time zero, 4 μmol L⁻¹ cold ligand was added, and the decrease in specific binding measured (A). A semilogarithmic plot of the data is shown in B. (Reproduced from reference 28 with permission)

(100 nmol L^{-1}), then a curvilinear plot is obtained (Figure 8.16 below) which may be resolved into high- and low-affinity receptor populations. The proportion of the total binding that is low affinity will determine the magnitude of the difference obtained in the analysis of the results shown in Figure 8.9 when compared with the values obtained in Figure 8.16. In NCB-20 membranes, the low-affinity binding represents a very small proportion of the total, and for most purposes the difference is trivial. However, if the proportion of the high-affinity sites is reduced (as in desensitization, cf. Figure 8.16), or if there is relatively more of the low affinity binding site (as in platelet[21] or lung homogenates[25]), then there is a possibility of a serious misinterpretation of the data. Hence, where appropriate, the contribution of the two receptor sub-types should be determined separately.

STRUCTURE-ACTIVITY RELATIONSHIPS OF AGONISTS AT PGI$_2$ RECEPTORS

There are many studies now comparing the capacities of numerous prostaglandins to activate PGI$_2$ receptors or displace [^{3}H]PGI$_2$ or [^{3}H]iloprost from membrane binding sites[16,21,22,25,26,28]. Table 8.1 is a composite from several such tables, and a comparison with Figure 8.10 reveals several structural elements within the PGI$_2$ molecule that are required for high-affinity binding. This topic has been dealt with very fully elsewhere[16], and lies beyond the scope of this review, except to highlight a few points. First, the intramolecular proton source (the C1 carboxyl group) renders the vinyl ether of PGI$_2$ very vulnerable to hydrolysis. The product of this hydrolysis is 6-oxo-PGF$_{1\alpha}$,

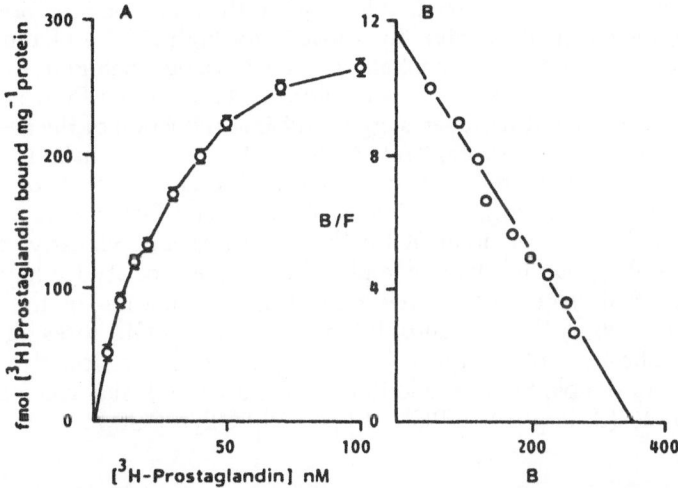

Figure 8.9 Binding of [^{3}H]iloprost to NCB-20 membranes. A, equilibrium binding of selected concentrations of [^{3}H]iloprost to NCB-20 membranes. Data are means ± SEM of triplicate determinations of specific binding, and are represented as a Scatchard plot (B). F is the free ligand concentration (nmol L^{-1}), and B is the [^{3}H]iloprost bound (fmol (mg protein)$^{-1}$). (Reproduced from reference 28 with permission)

Table 8.1 The relative potencies of prostaglandins that inhibit the binding of [^{3}H]PGI$_2$ or [^{3}H]iloprost to NCB-20 membranes

Prostaglandin	[^{3}H]agonist binding, K_i (nmol L^{-1})
PGI$_2$ analogues	
Iloprost	24.0
PGI$_2$	30.5
6α-carbacyclin	38.1
6β-PGI$_1$	654
ZK36375, (5Z)-iloprost	3 810
E-series prostaglandins	
PGE$_1$	37
13,14-dihydro-PGE$_1$	315
8-iso-PGE$_1$	735
5,6-trans-PGE$_2$	735
17-phenyl-PGE$_2$	4 370
13,14-dihydro-PGE$_2$	8 410
PGE$_2$	13 370
13,14-dihydro-15-oxo-PGE$_2$	> 100 000
15-epi-PGE$_2$	> 100 000
F and D series prostaglandins	
PGF$_{1α}$	> 100 000
6-oxo-PGF$_{1α}$	> 100 000
PGF$_{2α}$	> 100 000
PGD$_1$	> 100 000
PGD$_2$	> 100 000

which has little or no affinity for the PGI$_2$ receptor. The C1 carboxyl group is also a requirement for high-affinity binding, and esters at this position are biologically inactive. The 5–6 double bond (in the *trans* configuration) on the upper (α) side chain also confers the capacity for high-affinity binding, as 6β-PGI$_1$ and ZK36375 have substantially greater K_i values than PGI$_2$ or iloprost. In this respect, the relatively high affinity of PGE$_1$ for the PGI$_2$ receptor is not easily explained. It has been suggested[16] that reduction of the 5–6 double bond of the E-series prostaglandins allows the α side chain to adopt a configuration in solution that more closely resembles that of PGI$_2$. A comparison of the biological activities of the E- and F-series prostaglandins suggest an absolute requirement for the 11-OH group. Similarly, oxidation for the 15-OH group results in complete loss of the capacity for high-affinity binding to PGI$_2$ receptors. Furthermore, the configuration of the 15S-OH group is crucial, as the 15R-substituted analogue of PGE$_2$ loses all activity. Other modifications of the molecule may be less crucial, particularly reduction of the 13–14 double bond or additions to the lower (ω) side chain at carbon atoms 16–20 (cf. iloprost v. PGI$_2$; 17-phenyl-PGE$_2$ v. PGE$_2$).

CATION REQUIREMENT FOR HIGH-AFFINITY PGI$_2$ BINDING

The binding of [^{3}H]PGI$_2$ to its receptor is substantially increased by the addition of divalent cations in group 2A of the Periodic Table[29]. This effect is shown in Figure 8.11, and is mediated equally by Ca^{2+}, Ba^{2+}, Sr^{2+} or

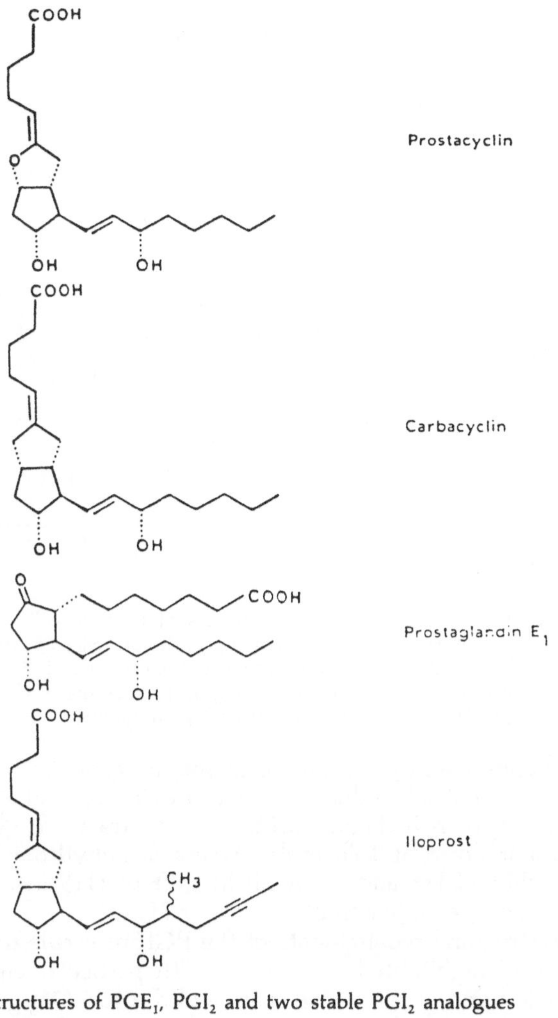

Figure 8.10 Structures of PGE$_1$, PGI$_2$ and two stable PGI$_2$ analogues

Mg^{2+} ions. The increase in binding shown in Figure 8.11 has been shown to be due to altered affinity of [^{3}H]PGI$_2$ binding without a change in the maximum binding capacity of the membranes. Concentration curves in the presence of 1 or 50 mmol L^{-1} MgSO$_4$ revealed values of 57.4 nmol L^{-1} and 21.9 nmol L^{-1} respectively, while the values for the receptor densities were 1014 and 1030 fmol mg^{-1} membrane protein.

The affinity of agonist binding to numerous receptors (e.g. α- or β-adrenoceptors) is increased by divalent cations. However, in the case of PGI$_2$ receptors, the possibility of a specific Ca^{2+}-binding site on the receptor or G-protein seemed unlikely as the effect of Ca^{2+} was mediated equally by several divalent cations, and was not inhibited by La^{3+} ions. We proposed that the cation might complex with the PGI$_2$ molecule in solution, and this

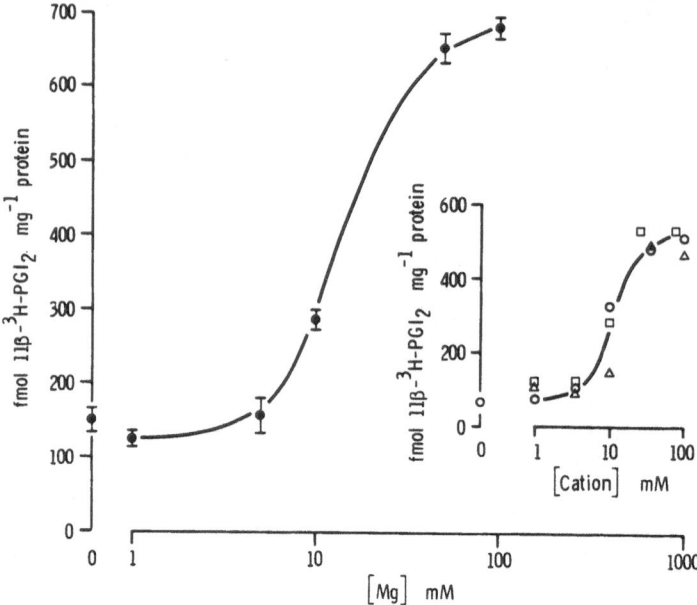

Figure 8.11 The binding of [³H]PGI₂ to membranes of NCB-20 cells. Results show the Mg²⁺-dependent increase in specific [³H]PGI₂ binding in the presence of 10 mmol L⁻¹ EDTA. Results are means ± SEM of triplicate determinations in the presence of 30 nmol L⁻¹ [³H]PGI₂. The inset shows a similar increase in [³H]PGI₂ binding in the presence of Ca²⁺ (○), Ba²⁺ (□) or Sr²⁺ (△) ions. (Reproduced from reference 30 with permission)

possibility was addressed by ¹H-nuclear magnetic resonance spectroscopy[30]. The spectrum was identical to that described previously, and a portion of the total spectrum is shown in Figure 8.12. The spectra were obtained in the absence or presence of a 50-fold molar excess of anhydrous MgCl₂. There was an upfield shift of H5 and a downfield shift of H15 in the presence of MgCl₂, with no corresponding shifts of H9 or H11.

Some of the structural requirements of the PGI₂ molecule for high-affinity binding have been highlighted previously, with particular emphasis placed on the 5,6-double bond of the α-side chain and the 15S-OH group of the ω-side chain. It is evident that the cation-dependent shifts in the ¹H-nmr spectrum occurred at sites that have been identified as critical for high-affinity binding, and it has been proposed[30] that PGI₂ may exist in at least 2 conformational states with different K_d values in the ligand–receptor interaction. It seems likely that the cation(s) forms an ion-pair with the C1 carboxyl group, and that the cation also interacts with remote sites of electron density within the PGI₂ molecule (i.e. the 5,6-double bond and the 15-OH group). We suggested then that the resultant change in the conformation of the PGI₂ molecule would more readily accommodate the geometric constraints of the receptor.

PGI₂ RECEPTOR STRUCTURE

A thorough analysis of receptor structure usually requires as a prerequisite that the receptor may be solubilized, and that it retains its capacity for ligand

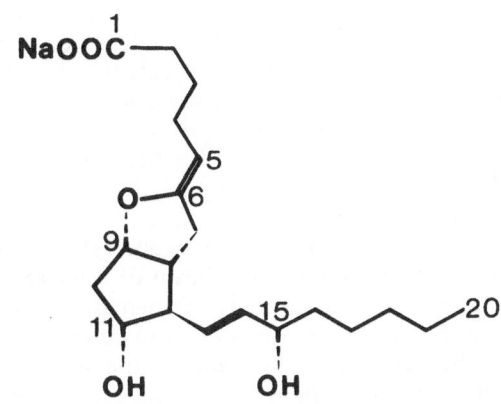

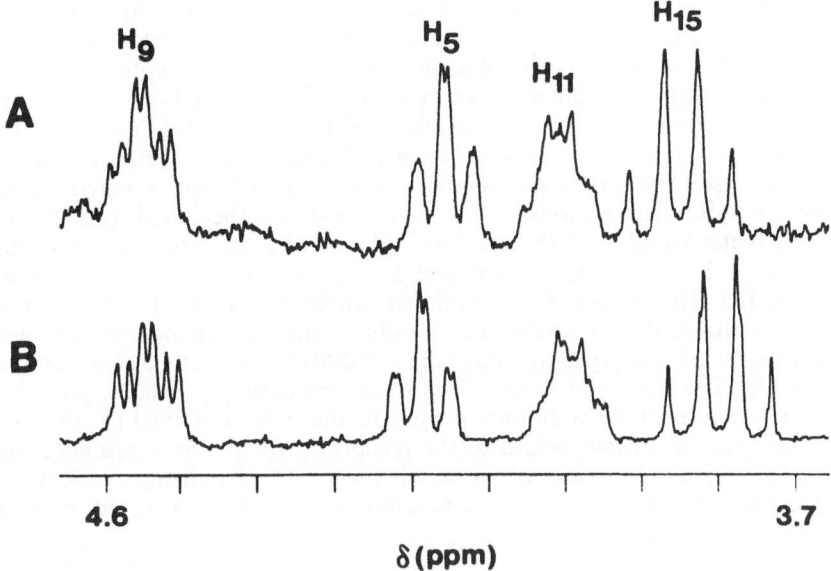

Figure 8.12 ¹H-NMR spectrum of PGI₂ (Na salt). The spectra were obtained from a solution of PGI₂ (5.3 mmol L⁻¹) in D₄-methanol. The spectra were obtained on a Varian XL 200 spectrometer at 200 MHz with the temperature maintained at 22°C. Chemical shifts are relative to the internal standard tetramethylsilane ($\delta = 0$). Results were obtained in the presence (A) of 300 mmol L⁻¹ MgCl₂ and absence (B) of MgCl₂. (Reproduced from reference 30 with permission)

binding. Despite numerous efforts by many groups, however, solubilization of the PGI₂ receptor in a state that permits ligand binding was unsuccessful until very recently (MacDermot, unpublished results). There is, however, no published data on the structure of the solubilized receptor, and our knowledge is at present confined to results obtained by the method of radiation inactivation[28].

The technique of radiation inactivation, and its application in the field of biochemistry, has been reviewed very extensively elsewhere[31]. In brief, proteins and other large molecules are susceptible to ionizing radiation, and a single 'hit' by an electron in the beam of a linear accelerator results in total loss of the structural integrity of the molecule. The identity of many proteins may be established (and quantified) by methods that do not require their purification, e.g. the catalytic activity of an enzyme, or the capacity of a polypeptide to bind antibody or specific ligand. The reduction in the amount of the measured protein placed in the beam of a linear accelerator is related to the radiation dosage, and a simple mathematical relationship[32] has been established which relates the 'target size' (and hence the molecular weight of the protein) to the exponential decline in the amount of a protein with increasing radiation dosage. Application of this method allows direct measurement of the molecular weight of a biologically active protein without prior purification. Furthermore, it is possible to estimate the total molecular weights of complexes of several proteins. Because of the known interactions between the receptor, the G protein and catalytic subunit of adenylate cyclase, this method was chosen for further examination of the PGI_2 receptor.

In preliminary experiments, the molecular weights of both soluble and membrane-bound enzymes were established to validate the method[28]. The enzymes chosen were lysozyme, N-acetyl-β-D-glucosaminidase and acetylcholinesterase. The molecular weight values obtained approximated closely to values published previously, and the method was then used to determine the molecular weights of the catalytic subunit of adenylate cyclase (E), the complex of E and the G protein and finally the complex of EG with the receptor (R). The experiment is outlined briefly in Table 8.2. Inspection of Table 8.2 shows that the molecular weight values for the individual protein constituents of the system were E, 112 000 Da; G, 88 000 Da; and R, 83 000 Da. The values of E and G approximate closely to values published elsewhere and provide additional weight to the value obtained for the PGI_2 receptor. The molecular weight of the receptor protein was determined also in similar experiments ($n = 3$), in which the effect of ionizing radiation on [³H]iloprost binding capacity was measured. The result is presented in Figure

Table 8.2 Identification of the PGI_2 receptor, the G_s regulatory protein and adenylate cyclase by the method of radiation inactivation

Substrate + ligands	Complex	Molecular weight
Mn^{2+}, ATP	E	112 000
Mg^{2+}, ATP, F^-	GE	200 000
Mg^{2+}, ATP, GTP or Gpp(NH)p, carbacyclin	RGE	283 000

NCB-20 membranes were prepared, resuspended in 25 mmol L⁻¹ Tris–HCl buffer, pH 8.5, containing 0.29 mol L⁻¹ sucrose, lyophilized and then irradiated. The surviving adenylate cyclase activity was measured using the substrate and ligands shown. The data were analysed as single exponential decay curves relating enzyme activity to irradiation dosage (M_{rad}). (Reproduced from reference 28 with permission)

8.13 and the molecular weight value of the receptor was 82 800 ± 12 900. This is in reasonable agreement with the value of R calculated as the difference in the molecular weights of the RGE and GE complexes.

DESENSITIZATION OF PGI₂ RESPONSIVENESS *IN VITRO*

Agonist-specific desensitization of prostacyclin-stimulated adenylate cyclase activity has been demonstrated in numerous systems, including human fibroblasts[33], and platelets *in vitro*[4] and *in vivo*[34]. We have examined the mechanism of desensitization in both human platelets[35] and in cells of the NCB-20 cell line[36,37]. Important and interesting differences have emerged which provide some insights into the events that follow agonist occupation of membrane receptors.

Prolonged culture of NCB-20 cells in the presence of carbacyclin results in a slow loss of sensitivity to subsequent challenge with PGI₂[36]. This is

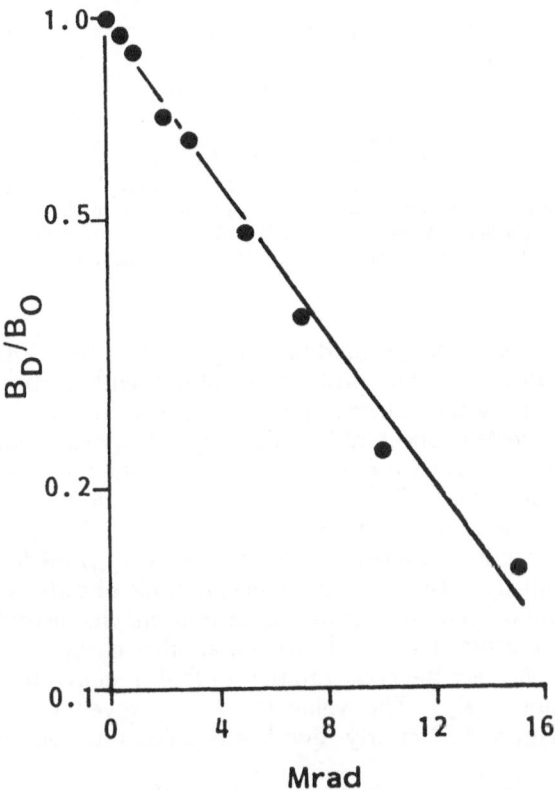

Figure 8.13 Radiation inactivation of the PGI₂ receptor. Lyophilized membranes were irradiated in triplicate at 4°C and the surviving specific binding of 25 nmol L⁻¹ [³H]iloprost was measured in duplicate (●). B_D was the surviving specific binding of [³H]iloprost, and B_0 the original binding. Results are presented as means ± SEM. (Reproduced from reference 28 with permission)

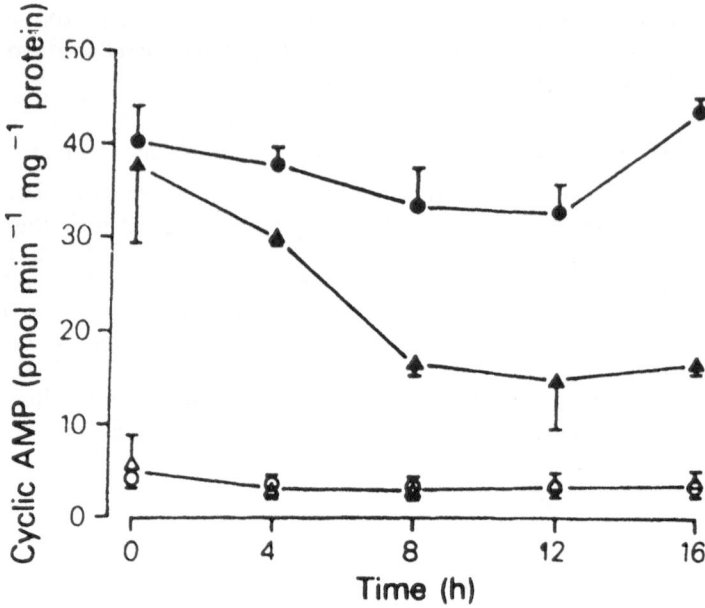

Figure 8.14 Basal and PGI$_2$-stimulated adenylate cyclase activity of NCB-20 homogenates from cells cultured in the absence or presence of carbacyclin. Cells were cultured for selected times in the absence (circles) or presence (triangles) of 1 μmol L^{-1} carbacyclin. Adenylate cyclase activity was determined in duplicate in homogenates of these cells in the absence ($\triangle$○) or presence ($\blacktriangle$●) of 4 μmol L^{-1} PGI$_2$. Results show means $\pm$ SEM of triplicate plates at each time point. (Reproduced from reference 36 with permission)

illustrated in Figure 8.14; it should be noted also that basal adenylate cyclase activity was unchanged by prolonged culture with carbacyclin. In later experiments, cells were cultured for 16 h in the absence or presence of carbacyclin at selected concentrations between 10 nmol L^{-1} and 10 μmol L^{-1}. Full concentration curves were then generated for the activation of adenylate cyclase by prostacyclin[37]. Eadie–Hofstee transformations of these concentration curves are shown in Figure 8.15, from which it is apparent that the maximum increase in adenylate cyclase activity (δv_{max}) mediated by PGI$_2$ is reduced sequentially with increasing concentrations of carbacyclin during the 16 h desensitization. The maximum increase in enzyme activity is given by the abscissa intercepts. There is, however, another change that accompanies desensitization, namely the concentration of PGI$_2$ required for half-maximum enzyme activation (K_{act}). The value for K_{act} is given by -1/slope, and inspection of Figure 8.15 clearly reveals a reduction in slope with increasing desensitization.

The first interesting anomaly was revealed at this stage when a comparison was made of the binding of [^{3}H]iloprost to NCB-20 membranes prepared from cells cultured under control conditions, or in the presence of 1 μmol L^{-1} carbacyclin[37]. The results of two concentration curves are presented in Figure 8.16 as the corresponding Scatchard plots. It will be apparent that the

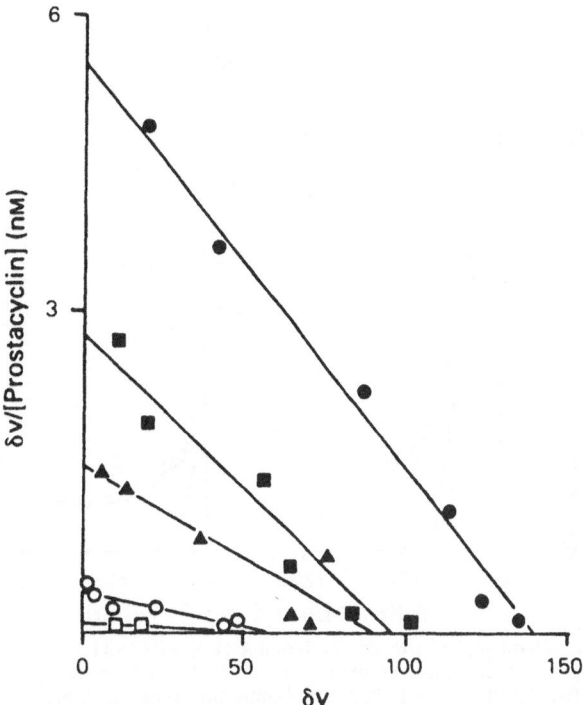

Figure 8.15 Activation of adenylate cyclase by 4-1000 nmol L^{-1} PGI_2 in control cells (●), and cells that had been cultured for 16 h with 0.01 μmol L^{-1} (■), 0.10 μmol L^{-1} (▲), 1.00 μmol L^{-1} (○) or 10 μmol L^{-1} (□) carbacyclin. An Eadie–Hofstee plot of the data is presented, where δv is the increase in adenylate cyclase activity stimulated by PGI_2. Data are means of triplicate determinations. (Reproduced from reference 37 with permission)

desensitization of NCB-20 cells is accompanied by a significant reduction in the binding capacity of the membranes, while the K_d for high-affinity binding (-1/slope) remains unchanged. Hence, the increase in the value of K_{act} for the PGI_2-dependent activation of adenylate cyclase that accompanies desensitization cannot be explained on the basis of a change in the affinity of PGI_2 for its membrane receptor.

A number of experiments were undertaken to investigate whether there was altered coupling between the receptor (R), the guanyl-nucleotide regulatory binding protein ($G_{\alpha\beta\gamma}$) or the catalytic subunit of adenylate cyclase (E) of NCB-20 cells. A schematic representation of these proteins within the lipid bilayer of the plasma membrane is shown in Figure 8.27. The arrowed solid lines represent the normal points of interaction between the proteins. Activation of the catalytic subunit E may be effected, in the absence of a specific agonist for surface receptors (R), by stimulation of the G-protein complex with fluoride ions. F^- ions probably produce their effect by facilitating dissociation of $G_{s\alpha}$ from $G_{s\beta\gamma}$, and $G_{s\alpha}$ is then free to complex with E. This association is an essential step in the activation of adenylate cyclase. The possibility that desensitization of PGI_2 receptors of NCB-20 cells might be

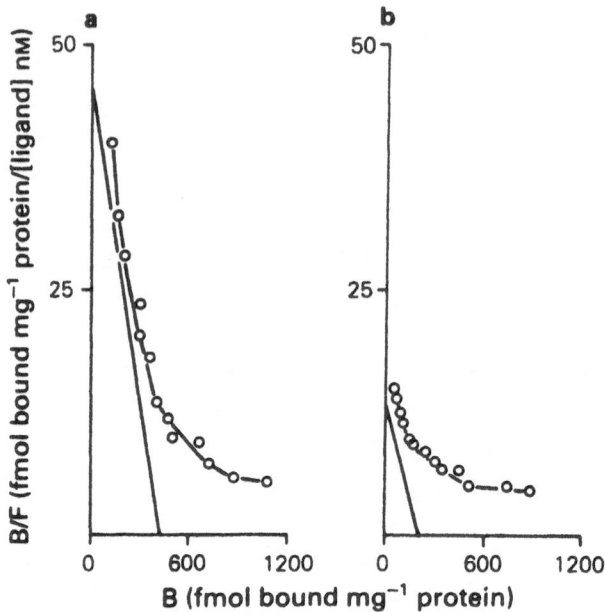

Figure 8.16 Scatchard plot of the specific binding of 3-200 nmol L^{-1} [^{3}H]iloprost to control NCB-20 membranes (a), and the membranes of cells that had been cultured with 1 μmol L^{-1} carbacyclin for 16 h (b). B is fmol [^{3}H]iloprost bound (mg protein)$^{-1}$, and F is the free ligand concentration (nmol L^{-1}). Data are means of triplicate determinations, and are analysed as a 3 parameter model identifying a single high-affinity binding site and a non-saturable binding component. The straight line defines the single high-affinity binding site, and was determined by iterative non-linear regression analysis for multi-compartment systems. (Reproduced from reference 37 with permission)

accompanied by an alteration in G$_s$ or E (or even altered coupling between them) was examined. Figure 8.17 shows F$^-$-dependent changes in adenylate cyclase activity of NCB-20 membranes, and it is quite clear that desensitization of these cells by prolonged culture in carbacyclin produces no alteration in F$^-$-sensitivity. Also considered was the possibility that the increase in K_{act} during desensitization might be due to stable coupling of the receptor (R) with some other membrane protein. The target size of the receptor was therefore examined before and after desensitization by the method of inactivation by ionizing radiation (described previously). Once again, however, the receptor size was unaltered, as shown in Figure 8.18 (82 800 Da in controls and 88 000 Da after desensitization)[37].

It is possible to explain a change in the K_{act} value for activation of adenylate cyclase by PGI$_2$ in the absence of a change in the K_d value for ligand binding by invoking the concept of spare receptors[38]. In a cell membrane in which there is a 1:1 stoichiometry between receptor numbers and 'affector systems', then 50% occupancy will result in 50% activation of the affector system. However, if there are (for example) twice as many receptors as affector systems, then a 50% increase in response may be mediated by occupancy of

194

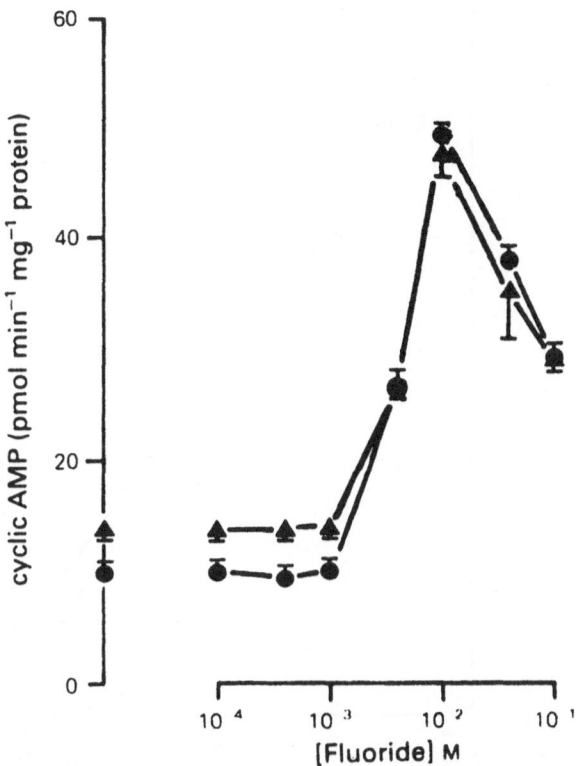

Figure 8.17 Activation of adenylate cyclase by NaF in control NCB-20 cells (●) and cells that had been cultured with 1 μmol L^{-1} carbacyclin for 16 h (▲). Data are means $\pm$ SEM of triplicate determinations. (Reproduced from reference 37 with permission)

only 25% of the total receptor number. The concept may be expressed numerically[37] if the following assumptions are made:

(1) The receptors (R) interact with a complex (GE) of the adenylate cyclase catalytic subunit (E) and the guanyl-nucleotide binding regulatory protein (G) with a 1:1 stoichiometry and (y) complexes of GE are activated when an equal number (y) of receptors are occupied.

(2) The probability of an interaction between any particular GE complex and any receptor molecule is equal.

(3) The enzyme (E) exists in a 'basal' or 'activated' state, but in no intermediate states, and gradual increases in enzyme activity are mediated by sequential activation of GE complexes.

(4) The level of activation of E is dependent on the number of occupied receptors per unit area of membrane, and not (necessarily) on the fractional occupancy of the receptors with agonist.

The number of occupied receptors (r) is given by $r = [R]_n/[1 + (K_D/L)]$ where $[R]_n$ is the total number (n) of receptors. Clearly, at 50% occupancy,

195

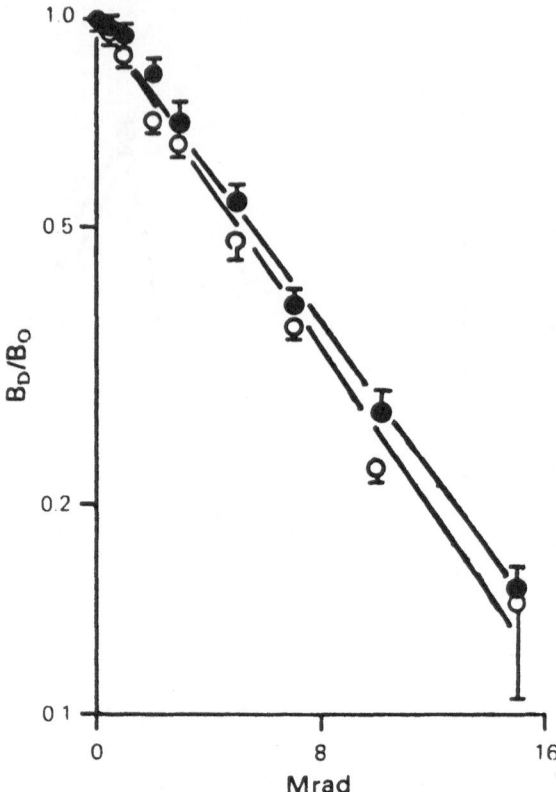

Figure 8.18 Radiation inactivation of the PGI_2 receptor from control (●) and desensitized cells (○). Desensitized cells had been cultured with 1 μmol L^{-1} carbacyclin for 16 h. Membranes were prepared, lyophilized and irradiated in triplicate at 4°C. The surviving specific binding at 25 nmol L^{-1} [³H]iloprost was measured in duplicate. B_D was the surviving specific binding of [³H]iloprost after selected irradiation dosages and B_0 was the original binding. (Reproduced from reference 37 with permission)

$r = [R]_n/2$. If $[R]_n$ exceeds the number of adenylate cyclase molecules (y) by a factor, x, then $[R]_n = xy$.

Further, if $[R]_y$ is the number of receptors equal to y enzyme molecules then $[R]_n = [R]_y x$, or $[R]_y = [R]_n/x$.

Now, 50% enzyme activation is produced when $r = [R]_y/2$,

$$\text{whence } r = \frac{[R]_n}{2x} \qquad (1)$$

In the general case, the concentration of ligand, [L], required to occupy r receptors is given by:

196

$$[L] = K_D \frac{r}{[R]_n - r} \tag{2}$$

Thus, to produce 50% enzyme activation, (1) may be substituted into (2) and:

$$[L] = K_{act} = \frac{\dfrac{K_D[R]_n}{2x}}{[R]_n - \dfrac{[R]_n}{2x}}$$

$$\text{or } K_{act} = \frac{K_D}{2x - 1} \tag{3}$$

Experiments were then performed[37] to test the validity of the concept of spare receptors as the explanation of the alteration in K_{act} value during desensitization in NCB-20 cells. It was shown first that desensitization to PGI$_2$ responsiveness was mediated by a relatively rapid loss of membrane receptors ($k = 5.08 \times 10^{-5}\,s^{-1}$). In other experiments, however, cells were cultured in the presence of cycloheximide (an inhibitor of ribosomal translation that arrests totally new protein synthesis) which resulted in a substantially slower loss of both adenylate cyclase molecules as measured by basal enzyme activity ($k = 1.94 \times 10^{-5}\,s^{-1}$), and PGI$_2$ receptors ($k = 0.92 \times 10^{-5}\,s^{-1}$).

The model proposed above clearly suggests that the relative proportion of [R] and [GE] per unit area of membrane (and hence the value of x) affects the value of K_{act}. This was tested by culture of NCB-20 cells in the absence or presence of carbacyclin, cycloheximide or both together. The cells were then harvested, and concentration curves generated for PGI$_2$-dependent activation of adenylate cyclase in homogenates of these cells. The results are shown in Figure 8.19 as the corresponding Eadie–Hofstee plots. Once again, desensitization is accompanied by an increase in the value of K_{act} (-1/slope) and a reduction in the maximum increase in enzyme activation. Further, when cells were cultured in cycloheximide, there was (predictably) a loss of the maximum enzyme activation as well as a reduction in basal enzyme levels. However, there was loss of both adenylate cyclase molecules and receptor molecules at broadly similar rates under these conditions, and there was, therefore, little or no change in the relative proportions of R and GE. Hence, the K_{act} value for PGI$_2$-dependent activation of adenylate cyclase was unchanged. When cells were cultured in the presence of both carbacyclin and cycloheximide (Figure 8.19), the differential rates of the effects mediated by the two compounds resulted in a total response not substantially different from the effect of carbacyclin alone[37].

The results support strongly the interpretation that the change in the value of K_{act} during desensitization is due to loss of spare PGI$_2$ receptors. Additional evidence was gained, however, to support this proposed mechanism when measurements were made of resensitization[37]. This is shown in Figure 8.20.

197

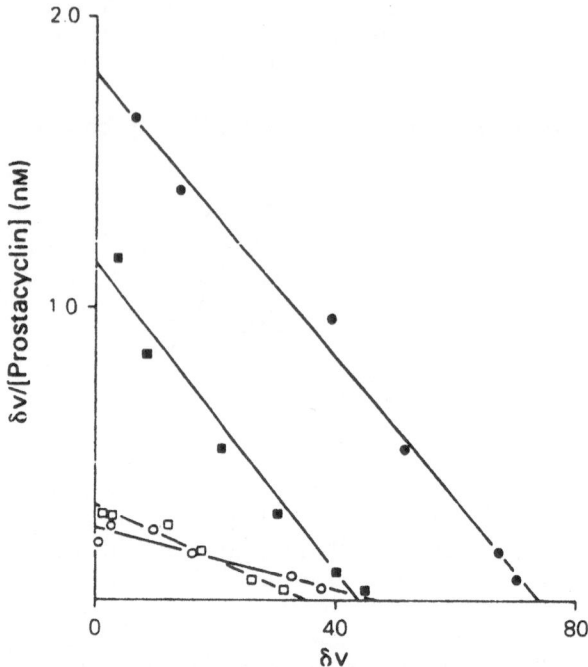

Figure 8.19 An Eadie–Hofstee plot for the activation of adenylate cyclase by 4–1000 nmol L^{-1} PGI$_2$ in control cells (●), and cells that had been cultured for 14 h with 1 μmol L^{-1} carbacyclin (○). 20 μg ml^{-1} cycloheximide (■) or 1 μmol L^{-1} carbacyclin + 20 μg ml^{-1} cycloheximide (□). Data are means of triplicate determinations. (Reproduced from reference 37 with permission)

Cell division was arrested with cytosine arabinoside to avoid the problem of receptor expression in the products of mitosis during the course of the experiment. It is quite apparent that resensitization of desensitized cells occurs in the absence of carbacyclin, and in further experiments (data not shown) the resensitization was shown to be dependent on *de novo* protein synthesis. There was no resensitization in the presence of cycloheximide or actinomycin D (an inhibitor of transcription). It is of particular significance that, when cells were desensitized and then allowed to resensitize, the synthesis of new receptor was accompanied by a restoration of the capacity for enzyme activation, and also by a return to the relatively high-affinity K_{act} for enzyme stimulation (Figure 8.21).

There are important differences in the events that accompany prolonged agonist occupation of PGI$_2$ receptors of human platelets when compared with NCB-20 cells. There are also several similarities, however. There is a similar reduction in high-affinity receptor sites (with no change in K_d), and also reduced PGI$_2$-mediated activation of adenylate cyclase[39]. Once again, the value for K_{act} is increased, suggesting the presence of spare receptors. In contrast to desensitization of NCB-20 cells, however, there is also a reduction in basal adenylate cyclase activity[35]. In 5 similar experiments, in which platelets

198

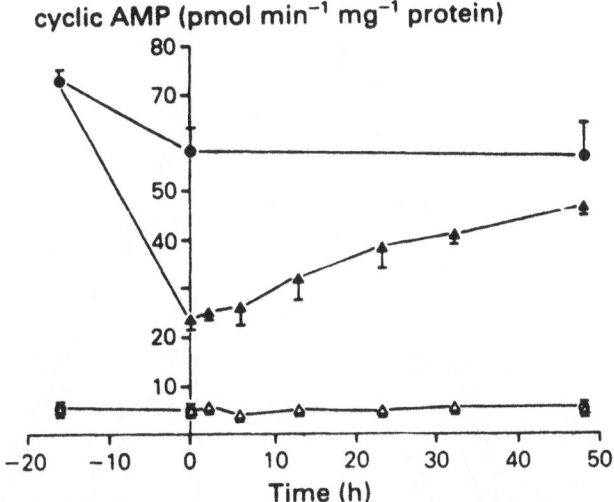

cyclic AMP (pmol min⁻¹ mg⁻¹ protein)

Figure 8.20 Resensitization of PGI$_2$-stimulated adenylate cyclase activity. NCB-20 cells were cultured with 10 μmol L^{-1} cytosine arabinoside for 24 h. They were then cultured with (▲△) or without (●○) 1 μmol L^{-1} carbacyclin for 16 h. The cells were washed with culture medium and allowed to resensitize for 48 h. Basal (open symbols) and 4 μmol L^{-1} PGI$_2$-stimulated (solid symbols) adenylate cyclase activity were measured. Values are means ± SEM of triplicate determinations. (Reproduced from reference 37 with permission)

were incubated *in vitro*, with 10 μmol L^{-1} iloprost, basal enzyme activity of control platelets was 24.9 ± 0.4 pmol cyclic AMP min^{-1} (mg protein)$^{-1}$, and in desensitized platelets was 15.1 ± 2.5 pmol cyclic AMP min^{-1} (mg protein)$^{-1}$. We were particularly interested to find also that responsiveness to the stable adenosine analogue, NECA (5'-(N-ethyl)-carboxamidoadenosine), which is mediated by the adenosine (A$_2$) receptor, was also reduced following iloprost pretreatment[35]. This example of heterologous desensitization is shown in Figure 8.22. The reduction in basal enzyme activity suggested changes in the system beyond those that could be explained on the basis of receptor loss alone. This was supported by the observations (Figures 8.23 and 8.24) that desensitization with iloprost resulted in reduced sensitivity to both NaF and Gpp(NH)p. These results suggested strongly that the heterologous desensitization mediated by iloprost was due to a change in the G$_s$-protein or in the coupling of G$_s$ with the catalytic subunit (E).

Further experiments (data not shown) revealed clearly that heterologous desensitization of adenosine (A$_2$) responses produced by iloprost were not accompanied by a reduction in the number of adenosine (A$_2$) surface receptors[35]. On the other hand, prolonged exposure to stable adenosine analogues resulted in homologous desensitization of adenosine responsiveness and loss of adenosine A$_2$ receptors[35].

The response to GTP was of particular interest, and Figure 8.25 shows measurement of adenylate cyclase over a range of GTP concentrations in the absence or presence of 10 μmol L^{-1} NECA. Enzyme activity was measured

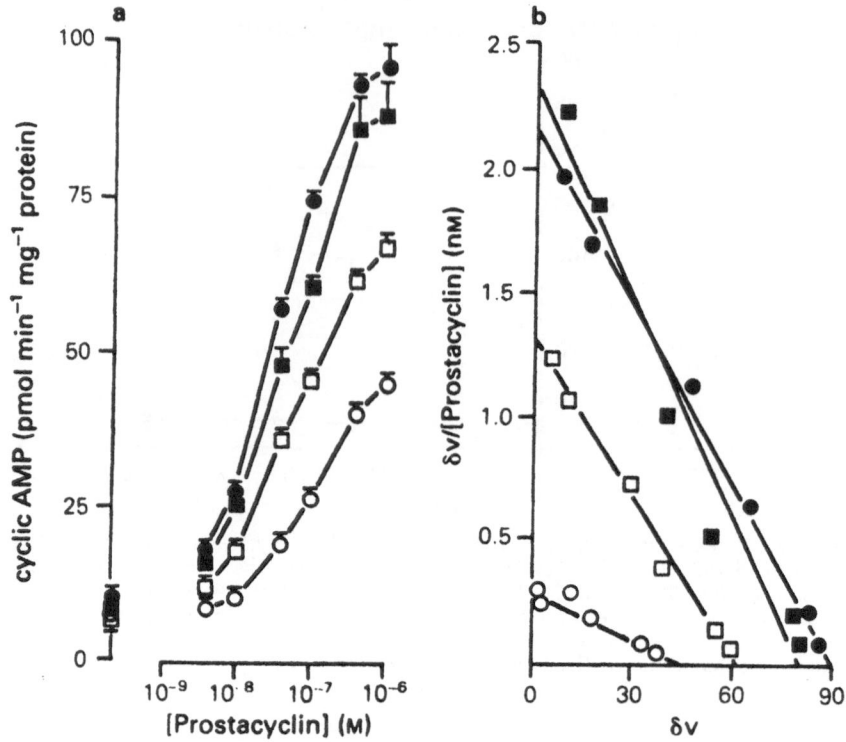

Figure 8.21 Activation of adenylate cyclase by PGI_2 in desensitized cells (○) and their controls (●), and resensitized cells (□) and their appropriate controls (■). NCB-20 cells were cultured with cystosine arabinoside for 24 h. They were then cultured with $1 \mu mol L^{-1}$ carbacyclin for a further 16 h and either harvested (desensitized cells) or allowed to resensitize for 48 h (resensitized cells). PGI_2-stimulated adenylate cyclase activity was measured (a). Data are means ± SEM of triplicate determinations. The data are presented as an Eadie–Hofstee plot (b) where δv is the increase in adenylate cyclase activity stimulated by PGI_2. (Reproduced from reference 37 with permission)

in membranes prepared from control or desensitized platelets, and it is apparent that GTP sensitivity is preserved in both membrane preparations. It was noted that the reduction in basal enzyme activity that accompanies desensitization was apparent only in the presence of GTP. Specifically, enzyme activity measured in the absence of GTP (shown on the ordinate intercepts of Figure 8.25) was the same in membranes of control and desensitized platelets. This result provides compelling evidence that the altered response of adenylate cyclase to NaF or Gpp(NH)p following desensitization with iloprost is produced by a change in the G_s-protein and not in the coupling of G_s to the catalytic subunit (E).

The underlying cause of the altered activity of the G_s-protein was further examined by the method of ADP-ribosylation of $G_{s\alpha}$ in the presence of cholera toxin[35]. The 45 000 Da $G_{s\alpha}$ subunit of the G_s complex may be ADP-ribosylated, a reaction which results in activation of adenylate cyclase. If

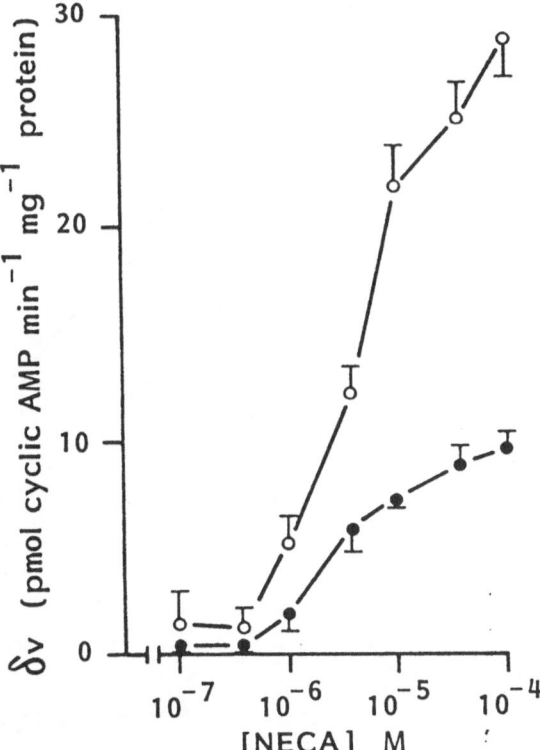

Figure 8.22 Heterologous desensitization of adenosine (A_2) receptors by iloprost. Platelets were incubated for 24 h in the absence (○) or presence (●) of $10\,\mu\text{mol}\,\text{L}^{-1}$ iloprost. Platelet membranes were prepared, and adenylate cyclase activity measured in the absence or presence of NECA ($0.1-100\,\mu\text{mol}\,\text{L}^{-1}$). Results show mean ± SEM values for the increase in enzyme activity (δv) (Reproduced from reference 35 with permission)

[^{32}P]NAD is employed as substrate in this reaction, the ADP-ribosylated protein may be identified by the method of polyacrylamide gel electrophoresis followed by autoradiography of the gel. This method was employed in an examination of the membrane proteins of control and desensitized platelets. Coomassie-blue staining of the gels revealed no differences following desensitization, but there was a >80% loss of the 45 000 Da protein as revealed by [^{32}P]ADP-ribosylation. The autoradiograph and scans are shown in Figure 8.26.

There is clearly a complex sequence of events that accompanies occupation of PGI$_2$ or adenosine (A_2) receptors by the appropriate agonists on human platelets. Both receptors are lost to a greater or lesser extent from the surface of the membrane, and the proportion of receptors lost may be shown to correspond closely to the proportion of receptors occupied by agonist. There are, however, effects due to agonist occupation of PGI$_2$ receptors which are not mirrored by similar changes after occupation of adenosine (A_2) receptors.

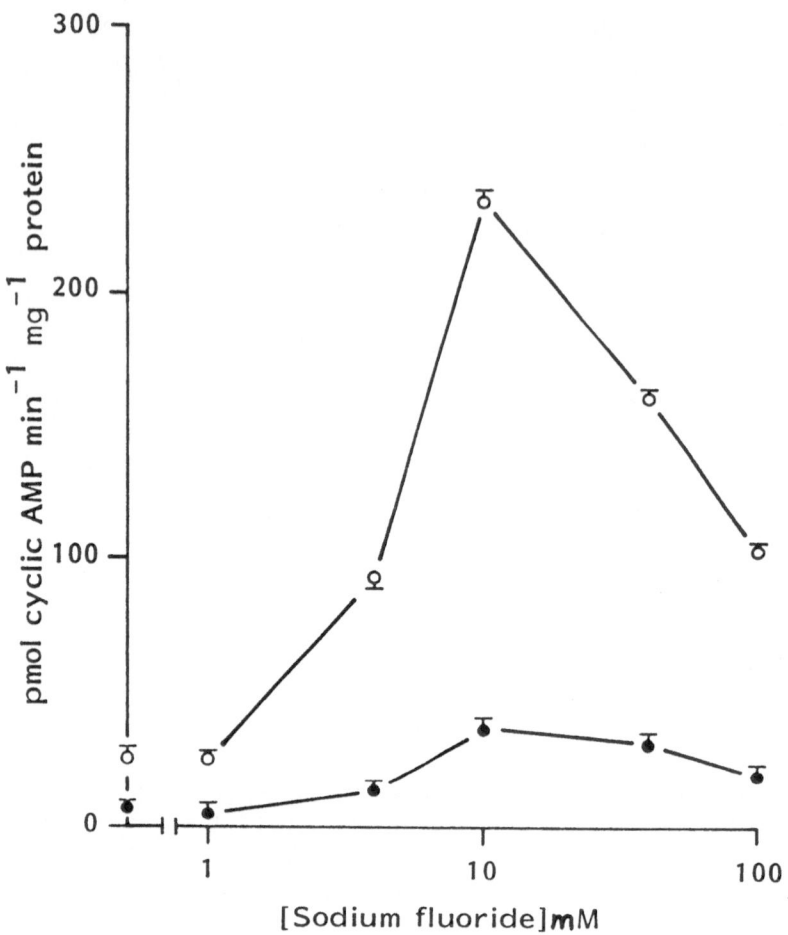

Figure 8.23 Adenylate cyclase activation by NaF after pretreatment with iloprost. Platelets were incubated for 24 h in the absence (○) or presence (●) of 10 μmol L^{-1} iloprost. Platelet membranes were prepared, and adenylate cyclase activity measured in the absence or presence of NaF (1–100 mmol L^{-1}). Results show means ± SEM of triplicate determinations. (Reproduced from reference 35 with permission)

Prolonged occupation of PGI$_2$ receptors results in a substantial (> 80%) reduction in the amount of G$_{s\alpha}$, and the possibility clearly exists that both the receptor and the G-protein (or part of the G-complex) are internalized together. There is no explanation at present for the lack of similar effect due to adenosine. Figure 8.27 shows a schematic representation of the proteins involved in the process.

DESENSITIZATION OF PGI$_2$ RESPONSIVENESS *IN VIVO*

The percentage of maximum desensitization of PGI$_2$ responsiveness that accompanies exposure to agonists *in vitro* parallels closely the calculated

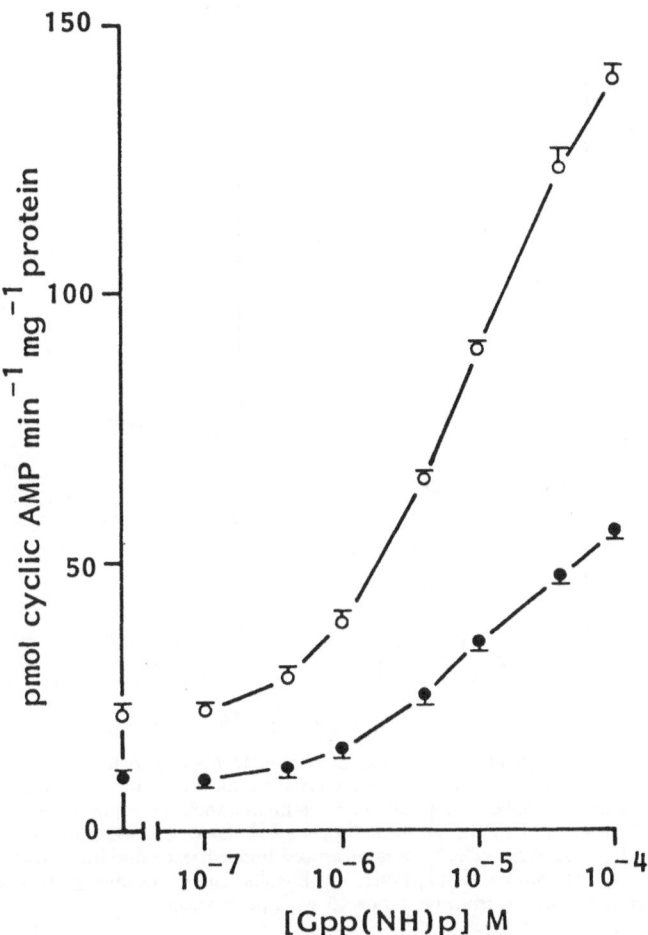

Figure 8.24 Adenylate cyclase activation by Gpp(NH)p after pretreatment with iloprost. Platelets were incubated for 24 h in the absence (○) or presence (●) of 10 μmol L^{-1} iloprost. Platelet membranes were prepared, and adenylate cyclase activity measured in the absence or presence of Gpp(NH)p (0.1–100 μmol L^{-1}). Results show means $\pm$ SEM of triplicate determinations. (Reproduced from reference 35 with permission)

fractional occupancy of surface receptors[37,39]. *In vivo*, however, such a clear relationship is not seen. An infusion of PGI$_2$ at a rate of 5 ng kg^{-1} min^{-1} results in a circulating concentration of 150–200 pg ml^{-1} PGI$_2$, at which concentration (approximately 0.5 nmol L^{-1}), the occupancy of PGI$_2$ receptors would be < 3% of the total (the K_d is taken as 20 nmol L^{-1} in this calculation). Nevertheless, under these circumstances, desensitization of up to 80% may be obtained in platelet PGI$_2$-dependent responses[34].

This anomaly has been addressed in a series of experiments[40] performed in collaboration with scientists at Schering AG (Berlin). Iloprost was infused

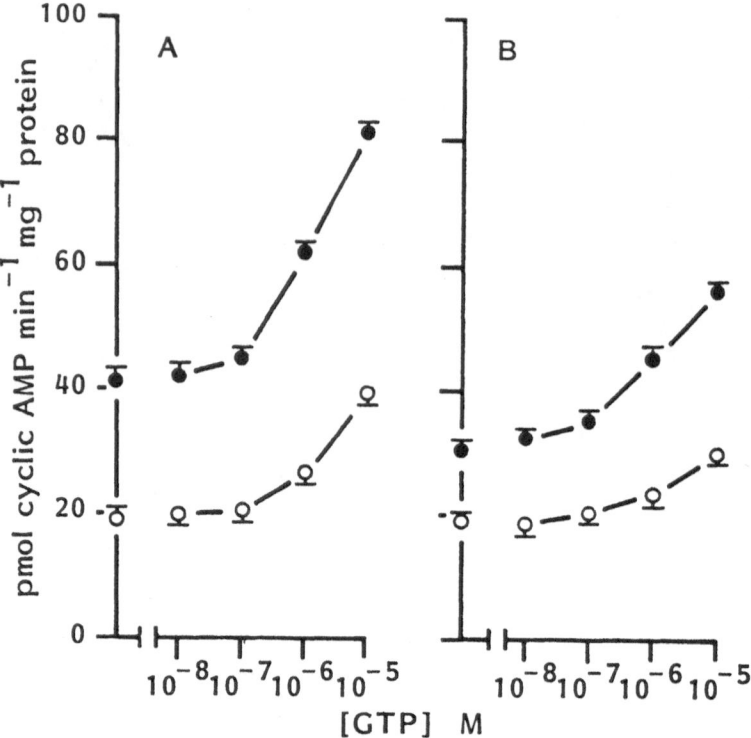

Figure 8.25 NECA-dependent activation of adenylate cyclase in the absence or presence of GTP, after pretreatment with iloprost. Platelets were incubated for 24 h in the absence (A) or presence (B) of $10 \mu mol L^{-1}$ iloprost. Platelet membranes were prepared, and adenylate cyclase activity measured in the absence (open symbols) or presence (closed symbols) of $10 \mu mol L^{-1}$ NECA. Enzyme activity was measured under these conditions in the absence or presence of GTP $(10 nmol L^{-1}-10 \mu mol L^{-1})$. Results show means $\pm$ SEM of triplicate determinations. (Reproduced from reference 35 with permission)

into a peripheral forearm vein of the right arm of a healthy volunteer at a rate of $1.5 ng kg^{-1} min^{-1}$. At this infusion rate, the subject became flushed secondary to peripheral vasodilatation. Blood samples were withdrawn from a remote vein (left arm), or 12 cm above the infusion site in the right arm (Figure 8.28). Measurements were made of the concentrations of iloprost in the two arms, and these are shown in the same figure. A comparison of the relative concentrations of iloprost in the syringe and in the vein draining the infusion site revealed a dilution factor of about 100. Since the infusion rate was at $5 ml h^{-1}$, it follows that the blood flow through the peripheral forearm vein *at rest* is very slow (about $500 ml h^{-1}$). This represents about 0.25% of cardiac output. It is proposed[40] that during the passage of platelets through the peripheral vein draining the infusion site in this experiment, the fractional occupancy of platelet PGI_2 receptors with iloprost was very high. The ambient concentration of prostacyclin was calculated as $40 nmol L^{-1}$. The high fractional occupancy of these receptors would be accompanied by substantial

PROSTACYCLIN RECEPTORS

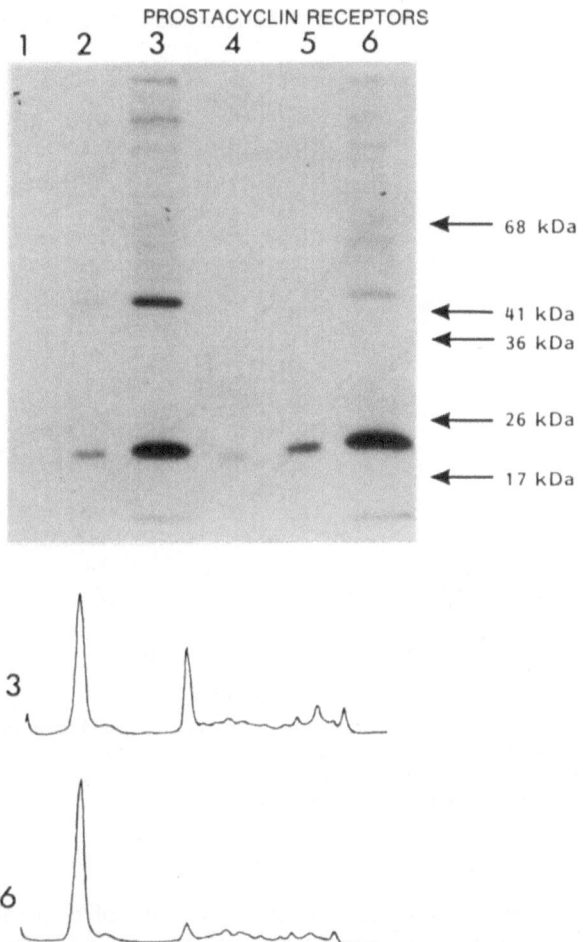

Figure 8.26 [^{32}P]ADP-ribosylation of platelet membrane proteins after pretreatment with iloprost. Platelets were incubated for 24 h in the absence (lanes 1–3) or presence (lanes 4–6) of 10 μmol L^{-1} iloprost. Platelet membranes were prepared, and ADP-ribosylation of membrane proteins performed in the presence of cholera toxin (A subunit). The gels were loaded with (lanes 1–6) 3.95, 9.88, 39.5, 3.05, 7.63, 30.5 μg protein. The figure shows the autoradiograph of the 6 lanes, and a densitometer scan of lanes 3 and 6. In a control experiment, there was no significant labelling of the platelet membrane proteins in an incubation from which cholera toxin had been omitted. (Reproduced from reference 35 with permission)

desensitization, with little or no capacity for recovery of that sensitivity (platelets having no capcity for *de novo* protein synthesis). The sequential passage of blood cells through this small portion of the total vascular bed would result in an exponential decline in the number of cells that retain their original sensitivity to iloprost.

It should be possible to validate or refute the proposed mechanism for *in vivo* desensitization of PGI$_2$ responsiveness following intravenous infusion. First, infusion of iloprost into a large central vein, with rapid mixing, would be predicted to result in little or no significant desensitization of platelet PGI$_2$

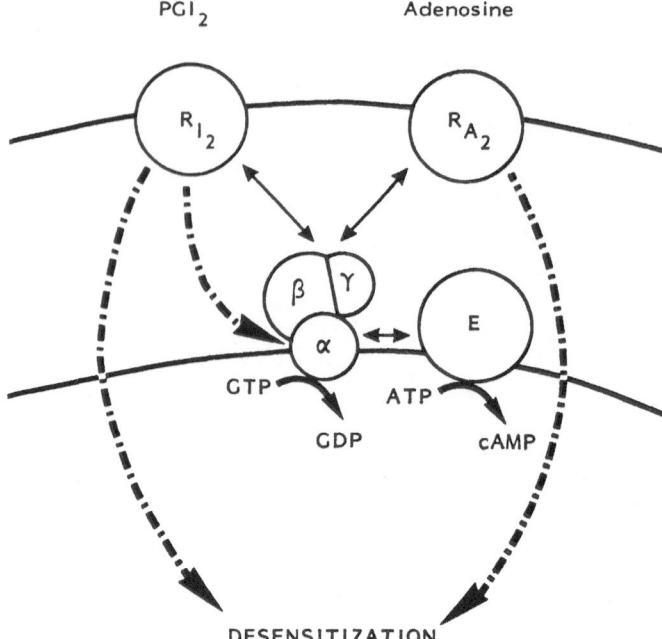

Figure 8.27 Arrangement of the constituent proteins in the lipid bilayer of a human platelet. The diagram shows a schematic representation of the receptors (R) for PGI_2 and adenosine (A_2), the catalytic subunit of adenylate cyclase (E), and the 3 subunits (α, β and γ) of the guanyl nucleotide-binding regulatory protein (G_s)

responses. Further, infusion at a much lower rate of a metabolically more stable PGI_2 analogue (with a plasma half-life substantially greater than that of iloprost) would result in a similar pharmacological response with correspondingly lower drug concentrations close to the infusion site. Once again, the prediction would be that there would be correspondingly less desensitization.

The problem of *in vivo* desensitization of platelet responsiveness appears at first sight to limit substantially the potential therapeutic benefit of this family of antiplatelet drugs, but an appreciation of the events involved may yet allow a sensible approach to long-term administration of prostacyclin. Finally, it should be emphasized that the case for prolonged infusions of PGI_2 in peripheral vascular disease is not yet firmly established by controlled clinical trials.

ACKNOWLEDGEMENTS

I wish to acknowledge the major contribution of many friends and colleagues in these studies, most particularly U. Alt, I.A. Blair, W.A. Cramp, T.M. Cresp, C.T. Dollery, P.J. Leigh and A.J. Wilkins. These studies were supported by grants from the Wellcome Trust (UK) and the Medical Research Council (UK).

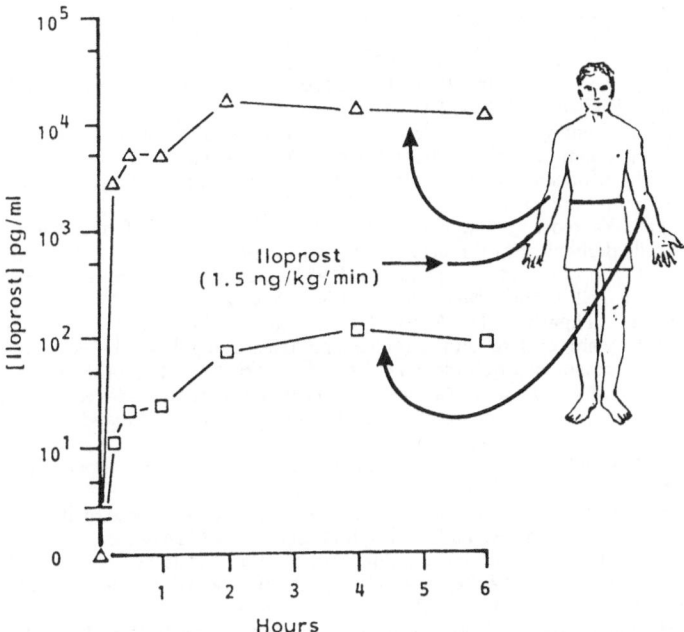

Figure 8.28 Plasma concentrations of iloprost during intravenous infusion. Blood samples were taken 12 cm above the infusion site or from the opposite arm. (Reproduced from reference 40 with permission)

REFERENCES

1. Moncada, S., Gryglewski, R.J., Bunting, S. and Vane, J.R. (1976). An enzyme isolated from arteries transforms prostaglandin endoperoxides to an unstable substance that inhibits platelet aggregation. *Nature (London)*, **263**, 663–665
2. Siegl, A.M., Smith, J.B., Silver, M.J., Nicolaou, K.C. and Ahern, D. (1979). Selective binding site for [³H]prostacyclin on platelets. *J. Clin. Invest.*, **63**, 215–220
3. Lombroso, M., Nicosia, S., Paoletti, R., Whittle, B.J.R., Moncada, S. and Vane, J.R. (1984). The use of stable prostaglandins to investigate prostacyclin (PGI₂)-binding sites and PGI₂-sensitive adenylate cyclase in human platelet membranes. *Prostaglandins*, **27**, 321–333
4. Miller, O.V. and Gorman, R.R. (1979). Evidence for distinct prostaglandin I₂ and D₂ receptors in human platelets. *J. Pharmacol. Exp. Ther.*, **210**, 134–140
5. Hall, J.M. and Strange, P.G. (1984). The use of a prostacyclin analogue, [³H]iloprost, for studying prostacyclin-binding sites on human platelets and neuronal hybrid cells. *Biosci. Rep.*, **4**, 941–948
6. Town, M-H., Schillinger, E., Speckenbach, A. and Prior, G. (1982). Identification and characterisation of a prostacyclin-like receptor in bovine coronary arteries using a specific and stable prostacyclin analogue, ciloprost, as radioactive ligand. *Prostaglandins*, **24**, 61–72
7. Rucker, W. and Schror, K. (1983). Evidence for high affinity prostacyclin binding sites in vascular tissue: radioligand studies with a chemically stable analogue. *Biochem. Pharmacol.*, **32**, 2405–2410
8. Garrity, M.J., Westcott, K.R., Eggerman, T.L., Andersen, N.H., Storm, D.R. and Robertson, R.P. (1983). Interrelationships between PGE₁ and PGI₂ binding and stimulation of adenylate cyclase. *Am. J. Physiol.*, **244**, E367–E372

207

9. Fassina, G., Froldi, G. and Caparrotta, L. (1985). A stable isosterically modified prostacyclin analogue, FCE-22176, acting as a competitive antagonist to prostacyclin in guinea-pig trachea and atria. *Eur. J. Pharmacol.*, **133**, 459–460

10. Salomon, Y., Londos, C. and Rodbell, M. (1974). A highly sensitive adenylate cyclase assay. *Anal. Biochem.*, **58**, 541–548

11. Gorman, R.R., Bunting, S. and Miller, O.V. (1977). Modulation of human platelet adenylate cyclase by prostacyclin (PGX). *Prostaglandins*, **13**, 377–388

12. Tateson, J.E., Moncada, S. and Vane, J.R. (1977). Effect of prostacyclin (PGX) on cyclic AMP concentrations in human platelets. *Prostaglandins*, **13**, 389–397

13. Minna, J.D., Yavelow, I. and Coon, H.G. (1975). Expression of phenotypes in hybrid somatic cells derived from the nervous system. *Genetics*, **79**, (Suppl.), 373–383

14. Minna, J., Glazer, D., and Nirenberg, M. (1972). Genetic dissection of neural properties using somatic cell hybrids. *Nature (London) New Biol.*, **235**, 225–231

15. MacDermot, J., Higashida, H., Wilson, S.P., Matsuzawa, H., Minna, J. and Nirenberg, M. (1979). Adenylate cyclase and acetylcholine release regulated by separate serotonin receptors of somatic cell hybrids. *Proc. Natl. Acad. Sci. USA*, **76**, 1135–1139

16. Blair, I.A., Hensby, C.N. and MacDermot, J. (1980). Prostacyclin-dependent activation of adenylate cyclase in a neuronal somatic cell hybrid: prostanoid structure-activity relationships. *Br. J. Pharmacol.*, **69**, 519–525

17. Rodbell, M. (1980). The role of hormone receptors and GTP-regulatory proteins in membrane transduction. *Nature (London)*. **284**, 17–22

18. MacDermot, J. (1979). Guanosine 5'-triphosphate requirement for activation of adenylate cyclase by serotonin in a somatic cell hybrid. *Life Sci.*, **25**, 241–246

19. Gilman, A.G. (1984). G-proteins and dual control of adenylate cyclase. *Cell*, **36**, 577–579

20. Helmreich, E.J.M. and Pfeuffer, T. (1985). Regulation of signal transduction by β-adrenergic hormone receptors. *TIPS Rev.*, **6**, 438–443

21. Shepherd, G.L., Lewis, P.J., Blair, I.A., de Mey, C. and MacDermot, J. (1983). Epoprostenol (Prostacyclin, PGI₂) binding and activation of adenylate cyclase in platelets of diabetic and control subjects. *Br. J. Clin. Pharmacol.*, **15**, 77–81

22. MacDermot, J. and Barnes, P.J. (1980). Activation of guinea pig pulmonary adenylate cyclase by prostacyclin. *Eur. J. Pharmacol.*, **67**, 419–425

23. MacDermot, J., Barnes, P.J. and Dollery, C.T. (1981). Distribution of prostacyclin-sensitive adenylate cyclase in guinea pig lung. In Lewis, P.J. and O'Grady, J. (eds.) *Clinical Pharmacology of Prostacyclin*, pp. 247–248. (New York: Raven Press)

24. Kadowitz, P.J., Chapnick, B.M., Feigen, L.P., Hyman, A.L., Nelson, P.K. and Spannhake, E.W. (1978). Pulmonary and systemic vasodilator effects of the newly discovered prostaglandin, PGI₂. *J. Appl. Physiol.*, **45**, 408–413

25. MacDermot, J., Barnes, P.J., Waddell, K.A., Dollery, C.T. and Blair, I.A. (1981). Prostacyclin binding to guinea pig pulmonary receptors. *Eur. J. Pharmacol.*, **75**, 127–130

26. Blair, I.A. and MacDermot, J. (1981). The binding of [³H]-prostacyclin to membranes of a neuronal somatic hybrid. *Br. J. Pharmacol.*, **72**, 435–441

27. Blair, I.A., Hensby, C.N. and MacDermot, J. (1981). Synthesis of [11β-³H]prostacyclin. *J. Label. Comp. Radiopharm.*, **18**, 361–370

28. Leigh, P.J., Cramp, W.A. and MacDermot, J. (1984). Identification of the prostacyclin receptor by radiation inactivation. *J. Biol. Chem.*, **259**, 12431–12436

29. Blair, I.A., Cresp, T.M. and MacDermot, J. (1981). Divalent cations increase [³H]-prostacyclin binding to membranes of neuronal somatic hybrid cells. *Br. J. Pharmacol.*, **73**, 691–694

30. MacDermot, J., Blair, I.A. and Cresp, T.M. (1981). Prostacyclin receptors of a neuronal hybrid cell line. Divalent cations and ligand-receptor coupling. *Biochem. Pharmacol.*, **30**, 2041–2044

31. Kempner, E.S. and Schlegel, W. (1979). Size determination of enzymes by radiation inactivation. *Anal. Biochem.*, **92**, 2–10

32. Kepner, G.R. and Macey, R.I. (1968). Membrane enzyme systems. Molecular size determination by radiation inactivation. *Biochim. Biophys. Acta*, **163**, 188–203

33. Gorman, R.R. and Hopkins, N.K. (1980). Agonist-specific desensitization of PGI₂-stimulated cyclic AMP accumulation by PGE₁ in human foreskin fibroblasts. *Prostaglandins*, **19**, 2–16

34. Sinzinger, H., Silberbauer, K., Horsch, A.K. and Gall, A. (1981). Decreased sensitivity of human platelets to PGI₂ during long-term intraarterial prostacyclin infusion in patients with peripheral vascular disease – a rebound phenomenon? *Prostaglandins*, **21**, 49–51

208

35. Edwards, R.J., MacDermot, J. and Wilkins, A.J. (1987). Prostacyclin analogues reduce ADP-ribosylation of the α-subunit of the regulatory G_s-protein and diminish adenosine (A_2) responsiveness of platelets. *Br. J. Pharmacol.* (In press)
36. Blair, I.A., Leigh, P.J. and MacDermot, J. (1982). Desensitization of prostacyclin receptors in a neuronal hybrid cell line. *Br. J. Pharmacol.*, **77**, 121–127
37. Leigh, P.J. and MacDermot, J. (1985). Desensitization of prostacyclin responsiveness in a neuronal hybrid cell line: selective loss of high affinity receptors. *Br. J. Pharmacol.*, **85**, 237–247
38. Homburger, V., Lucas, M., Cantau, B., Barabe, J., Penit, J. and Bockaert, J. (1980). Further evidence that desensitization of β-adrenergic-sensitive adenylate cyclase proceeds in two steps. *J. Biol. Chem.*, **255**, 10436–10444
39. Alt, U., Leigh, P.J., Wilkins, A.J., Morris, P.K. and MacDermot, J. (1986). Desensitization of iloprost responsiveness in human platelets follows prolonged exposure to iloprost *in vitro. Br. J. Clin. Pharmacol.*, **22**, 118–119
40. MacDermot, J. (1986). Desensitization of prostacyclin responsiveness in platelets. Apparent differences in the mechanism *in vitro* or *in vivo. Biochem. Pharmacol.*, **35**, 2645–2649

9
Platelet and vascular smooth muscle thromboxane A$_2$/prostaglandin H$_2$ receptors

D. E. Mais, P. V. Halushka and D. L. Saussy Jr.

INTRODUCTION

While thromboxane A$_2$ (TxA$_2$) and prostaglandin H$_2$ (PGH$_2$) are produced by a large number of mammalian cell types and influence their function, the focus of this review will be primarily on their receptors in vascular smooth muscle and platelets. The potential role of these compounds in mediating physiological and pathophysiological processes in the cardiovascular system and platelets is covered in other chapters of this book.

In 1974, Samuelsson and co-workers[1] described the synthesis of prostaglandin G$_2$ and H$_2$ from arachidonic acid using cyclo-oxygenase derived from sheep seminal vesicle microsomes. PGH$_2$ was found to have a half-life of about five minutes in aqueous media. One year later, the same group[2,3] showed that platelets further metabolized PGH$_2$ into a substance they named thromboxane A$_2$. TxA$_2$ was also very unstable with a half-life of approximately 30 s in aqueous media. Its hydrolysis product, TxB$_2$, is stable but devoid of biological activity. Because of its extreme lability, the structure for TxA$_2$ had to be postulated and was based on quenching experiments with various nucleophiles. Recently, the proposed structure has been confirmed as a result of the total synthesis of TxA$_2$ and its pharmacological evaluation[4]. Both TxA$_2$ and PGH$_2$ constrict vascular smooth muscle and aggregate platelets. TxA$_2$ appears, however, to be approximately ten times more potent as a stimulator of platelet aggregation[4]. Since platelet and blood vessels respond to both PGH$_2$ and TxA$_2$, the receptors have been referred to as TxA$_2$/PGH$_2$ receptors.

The study of these receptors has progressed slowly since the discovery of these two natural products for several reasons. The first is that the labile nature of these compounds precluded their use in pharmacological and receptor ligand binding studies except in a qualitative or semiquantitative manner for the former type of studies. The synthesis of stable analogues, which act as either mimetics or antagonists, has allowed for more careful and quantitative pharmacological evaluations to be conducted. Secondly, until recently, there were no stable analogues that could be radiolabelled and used for radioligand binding studies[5-8].

The third reason was that, shortly after the discovery of TxA$_2$, it was postulated that it could act as a calcium ionophore[9]. It was speculated that TxA$_2$ could translocate Ca^{2+} from its storage site within platelets to the cytosol. This event could be envisioned to occur without a receptor. This notion was dismissed, however, with the discovery of 13-azaprostanoic acid[10], the first TxA$_2$/PGH$_2$ receptor antagonist, which had no effect on thromboxane synthetase.

BIOSYNTHESIS OF TxA$_2$ AND PGH$_2$ IN PLATELETS

A wide variety of platelet aggregating agents can stimulate the enzymes, phospholipase C and phospholipase A$_2$, leading to the release of arachidonic acid from membrane phospholipid sites and subsequent metabolism to PGH$_2$ and TxA$_2$[11]. Arachidonic acid is stored at the 2 position of membrane phospholipids and its release is specifically catalysed by phospholipase A$_2$. Once released, it is rapidly metabolized by cyclo-oxygenase to form initially PGG$_2$ which is further metabolized to PGH$_2$. Aspirin and other non-steroidal anti-inflammatory drugs inhibit cyclo-oxygenase to prevent the synthesis of PGG$_2$. PGH$_2$ is metabolized by a cytochrome P$_{450}$-dependent enzyme thromboxane synthase to produce TxA$_2$[12]. This enzyme may be inhibited by a variety of imidazole[13,14] and pyridine[15] derivatives or structural analogues of PGH$_2$ and TxA$_2$[16].

STABLE TxA$_2$/PGH$_2$ AGONISTS AND ANTAGONISTS

The discovery of both the endoperoxides (PGG$_2$ and PGH$_2$) and TxA$_2$, stimulated the efforts of synthetic chemists to provide related compounds. The review of the chemistry of these stable analogues has been covered previously[17-19]. However, these stable agonists and antagonists have been very important in the development of this field because of their use in pharmacological and radioligand binding studies; a brief description of the chemistry should prove useful.

PGH$_2$ analogues

The first stable analogues of PGH$_2$ were reported shortly after its discovery (Figure 9.1)[20,21]. All three of these stable analogues proved to be mimetics of PGH$_2$ since they induced platelet aggregation and contracted vascular smooth muscle. Both U46619 and U44069 have been particularly useful since they were made readily available by the Upjohn Company to researchers worldwide ever since their synthesis. U46619 has been shown[22] to possess a spectrum of activity very similar to the natural endoperoxide and TxA$_2$. All of these

211

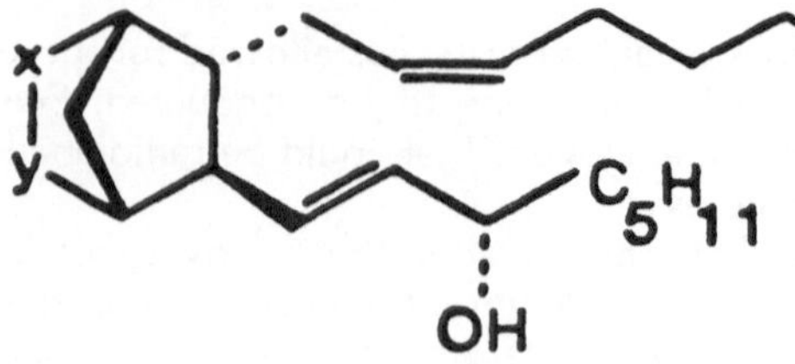

	X - Y
1	O - O
2	CH2 - O
3	O - CH2
4	N = N

Figure 9.1 Chemical structure of PGH$_2$ analogues: <u>1</u>, PGH$_2$; <u>2</u>, U46619; <u>3</u>, U44069; and <u>4</u>, 9,11-azo-PGH$_2$

endoperoxide derivatives which possessed the usual prostanoid side-chain substituents were agonists in platelet and vascular smooth muscle preparations. In addition, some also inhibited thromboxane synthase[16,23].

The studies of the structure–activity relationships indicate that the 5,6-double bond is essential for mimetic activity in platelets but not as critical in smooth muscle preparations[16]. Also, the 15(S) orientation of the hydroxy group is necessary for agonist activity in platelets, and inverting this group to 15(R) leads to antagonist activity in some cases[23,24] or loss of activity entirely[25]. TxA$_2$/PGH$_2$ antagonists are generally characterized by ω or bottom side-chain modifications, which will be considered under TxA$_2$ analogues.

TxA$_2$ analogues

The first stable analogues of TxA$_2$ were synthesized in 1979 and 1980 and were pinane TxA$_2$[26] and carbocyclic TxA$_2$[27] (Figure 9.2). The pinane analogue was a competitive antagonist of the TxA$_2$/PGH$_2$ receptor in both platelets and vascular smooth muscle. The carbocyclic analogue was a potent vasoconstrictor[28,29] but lacked any agonist effects on human platelets[27–29]. This analogue, in fact, had antagonistic properties against stable TxA$_2$/PGH$_2$ mimetic-induced platelet aggregation[29]. This inhibitory effect on platelet aggregation, however, may not be due entirely to competitive antagonism since it has been reported[30] that carbocyclic TxA$_2$ may increase cAMP levels within the platelet which will result in inhibition of platelet aggregation. The mono and dithia analogues of TxA$_2$ have also been prepared[31,32]. Both of these derivatives of TxA$_2$ were stable to hydrolysis and were agonists in both platelets and various smooth muscle preparations.

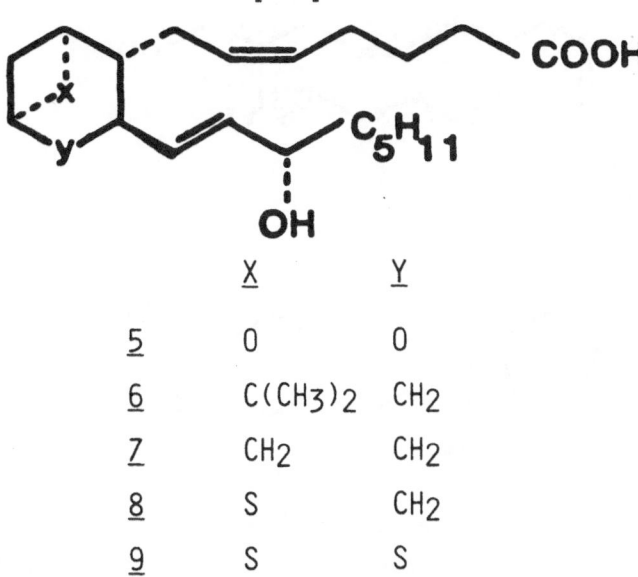

Figure 9.2 Chemical structures of TxA₂ analogues: **5**, TxA₂; **6**, pinane-TxA₂, PTA₂; **7**, carbocyclic TxA₂, CTA₂; **8**, monothia-TxA₂, ONO-11113; and **9**, dithiathromboxane A₂, STA₂

A large group of 7-oxabicyclo[2.2.1]heptane analogues have also been synthesized and evaluated[33]. Of the two possible orientations for the bridgehead oxygen, the α orientation, as shown in Figure 9.3, proved more potent than the corresponding β[33]. All possible permutations at the 8, 12 and 15 positions have been evaluated for activity. Curiously, some of the analogues possessing the unnatural *cis* orientation of the side chains at the 8 and 12 positions proved to be potent compounds.

As these modifications of the basic bicyclic nucleus were being made, a variety of analogues were being synthesized with altered side chains. For the most part, these changes were carried out on the bottom or ω side chain, since earlier studies with the 'classical' prostaglandins had shown that modifications distal to the C-15 position could be made without loss of activity[34]. In particular, some changes in the ω side chain resulted in compounds which were selective and potent TxA₂/PGH₂ receptor antagonists. The first such compound was 13-azaprostanoic acid (Figure 9.3)[35]. This analogue was an inhibitor of U46619-induced platelet aggregation and vascular smooth muscle contraction[10,36]. The structural features of both 13-azaprostanoic acid and pinane thromboxane A₂ were combined to produce a series of 13-azapinane thromboxane A₂ analogues, (Figure 9.3)[37]. These analogues proved to be selective TxA₂/PGH₂ antagonists, did not inhibit thromboxane synthase and in addition provided a useful molecule for radioligand binding studies[8,38]. Other examples, which include semicarbazone (EP045), hydrazine (SQ29,548) and substituted phenoxy (EP171) derivatives, have also been characterized and shown to possess either antagonist or agonist properties[39-41].

213

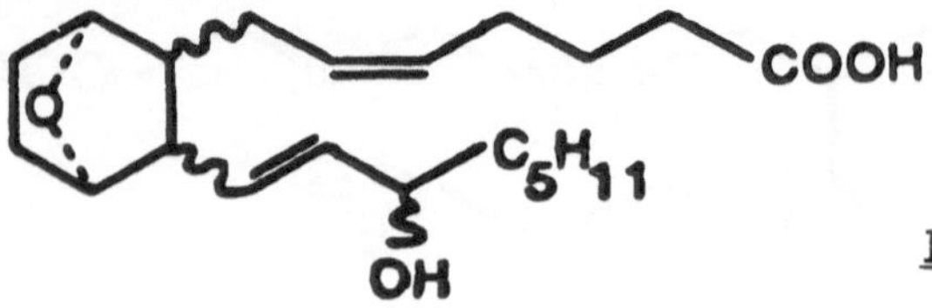

Figure 9.3 Chemical structure of: 10, 7-oxabicylo[2.2.1]heptane analogues; 11, 13-azapro-stanoic acid; and 12, 13-azapinane thromboxane A_2 analogues

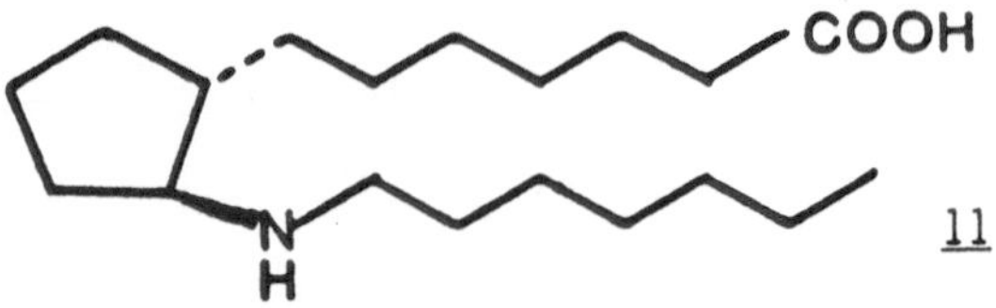

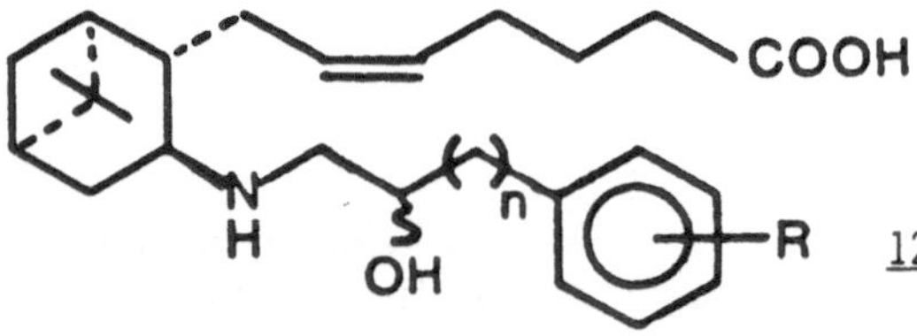

As these novel compounds were synthesized and their pharmacology evaluated, certain structure–activity relationships emerged and the reader is referred to other reviews which discuss these relationships in detail[17–19,42].

PHYSIOLOGICAL AND PHARMACOLOGICAL EFFECTS

Platelets

Arachidonic acid induces platelets to change shape, aggregate, secrete their granular contents, activate phospholipase C, phosphorylate a 40 kDa protein and myosin light chain and expose fibrinogen receptors. All of these events may or may not be independent of each other, but all require the conversion of arachidonic acid to either PGG_2, PGH_2 or TxA_2[43,44]. The formation of TxA_2 from PGH_2 does not appear to be necessary for platelet aggregation to occur, since PGH_2 aggregates platelets[45–47]. Shape change and aggregation can be induced either directly by metabolites of arachidonic acid or indirectly through the release of endogenously stored ADP[48–50]. Kinlough-Rathbone et al.[49] originally demonstrated that arachidonic acid could aggregate degranulated rabbit or human platelets. Since these platelets did not contain ADP,

214

they concluded that arachidonic acid-induced platelet aggregation was independent of secreted ADP. Recently, Cerletti *et al.* confirmed these observations[51]; however, they also showed that ADP was not required for arachidonic acid-induced platelet aggregation if TxA$_2$ was synthesized. When platelets were treated with a thromboxane synthase inhibitor and ADP removed by treatment with either apyrase or CP/CPK, the platelets did not aggregate in response to arachidonic acid. Similarly, U46619-induced platelet aggregation was inhibited by treatment of the platelets with CP/CPK or apyrase. They concluded that ADP was not required for arachidonic acid-induced platelet aggregation provided TxA$_2$ is generated, but ADP is required for PGH$_2$ to induce aggregation.

The platelet response to U46619 does not appear to be the same as that elicited by arachidonic acid or PGH$_2$[52]. At intermediate concentrations, U46619 induces a biphasic aggregation with secretion occurring after a lag phase and in parallel with the second wave of aggregation. In contrast to this, PGG$_2$, PGH$_2$ or TxA$_2$-like material used at intermediate concentrations produced reversible aggregation accompanied by secretion[52]. Arachidonic acid differed from all the above because aggregation was always accompanied by secretion. These results raise some interesting unanswered questions:

(1) Is there more than one intracellular site for the platelet receptors for these substances?

(2) Do the exogenously added compounds have access to the same receptor sites?

(3) Is there a separate receptor for the endoperoxides and thromboxane A$_2$?

Finally, in the platelet, the endoperoxide analogues may not be true mimetics of the actions of TxA$_2$ and/or PGH$_2$.

Vascular smooth muscle

PGH$_2$ and TxA$_2$ and their stable analogues contract vascular smooth muscle from many vascular beds. As with platelets, PGH$_2$ can contract vascular smooth muscle without being converted to TxA$_2$[22,53]. Recent work utilizing carbocyclic TxA$_2$ in coronary arteries demonstrated that it was most potent in dog, followed closely by monkey, then human[54]. These effects were similar in small, medium or large vessels in the same species[55]. The contractile effect of CTA$_2$ was antagonized by calcium antagonists or a reduction in extracellular calcium[56,57]. The intracellular calcium antagonist, TMB-8, had no effect on the canine pulmonary artery vasoconstrictor response to U46619 *in vivo*[58]. Taken together, these observations raise the possibility that an extracellular source of calcium is necessary to mediate the contractile response to U46619.

A wide variety of other vascular tissues are sensitive to PGH$_2$, TxA$_2$ and their stable mimetics. These include rat[59,60] and rabbit[61,62] aorta, and human umbilical vessels[63]. The dog saphenous vein has been commonly used to study the pharmacology of stable TxA$_2$/PGH$_2$ agonists and antagonists[22,38,64] since it appears to be one of the most sensitive vascular tissues to these compounds.

215

SPECIES DIFFERENCES IN PLATELET RESPONSES TO PGH_2, TxA_2, THEIR MIMETICS AND ANTAGONISTS

Guinea-pig

Of all species that have been studied, guinea-pig platelets appear to be the most similar to human platelets. Irreversible aggregation results from the addition of either sodium arachidonate or the endoperoxide analogue, 9,11-azo-PGH_2[65]. Guinea-pig platelets appear to be more sensitive than human platelets to sodium arachidonate[65]. Like human platelets, guinea-pig platelet aggregation induced by sodium arachidonate or 9,11-azo-PGH_2 is blocked by the prior addition of either pinane TxA_2 or carbocyclic TxA_2[65]. Thus, it appears that, like human platelets, guinea-pig platelets possess an active pathway converting arachidonic acid to the endoperoxides and TxA_2 and that guinea-pig platelet TxA_2/PGH_2 receptors are similar to those in human platelets. Radioligand binding studies have recently been performed on washed guinea-pig platelets and the results support a similarity between human and guinea-pig platelets[66]. While differences are apparent in comparing the competition of the radioligand with a series of agonists and antagonists, the similarities outweigh the differences. Collectively, the pharmacological and radioligand binding studies would suggest that the guinea-pig platelets may be a useful model for studying the role of platelet TxA_2/PGH_2 receptors in disease states.

Rabbit

Rabbit platelets respond to the addition of arachidonic acid with irreversible aggregation which can be blocked by indomethacin[66]. Aggregation induced by low doses of arachidonic acid can be blocked by a thromboxane synthase inhibitor but this inhibition can be overcome by addition of higher concentrations of arachidonic acid in the absence of TxA_2 generation[67]. PGH_2 stimulates reversible rabbit platelet aggregation which is only partially blocked by a thromboxane synthetase inhibitor[67]. Neither pinane TxA_2 nor ONO-11120, a more potent TxA_2/PGH_2 antagonist, blocked the aggregation responses of rabbit platelets to either sodium arachidonate[65,68] or 9,11-azo-PGH_2[65] as they do in human platelets. Indeed, recent radioligand binding studies[68] with a competitive TxA_2/PGH_2 receptor antagonist failed to show any specific binding to washed rabbit platelets, suggesting either the absence of TxA_2/PGH_2 receptors in rabbit platelets, or, more likely, that they are very different from human platelets.

Rat

There exists some controversy over whether or not TxA_2 and the endo-peroxides play a role in arachidonic acid-induced platelet aggregation in the rat. Early studies in PRP showed that arachidonic acid, but not PGH_2, was capable of inducing rat platelet aggregation, even though both agents

216

produced sufficient TxA$_2$ to produce aggregation[69]. In addition, U46619 did not produce an aggregatory response[70].

Further studies comparing responses in washed platelets with those in PRP demonstrated that arachidonic acid gives variable responses in rat platelets, depending upon the concentration used and whether the aggregation responses occur in PRP or washed platelets[70]. In washed rat platelets three types of responses to added arachidonic acid were observed:

(1) 2–10 μmol L^{-1} arachidonic acid produced shape change and irreversible aggregation. These effects were abolished by the cyclooxygenase inhibitor, flurbiprofen, and the TxA$_2$/PGH$_2$ receptor antagonist, EP092. Addition of the thromboxane synthase inhibitor, dazoxiben, produced only partial inhibition of these responses.

(2) 20–200 μmol L^{-1} arachidonic acid produced suppressed aggregatory responses, and inhibited the aggregation response to ADP added 2 min after arachidonic acid.

(3) 250–1000 μmol L^{-1} arachidonic acid produced irreversible aggregation which was insensitive to flurbiprofen, EP092, and dazoxiben. The TxA$_2$/PGH$_2$ mimetics, U44619 and EP171, produced shape change and irreversible aggregation responses.

Thus, it appears that low doses of arachidonic acid aggregate washed rat platelets by a mechanism dependent upon TxA$_2$ and/or PGH$_2$. Moderate doses appear to stimulate the production of an antiaggregatory metabolite, which is probably not PGD$_2$[71], since rat platelets are unresponsive to PGD$_2$[71]. Higher doses stimulate aggregation which is independent of thromboxane A$_2$ and the endoperoxides. This may represent the detergent effect of the high concentrations of arachidonic acid used.

Thus, while rat platelets produce the proaggregatory endoperoxides and TxA$_2$ and appear to be capable of responding to them, it is not clear that the rat platelet TxA$_2$/PGH$_2$ receptor is similar to that found in human platelets.

Dog

Canine platelets present a unique problem when studying the TxA$_2$/PGH$_2$-dependent pathway of aggregation. Canine platelets appear to fall into two distinct groups: one which responds to arachidonic acid, and another group which does not respond to arachidonic acid or stable TxA$_2$ mimetics, even though they respond normally to ADP and collagen[72]. The unresponsive platelets can be converted to responsive platelets upon addition of subaggregatory doses of agents, such as epinephrine, which act to decrease elevated cyclic AMP. The role of cyclic AMP in contributing to the lack of response is uncertain since both groups of platelets have the same basal cAMP levels[73]. The differences between the two groups cannot be ascribed to lack of PGH$_2$/TxA$_2$ synthesis, since non-responders also synthesize TxA$_2$[73]. Furthermore, non-responders do not aggregate in the presence of stable TxA$_2$ mimetics which bypass TxA$_2$/PGH$_2$ synthesis[65].

The mechanism of conversion of non-responders is uncertain, but could involve either an unmasking of receptors for TxA_2/PGH_2, or loss of some inhibitory factor between receptor occupancy and the aggregatory response. The latter seems more likely, since neither epinephrine nor ADP, in concentrations which convert non-responsive platelets to responsive platelets, changed the density of the TxA_2/PGH_2 receptors or their affinity for U46619 in washed canine platelets[68,74]. Thus, it appears that both agonists and antagonists can bind to the receptor in non-responsive platelets, both agonists are incapable of rendering a response unless cyclic AMP levels have been previously lowered.

Further differences between human and canine platelet receptors have also been noted, in that the rank orders of potency for a series of receptor antagonists and two agonists were different in the two species[38].

Other species

Feline platelets aggregate in response to arachidonic acid or 9,11-azo-PGH_2.[65] The aggregation response may be blocked by the TxA_2/PGH_2 antagonist, pinane TxA_2, but differences when compared with human platelets have been noted[65].

Platelets from cows, mink, and pigs change shape but do not aggregate in response to sodium arachidonate[75]. This lack of response may be due to the low activity of thromboxane synthase in platelets from these animals compared with human platelets[75]. Sheep platelets do not aggregate in response to either sodium arachidonate or 9,11-azo-PGH_2.[65] Thus, their platelets may not possess TxA_2/PGH_2 receptors.

DO TxA_2/PGH_2 RECEPTOR SUBTYPES EXIST?

The first suggestion that vascular TxA_2/PGH_2 receptors were different from those of the platelet was made by Needleman et al.[76] and was based upon the pharmacological effects of α and ω side-chain-modified TxA_2 and PGH_2 analogues in washed human platelets and isolated rabbit aorta. A similar conclusion was reached by Fitzpatrick et al.[77] and Gorman et al.[78] studying a series of TxA_2/PGH_2 antagonists in human platelets and rat aorta. In addition, carbocyclic TxA_2 has been found to be an antagonist in human platelets, but an agonist in cat coronary arteries[79]. All of these studies provided evidence suggesting that a distinction between the receptors for these two tissues could be made. However, in all cases, the tissues were obtained from different species which could have accounted for the apparent differences.

Mais et al.[38] have provided further evidence for the existence of distinct classes of receptors in platelets and blood vessels. They studied the activity of a series of 13-azapinane TxA_2 antagonists in human and canine platelets and saphenous vein. The structure–activity relationship for the series of antagonists for the human platelet receptor was found to be significantly different from that for the human vascular receptor and the canine platelet receptor[38]. The canine vascular receptor was the same as the human vascular receptor but different from the canine platelet receptor. They chose to name the platelet receptors [TxA$_2$/PGH$_2$]$_\alpha$, α for aggregation, and [TxA$_2$/PGH$_2$]$_\tau$, τ for tone[38]. Mais et al. also found that the orientation of the 15-hydroxy group did not influence the activity of a series of 13-azapinane TxA$_2$ antagonists in the platelet but did in the saphenous vein[64].

These structure–activity relations have recently been extended to a related series of 13-azapinane analogues, which possess a variety of substitutions on the ω side chain[80]. In this series of analogues, not only was the rank order between platelets and vessels significantly different for the antagonists, but several of the analogues were agonists in the vessels but all were competitive antagonists in the platelets[80]. Akbar et al.[81] have found a different rank order of potency for a series of 13-azaprostanoic acid analogues in rat thoracic aorta and human platelets. However, interestingly they concluded that the receptors were not different[81]. A series of 16-phenoxy PGE$_1$ analogues have been prepared by Banerjee et al.[61] which possess TxA$_2$/PGH$_2$-like activity in rabbit aortic strips and rat platelet-rich plasma. These workers noted a correlation between agonist activity in the aorta and the rat platelets[61]. However, analysis of the same data by the Spearman's rank order correlation shows distinct rank order differences for the compounds between the two tissues. Ogletree et al.[82] have also provided evidence recently for the existence of TxA$_2$/PGH$_2$ receptor subtypes based on relative affinities and stimulatory potencies for U46619, PGD$_2$, PGE$_2$ and PGF$_{2\alpha}$ in human platelets and rat aorta.

Thus, the current evidence strongly supports the notion that the TxA$_2$/PGH$_2$ receptor in platelets is distinct from that in blood vessels. In addition, the possibility has been raised that there may be subsets of receptors within the platelet[83–85].

SECOND MESSENGER SYSTEMS

Platelets

Since 1977, various potential second messengers for the platelet TxA$_2$/PGH$_2$ receptor have been proposed. Among the earliest was a role for cyclic AMP. It was originally reported that PGG$_2$ inhibited PGE$_1$-stimulated adenylate cyclase in platelets[86]. However, this effect was claimed to be the result of released ADP. Subsequent work by Miller et al.[87] and Miller and Gorman[88] demonstrated that PGH$_2$ and TxA$_2$ had no effect on basal adenylate cyclase activity. The calcium antagonist, TMB-8, inhibited the capacity of TxA$_2$ to decrease cAMP levels[89]. Collectively, these observations led to the conclusion that the inhibition of PGE$_1$-stimulated adenylate cyclase by TxA$_2$ was not a direct effect but was secondary to an increase in intracellular free calcium and/or release of ADP. Arachidonic acid and PGH$_2$ decreased platelet cAMP levels previously elevated by PGI$_2$[90]. Indomethacin blocked the former effect; however, a thromboxane synthase inhibitor did not prevent this effect. Neither U44069 nor U46619 had any effect on basal or PGE$_1$-stimulated adenylate cyclase[91]. Thus, in the platelet, the TxA_2/PGH_2 receptor does not appear to be directly linked to inhibition of adenylate cyclase.

Arachidonic acid, TxA_2, PGH_2 and their stable mimetics produce an increase in intracellular free calcium in human platelets or alter the binding or flux of calcium in platelet membrane vesicles[92-94]. These effects were blocked by the receptor antagonist, 13-azaprostanoic acid[94,95]. The dense tubular system is believed to be the source of calcium. The mechanism by which calcium is elevated in platelets by TxA_2/PGH_2 or their mimetics remains unknown. However, much recent evidence suggests that turnover of phophatidyl inositol polyphosphates plays an important intermediary role[96-99].

Stimulation of phospholipase C by a variety of agonists, including PGH_2, TxA_2 and their stable mimetics, results in the formation of inositol trisphosphate, cyclic inositol trisphosphate and diacylglycerol[100-105]. The inositol polyphosphates can act, presumably at their receptors, to cause an increase in intraplatelet free calcium resulting in aggregation. However, this does not appear to be the entire story. Authi et al.[99] have recently demonstrated that, when inositol trisphosphate was introduced into saponin permeabilized platelets, aggregation resulted. This could be blocked by cyclo-oxygenase inhibitors or TxA_2/PGH_2 receptor antagonists. They concluded that the calcium released by inositol triphosphates, whatever its source, acts to stimulate calcium-dependent phospholipase A_2 releasing arachidonic acid from membrane phospholipids. Arachidonic acid is then converted to PGH_2 and TxA_2, resulting in aggregation. Thus, the exact role of inositol polyphosphates in platelet aggregation, in particular their role as a second messenger, remains to be determined.

Coupled to the release of inositol polyphosphates is the release of diacylglycerol with subsequent stimulation of protein kinase C. This enzyme, upon activation, results in the phosphorylation of various platelet proteins. Arachidonic acid, U46619 and 9,11-azo-PGH_2 have been shown to induce the phosphorylation of at least three different proteins[106-108]. One protein was actin binding protein of molecular weight 260 kDa, and a second of molecular weight 20 kDa was myosin light chain. Myosin light chain phosphorylation precedes shape change and aggregation, and probably plays an important role in the platelet reponse to aggregating agents[109]. A third protein, of molecular weight 40 kDa, had been unidentified until very recently. This protein has been purified and shown to dephosphorylate inositol triphosphate or cyclic inositol triphosphate at the 5-position[110]. Upon phosphorylation by protein kinase C, the enzyme becomes active[110]. The enzyme and its activation by kinase C provides the platelet (and other cells) with a mechanism to limit the consequences of the synthesis of the inositol polyphosphates.

It appears that phosphatidylinositol metabolism may be coupled to the platelet TxA_2/PGH_2 receptor. In addition, there has been recent evidence that this metabolism may involve a novel form of guanine nucleotide regulatory protein, termed N_p[111]. It has been shown that U44069 can stimulate a GTPase activity in human platelet membranes which is not sensitive to cholera or pertussis toxins, thereby providing evidence that this regulatory protein may be distinct from N_s and N_i[112].

220

Vascular smooth muscle

In vascular smooth muscle, the second messenger(s) for the TxA_2/PGH_2 receptor remain uncertain. Both U46619 and U44069 alter $^{45}Ca^{2+}$ fluxes in canine pulmonary artery and vein[113]. Loutzenhiser and vanBreemen also found that U44069 enhanced $^{45}Ca^{2+}$ efflux from rabbit aorta[114]. The cellular site(s) of calcium affected by agonists is (are) unknown. It has been postulated that mitochondria may be a possible site, since U46619 and prostaglandins have been shown to influence calcium fluxes in mitochondria[115]. However, the endoplasmic reticulum has not been ruled out as a source of the calcium that is released in response to TxA_2/PGH_2.

Recently, it was shown that inositol trisphosphate could induce calcium release and vasoconstriction in permeabilized rabbit pulmonary artery[116]. Perhaps, as in the platelet, the TxA_2/PGH_2 receptor is coupled to phosphatidyl-inositol polyphosphate turnover.

RADIOLIGAND BINDING STUDIES

The first studies using radiolabelled binding techniques involved [³H]13-azaprostanoic acid ([³H]13-APA)[6]. These studies used human platelet membranes and demonstrated that binding of this ligand was saturable, stereo-specific and displaceable by a series of compounds believed to interact at the TxA_2/PGH_2 receptor[6]. Two binding sites were noted, one of high affinity (100 nmol L⁻¹) and one of low affinity (3.5 μmol L⁻¹). At saturation[6], the B_{max} for the high-affinity site was 1 pmol (mg protein)⁻¹.

Radiolabelled ligand binding studies have been conducted using the tritium labelled agonist, U44069, in intact washed human platelets[5]. Using this ligand, two binding compartments were found which competed for cold ligand, along with a third undefined compartment. No K_d values were noted. A series of TxA_2/PGH_2 agonists, partial agonists and antagonists competed with the ligand with potency ratios similar to those found for their pharmacological activities in platelets. More recently, the same group used this ligand to correlate receptor occupancy by the ligand with induction of phosphatidate formation and elevation of cytosolic free calcium levels in human platelets[101]. In that study, they reported a K_d of 70 nmol L⁻¹ for [³H]U44069 and only a single class of binding sites[101].

Recently, the first ¹²⁵I-labelled radioligand for study of eicosanoid receptors has been described[7]. An analogue of 13-APA was synthesized with insertion of a phenol moiety in the ω side chain for subsequent incorporation of ¹²⁵I. The analogue, I-cis-APO, was utilized in binding experiments with human platelet membranes[7]. This compound was not of sufficient potency to be useful for more extensive investigations, but indicated that the concept of synthesizing and using [¹²⁵I]-labelled eicosanoid analogues for binding studies was tenable. Therefore, a series of compounds that were derivatives of 13-azapinane-TxA_2, a more potent series of TxA_2/PGH_2 receptor antagonists, were synthesized[117]. One of these compounds, PTA-OH, was iodinated to yield [¹²⁵I]PTA-OH, which proved suitable for binding studies in canine and human washed platelets and human platelet membranes[8,68,74,118].

I-PTA-OH was a competitive antagonist of U46619-induced platelet aggregation in washed human platelets. The pharmacologically derived K_d of $8\,\mathrm{nmol\,L^{-1}}$ agreed well with the kinetically determined K_d of $27\,\mathrm{nmol\,L^{-1}}$ in the binding studies. Scatchard analysis of equilibrium binding gave a K_d of $21\,\mathrm{nmol\,L^{-1}}$ and a B_{max} of $0.89\,\mathrm{pmol\,(mg\ protein)^{-1}}$ (2530 binding sites/platelet) and revealed the presence of a single class of binding sites[8] (Figure 9.4). The B_{max} derived from these studies agreed well with the $1\,\mathrm{pmol\,(mg\ protein)^{-1}}$ obtained using [³H]13-APA[6] and the 1700 sites/platelet obtained from the [³H]U44069 studies[5]. [¹²⁵I]PTA-OH could be displaced from its binding site by a series of antagonists and agonists. For the antagonists, the rank order of potency for displacing the ligand from its binding site correlated ($r = 0.93$) with the rank order of potency for their ability to inhibit U46619-induced aggregation in human platelet-rich plasma[8]. In addition, $PGF_{2\alpha}$, PGD_2 and the

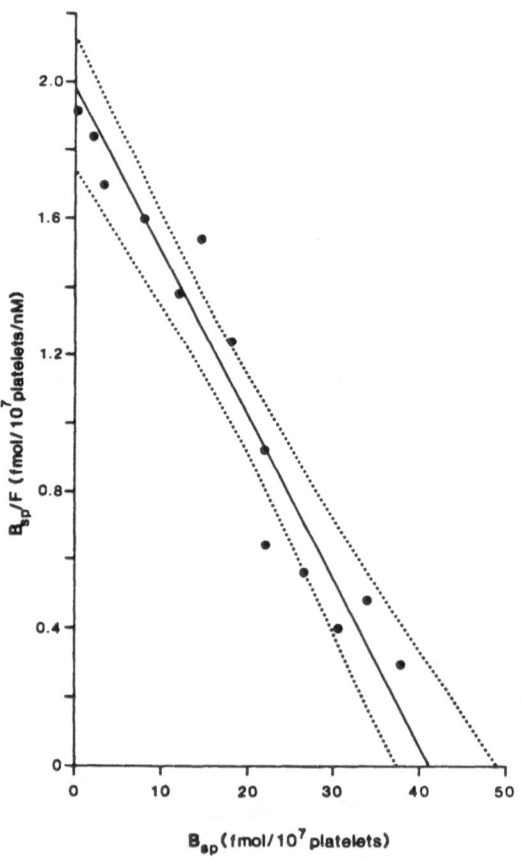

Figure 9.4 Scatchard plot for equilibrium binding data of [¹²⁵I]PTA-OH to washed human platelets. The data are the result of five separate experiments and are expressed as the line of best fit and the 95% confidence band around that line. $K_d = 21\,\mathrm{nmol\,L^{-1}}$; $B_{max} = 890\,\mathrm{fmol}$ (mg protein)$^{-1}$. Reprinted from *J. Pharmacol. Exp. Ther.* by permission of the publisher

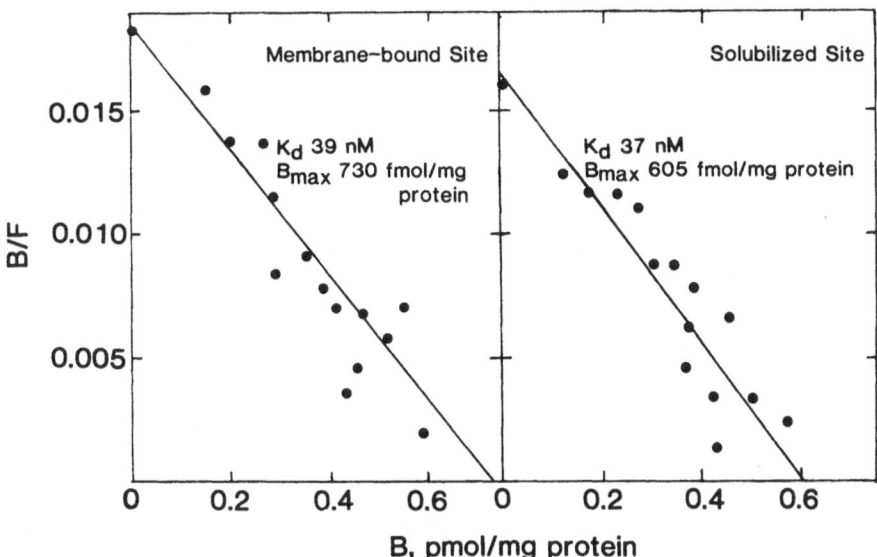

Figure 9.5 Scatchard plot for equilibrium binding of [^{125}I]PTA-OH to intact and CHAPS solubilized membranes from a single subject. (left) Membrane bound site: $K_d = 39$ nmol L^{-1}; $B_{max} = 730$ fmol (mg protein)$^{-1}$. (right) Solubilized site: $K_d = 37$ nmol L^{-1}; $B_{max} = 605$ fmol (mg protein)$^{-1}$. Reprinted from ref. 121 by permission of the authors

stable PGI$_2$ analogue iloprost, competed with the ligand, but only at concentrations much higher than those required to produce their pharmacological effects. These results have been recently confirmed by Narumiya *et al.*[68].

A similar set of results have been obtained in human platelet membranes[118]. However, notable differences were observed in the displacement of [^{125}I]PTA-OH by TxA$_2$/PGH$_2$ mimetics such as U46619. Indeed, the IC$_{50}$ values obtained in membranes were nearly two orders of magnitude greater than that observed in washed human platelets[118]. Since antagonists were not affected, these results suggest that the preparation of platelet membranes is altering the receptor affinity for agonists, but not antagonists. Possibly, the platelet is releasing a substance which is altering the TxA$_2$/PGH$_2$ receptor. Recent work suggests that platelets release a protein during lysis which alters the receptors' affinity for agonists[119]. Release of this material may offer an explanation for the desensitization of platelets by TxA$_2$/PGH$_2$ mimetics[85].

Recently, [^{3}H]U46619 has been made commercially available and the binding of this agonist to washed human platelets has been reported[120]. The K_d for U46619 binding was 109 nmol L^{-1} and the B_{max} was 350 fmol/10^8 platelets (2000 sites per platelet)[120]. The number of sites per platelet agrees well with that reported for [^{125}I]PTA-OH and [^{3}H]U44069 binding.

Binding studes have been carried out with [^{125}I]PTA-OH in washed canine platelets[68,74] and washed guinea-pig platelets[66]. The results were qualitatively similar to that obtained in washed human platelets.

The TxA$_2$/PGH$_2$ receptor has been solubilized in active form using the detergent, CHAPS[121]. Studies of radioligand binding to the solubilized

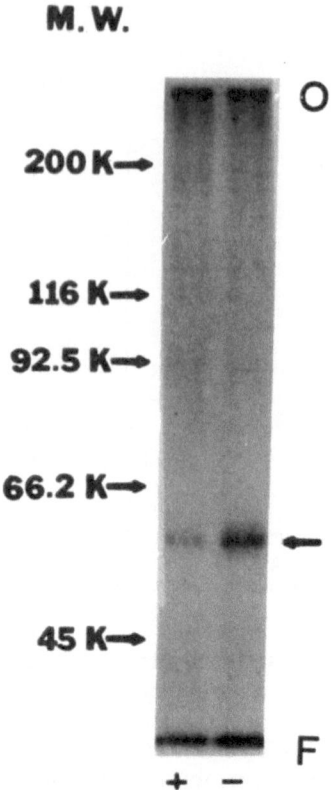

Figure 9.6 Autoradiogram of photoaffinity labelled TxA_2/PGH_2 receptor. Solubilized membranes were incubated with 5 μCi of an ^{125}I-labelled photoaffinity ligand either in absence (−) or presence (+) of non-photolysable TxA_2/PGH_2 agonist SQ26655 (50 μmol L^{-1} final). Protein was subjected to SDS-PAGE (7% acrylamide) under non-reducing conditions. The molecular weight markers are indicated on the left and the specifically labelled band is shown by arrow on right. Molecular weight was approximately 60 000 Daltons

receptor compared favourably with those in intact membranes[121] (Figure 9.5). Hydrodynamic studies have provided an estimate of the molecular weight of the receptor–detergent complex of 140 000 Da[122]. In addition, a photoaffinity ligand has been described and its irreversible incorporation into human platelet membranes and solubilized membranes documented[123]. The results with an ^{125}I-labelled photoaffinity ligand and SDS-polyacrylamide gel electrophoresis suggest a molecular weight of approximately 60 000 Da (Figure 9.6) (unpublished observations).

With the advent of radioligands and photoaffinity probes of high affinity and high specific activity for the TxA$_2$/PGH$_2$ receptor, greater understanding into the nature of this receptor in platelets and other tissues should be forthcoming. In particular, information on receptor number, regulation, structure and function will surely be obtained in the future.

FUTURE DIRECTIONS

Future studies of the TxA$_2$/PGH$_2$ receptors should prove interesting and exciting. Purification of the receptor to homogeneity will allow structure–function studies to progress by means of reconstitution experiments and peptide mapping. Purification and sequencing of a small peptide fragment of the receptor should allow for the cloning and total sequencing of the receptor.

Another area of study should involve determining the manner of regulation of the receptor in the platelet and other tissues and the mechanisms of desensitization of the receptor to TxA$_2$/PGH$_2$ mimetics. While desensitization by arachidonic acid has been noted[85] in the platelet, its mechanism is not known.

Finally, there is a need to develop radioligand binding assays, either in a vascular tissue preparation or a cell line derived from vascular smooth muscle. This would allow for the further characterization of the vascular TxA$_2$/PGH$_2$ receptor and its comparison with the receptor in the platelet.

ACKNOWLEDGEMENTS

Supported in part by NIH grants HL36838 and HL29566. Perry V. Halushka is a Burroughs–Wellcome Scholar in Clinical Pharmacology. The secretarial assistance of Ms. Virginia Minchoff and Ms. Connie Hill is gratefully acknowledged.

REFERENCES

1. Hamberg, M., Svensson, J., Wakabayashi, T. and Samuelsson, B. (1974). Isolation and structure of two prostaglandin endoperoxides that cause platelet aggregation. *Proc. Natl. Acad. Sci. USA*, **71**, 345–349
2. Hamberg, M., Svensson, J. and Samuelsson, B. (1975). Thromboxanes: A new group of biologically active compounds derived from prostaglandin endoperoxides. *Proc. Natl. Acad. Sci. USA*, **72**, 2994–2998
3. Hamberg, M. and Samuelsson, B. (1974). Prostaglandin endoperoxides. Novel transformations of arachidonic acid in human platelets. *Proc. Natl. Acad. Sci. USA*, **71**, 3400–3404
4. Bhagwat, S.S., Hamann, P.R., Still, W.C., Bunting, S. and Fitzpatrick, F.A. (1985). Synthesis and structure of the platelet aggregation factor thromboxane A$_2$. *Nature (London)*, **315**, 511–513
5. Armstrong, R.A., Jones, R.L. and Wilson, N.H. (1983). Ligand binding to thromboxane receptors on human platelets: Correlation with biological activity. *Br. J. Pharmacol.*, **79**, 953–964
6. Hung, S.C., Ghali, N.I., Venton, D.L. and LeBreton, G.C. (1983). Specific binding of the thromboxane A$_2$ antagonist 13-azaprostanoic acid to human platelet membranes. *Biochim. Biophys. Acta*, **728**, 171–178

7. Halushka, P.V., MacDermot, J., Knapp, D.R., Eller, T., Saussy, D.L. Jr., Mais, D., Blair, I.A. and Dollery, C.T. (1985). A novel approach for the study of thromboxane A_2 and prostaglandin H_2 receptors using an ^{125}I-labeled ligand. Biochem. Pharmacol., **34**, 1165–1170

8. Mais, D.E., Burch, R.M., Saussy, D.L. Jr., Kochel, P.J. and Halushka, P.V. (1985). Binding of a thromboxane A_2/prostaglandin H_2 receptor antagonist to washed human platelets. J. Pharmacol. Exp. Ther., **235**, 729–734

9. Gerrard, J.M. and White, J.G. (1978). Prostaglandins and thromboxanes: "Middlemen" modulating platelet function in hemostasis and thrombosis. In Spaet, T.H. (ed.) Progress in Hemostasis and Thrombosis, Vol. 4. pp. 87–125. (New York: Grune and Stratton)

10. LeBreton, G.C., Venton, D.L., Enke, S.E. and Halushka, P.V. (1979). 13-Aza-prostanoic acid: A specific agonist of the human blood platelet thromboxane/endoperoxide receptor. Proc. Natl. Acad. Sci. USA, **76**, 4097–4101

11. Lapetina, E.G. (1982). Regulation of arachidonic acid production: role of phospholipases C and A_2. Trends Pharmacol. Sci., **3**, 115–118

12. Ullrich, V. and Graf, H. (1984). Prostacyclin and thromboxane synthase as P-450 enzymes. Trends Pharmacol. Sci., 353–355

13. Needleman, P., Raz, A., Ferrendelli, J.A. and Minkes, M. (1977). Application of imidazole as a selective inhibitor of thromboxane synthase in human platelets. Proc. Natl. Acad. Sci. USA, **74**, 1716–1720

14. Iizuka, K., Akahane, K., Momose, D. and Nakazawa, M. (1981). Highly selective inhibitors of thromboxane synthase. 1. Imidazole derivatives. J. Med. Chem., **24**, 1139–1148

15. Tai, H., Lee, N. and Tai, C. (1980). Inhibition of thromboxane synthesis and platelet aggregation by pyridine and its derivatives. Adv. Prostagl. Thrombox. Res., **6**, 447–452

16. Gorman, R.R., Bundy, G.L., Peterson, D.C., Sun, F.F., Miller, O.J. and Fitzpatrick, F.A. (1977). Inhibition of human platelet thromboxane synthase by 9,11-azaprosta-5,13-dienoic acid. Proc. Natl. Acad. Sci. USA, **74**, 4007–4011

17. Saussy, D., Mais, D., Knapp, D. and Halushka, P. (1985). Thromboxane A_2 and prostaglandin endoperoxide receptors in platelets and vascular smooth muscle. Circulation, **72**, 1202–1207

18. Halushka, P., Mais, D. and Saussy, D. (1986). Platelet and vascular smooth muscle thromboxane A_2/prostaglandin H_2 receptors. Atherosclerosis Rev. (In press)

19. Wilson, N. and Jones, R. (1985). Prostaglandin endoperoxides and thromboxane A_2 analogs. In Pike, J. and Morton, D. (eds.) Advances in Prostaglandin, Thromboxane and Leukotriene Research, pp. 393–426. (New York: Raven Press)

20. Bundy, G. (1975). The synthesis of prostaglandin endoperoxide analogs. Tetrahedron Lett., **24**, 1957–1960

21. Corey, E., Nicolaou, K., Machedra, Y., Malmsten, C. and Samuelsson, B. (1975). Synthesis and biological properties of a 9,11-azo-prostanoid: Highly active biochemical mimic of prostaglandin endoperoxides. Proc. Natl. Acad. Sci. USA, **72**, 3355–3358

22. Coleman, R., Humphrey, P., Kennedy, I., Levy, G. and Lumley, P. (1981). Comparison of the actions of U-46619, a prostaglandin H_2 analogue, with those of prostaglandin H_2 and thromboxane A_2 on some isolated smooth muscle preparations. Br. J. Pharmacol., **73**, 773–778

23. Sun, F. (1977). Biosynthesis of thromboxane in human platelets. I. Characterization and assay of thromboxane synthase. Biochem. Biophys. Res. Commun., **74**, 1432–1440

24. Wilson, N., Peesapati, V., Jones, R. and Hamilton, K. (1982). Synthesis of prostanoids with bicyclo[2.2.1]heptane, and bicyclo[2.2.2]octane ring systems. Activities of 15-hydroxyepimers on human platelets. J. Med. Chem., **25**, 495–500

25. Corey, E., Narasaka, K. and Shibasaki, M. (1976). A direct stereocontrolled total synthesis of the 9,11-azo analogue of the prostaglandin endoperoxide PGH_2. J. Am. Chem. Soc., **98**, 6417–6418

26. Nicolaou, K., Magolda, R., Smith, J., Aharony, D., Smith, E. and Lefer, A. (1979). Synthesis and biological properties of pinane-thromboxane A_2, a selective inhibitor of coronary artery constriction, platelet aggregation, and thromboxane formation. Proc. Natl. Acad. Sci. USA, **76**, 2566–2570

27. Nicolaou, K., Magolda, R. and Claremon, D. (1980). Carbocyclic thromboxane A_2. J. Am. Chem. Soc., **102**, 1404–1409

226

28. Nicolaou, K., Smith, J. and Lefer, A. (1982). Chemistry and pharmacology of a series of new thromboxane analogs. *Drugs Future*, **7**, 331–340
29. Ohuchida, S., Hamanaka, N. and Hayashi, M. (1983). Synthesis of thromboxane A₂ analogs -1. *Tetrahedron*, **39**, 4257–4261
30. Armstrong, R., Jones, R., Peesapati, V., Will, S. and Wilson, N. (1985). Competitive antagonism at thromboxane receptors in human platelets. *Br. J. Pharmacol.*, **84**, 595–607
31. Ohuchida, S., Hamanaka, N. and Hayashi, M. (1983). Synthesis of thromboxane A₂ analogs-2. *Tetrahedron*, **39**, 4263–4268
32. Ohuchida, S., Hamanaka, N. and Hayashi, M. (1983). Synthesis of thromboxane A₂ analogs-4. *Tetrahedron*, **39**, 4273–4280
33. Sprague, P., Heikes, J., Harris, D. and Greenberg, R. (1983). 7-oxa-bicyclo[2.2.1]heptane analogs as modulators of the thromboxane A₂ and prostacyclin receptors. *Adv. Prostgl. Thrombox. Leuk. Res.*, **11**, 337–343
34. Nelson, N., Kelly, R. and Johnson, R. (1982). Prostaglandins and the arachidonic acid cascade. *Chem. Eng. News.*, **60**(33), 30–42
35. Venton, D., Enke, S. and LeBreton, G. (1979). Azaprostanoic acid derivatives. Inhibitors of arachidonic acid induced platelet aggregation. *J. Med. Chem.*, **22**, 824–830
36. Horn, P., Kohli, J., LeBreton, G. and Venton, D. (1984). Antagonism of prostanoid-induced vascular contraction by 13-azaprostanoic acid (13-APA). *J. Cardiovasc. Pharmacol.*, **6**, 609–613
37. Katsura, M., Miyamoto, T., Hamanaka, N., Kondo, K., Terada, T., Ohgaki, Y., Kawasaki, A. and Tsuboshima, M. (1983). *In vitro* and *in vivo* effects of new powerful thromboxane antagonists (3-alkylamino pinane derivatives). *Adv. Prostgl. Thrombox. Leuk. Res.*, **11**, 351–357
38. Mais, D., Saussy, D., Chaikhouni, A., Kochel, P.D., Hamanaka, N. and Halushka, P. (1985). Pharmacologic characterization of human and canine thromboxane A₂/prostaglandin H₂ receptors in platelets and blood vessels: Evidence for different receptors. *J. Pharmacol. Exp. Ther.*, **233**, 424–428
39. Jones, R. and Wilson, N. (1981). Thromboxane receptor antagonism shown by a prostanoid with a bicyclo[2.2.1]heptane ring. *Br. J. Pharmacol.*, **73**, 220–221P
40. Ogletree, M., Harris, D., Greenberg, R., Haslanger, M. and Nakane, M. (1985). Pharmacological actions of SQ 29,548, a novel selective thromboxane antagonist. *J. Pharmacol. Exp. Ther.*, **234**, 435–441
41. Jones, R., MacIntyre, D., Pollock, W., Shaw, A. and Wilson, N. (1985). An extreme of thromboxane-like activity. *Br. J. Pharmacol.*, **84**, 148P
42. Jones, R., Wilson, N. and Armstrong, R. (1985). Characterization of thromboxane receptors in human platelets. In Westwick, J., Scully, M., MacIntyre, D. and Kakkar, V. (eds.) *Mechanisms of Stimulus-Response Coupling in Platelets*, pp. 67–82. (New York and London: Plenum Press)
43. Smith, J.B. and Willis, A.L. (1971). Aspirin selectively inhibits prostaglandin production in human platelets. *Nature (London) New Biol.*, **231**, 237–239
44. Willis, A.L. (1974). An enzymatic mechanism for the antithrombotic effect of aspirin. *Science*, **183**, 325–327
45. Grimm, L.J., Knapp, D.R., Senator, D. and Halushka, P.V. (1981). Inhibition of platelet thromboxane synthesis by 7-(1-Imidazolyl) hetanoic acid: dissociation from inhibition of aggregation. *Thrombosis Res.*, **24**, 307–317
46. Bertele, V., Cerletti, C., Schieppati, A., DiMinno, G. and de Gaetano, G. (1981). Inhibition of thromboxane synthase does not necessarily prevent platelet aggregation. *Lancet*, **1**, 1057–1058
47. Hornby, E.J. and Skidmore, J.F. (1982). Evidence that prostaglandin endoperoxides can induce platelet aggregation in the absence of thromboxane A₂ production. *Biochem. Pharmacol.*, **31**, 1158–1160
48. Parise, L., Venton, D. and LeBreton, G. (1982). Thromboxane A₂/prostaglandin H₂ directly stimulates platelet shape change independent of secreted ADP. *J. Pharmacol. Exp. Ther.*, **222**, 276–281
49. Kinlough-Rathbone, R.L., Neimes, H.J., Mustard, J.F. and Pakham, M.A. (1976). Sodium arachidonate can induce platelet shape change and aggregation which are independent of the release reaction. *Science*, **192**, 1011–1012

227

50. Morinelli, T.A., Niewiarowski, S., Kornecki, E., Figures, W.R., Wachtfogel, Y. and Colman, R.W. (1983). Platelet aggregation and exposure of fibrinogen receptors by prostaglandin endoperoxide analogues. *Blood*, **61**, 41–49
51. Cerletti, C., Minoldo, S., Burchi, F., Maschio, A. and Gaetano, G. (1986). Requirement of ADP for arachidonic acid-induced platelet aggregation: Studies with selective thromboxane-synthase inhibitors. *Biochem. Pharmacol.*, **35**, 1201–1203
52. Charo, I., Feinman, R., Detwiler, T., Smith, J., Ingerman, C. and Silver, M. (1977). Prostaglandin endoperoxides and thromboxane A_2 can induce platelet aggregation in the absence of secretion. *Nature (London)*, **269**, 66–69
53. Smith, III, E.F., Rücker, W. and Schrör, K. (1983). RCS from human platelets: Is it only thromboxane? *Eur. J. Pharmacol.*, **95**, 121–124
54. Toda, N. (1984). Responses of human, monkey and dog coronary arteries *in vitro* to carbocyclic thromboxane A_2 and vasodilators. *Br. J. Pharmacol.*, **83**, 399–408
55. Miwa, K. and Toda, N. (1984). Regional differences in the response to vasoconstrictor agents of dog and monkey isolated coronary arteries. *Br. J. Pharmacol.*, **82**, 295–301
56. Smith, III., E.F., Lefer, A.M. and Nicolaou, K.C. (1981). Mechanisms of coronary vasoconstriction induced by carbocyclic thromboxane A_2. *Am. J. Physiol.*, **9**, H493–H497
57. Twoard, R. and Perzborn, E. (1982). Relaxation of carbocyclic thromboxane A_2-induced contractions of isolated coronary arteries by nifedipine. *Naunyn Schmeidebergs Arch. Pharmacol.*, **318**, 249–251
58. Angerio, A.D., Fitzpatrick, T.M., Kot, P.A., Ramwell, P.W., Rose, J.C. and Santoian, E.C. (1982). Effect of TMB-8 on the pulmonary vasoconstrictor action of prostaglandin $F_{2\alpha}$ and the thromboxane mimic, U46619. *Br. J. Pharmacol.*, **77**, 55–58
59. McGlynn, S., Mallarkey, G. and Smith, G.M. (1984). Comparison of the actions of 11,9 epoxymethano PGH_2 and 9,11 azo PGH_2 on rat aorta and stomach strip preparations. *Prostaglandins*, **27**, 105–110
60. Jones, R.L. and Wilson, N.H. (1978). A 17-p-fluorophenoxy prostanoid with potent and long-lasting thromboxane-like actions. *Br. J. Pharmacol.*, **63**, 362P
61. Banerjee, A., Tuffin, D. and Walker, J. (1985). Pharmacological effects of ($\pm$)-11-deoxy, 16-phenoxyprostaglandin E_1 derivatives in the cardiovascular system. *Br. J. Pharmacol.*, **84**, 71–80
62. Piper, P.J. and Vane, J.V. (1969). Release of additional factors in anaphylaxis and its antagonism by anti-inflammatory drugs. *Nature (London)*, **223**, 29–35
63. Tuvemo, T., Strandberg, K. and Hamberg, M. (1978). Contractile action of a stable prostaglandin endoperoxide analogue on the human umbilical artery. *Acta Physiol. Scand.*, **102**, 495–496
64. Mais, D., Dunlap, C., Hamanaka, N. and Halushka, P. (1985). Further studies on the effects of epimers of thromboxane A_2 antagonists on platelets and veins. *Eur. J. Pharmacol.*, **111**, 125–128
65. Burke, S.E., Lefer, A.M., Nicolaou, K.C., Smith, G.M. and Smith, J.B. (1983). Responsiveness of platelets and coronary arteries from different species to synthetic thromboxane and prostaglandin endoperoxide analogues. *Br. J. Pharmacol.*, **78**, 287–292
66. Halushka, P., Mais, D. and Garvin, M. (1986). Binding of a thromboxane A_2/prostaglandin H_2 receptor antagonist to guinea pig platelets. *Eur. J. Pharmacol.*, **131**, 49–54
67. Lewis, G.P. and Watts, I.S. (1982). Prostaglandin endoperoxides, thromboxane A_2 and adenosine diphosphate in collagen-induced aggregation of rabbit platelets. *Br. J. Pharmacol.*, **75**, 623–631
68. Narumiya, S., Okuma, M. and Ushikubi, F. (1986). Binding of a radioiodinated 13-azapinane thromboxane antagonists to platelets: Correlation with antiaggregatory activity in different species. *Br. J. Pharmacol.*, **88**, 323–331
69. Nishizawa, E.E., Williams, D.J. and Connell, C.L., (1983). Arachidonate induced aggregation of rat platelets may not require prostaglandin endoperoxides or thromboxane A_2. *Thrombosis Res.*, **30**, 289–296
70. Armstrong, R.A., Jones, R.L. and Tymkewycz, P.M. (1985). The nature of arachidonic acid-induced aggregation of rat platelets. *Br. J. Pharmacol.*, **84**, 147P
71. Smith, J.B., Silver, M.J., Ingerman, C.M. and Kocsis, J.J. (1974). Prostaglandin D_2 inhibits the aggregation of human platelets. *Thrombosis Res.*, **5**, 291–299
72. Johnson, G.J., Leis, L.A., Rao, G.H.R. and White, J.G. (1979) Arachidonate-induced platelet aggregation in the dog. *Thrombosis Res.*, **14**, 147–154

228

73. Johnson, G.J., Rao,. G.H.R., Leis, L.A. and White, J.G. (1980). Effect of agents that alter cyclic AMP on arachidonate-induced platelet aggregation in the dog. *Blood*, **55**, 722–729

74. Mais, D.E., Kochel, P.J. Saussy, D.L. Jr. and Halushka, P.V. (1985). Binding of an ^{125}I-labeled thromboxane A₂/prostaglandin H₂ receptor antagonist to washed canine platelets. *Mol. Pharmacol.*, **28**, 163–169

75. Meyers, K.M., Katz, J.B., Clemmons, R.M., Smith, S.B. and Holmsen, H. (1980). An evaluation of the arachidonate pathway of platelets from companion and food-producing animals, mink, and man. *Thrombosis. Res.*, **20**, 13–24

76. Needleman, P., Minkes, M. and Raz, A. (1976). Thromboxanes: Selective biosynthesis and distinct biological properties. *Science*, **193**, 163–165

77. Fitzpatrick, F.A., Bundy, G.L., Gorman, R.R. and Honohan, T. (1978). 9,11-Epoxyimino-prosta-5,13-dienoic acid is a thromboxane A₂ antagonist in human platelets. *Nature (London)*, **275**, 764–766

78. Gorman, R., Maxey, K. and Bundy, G. (1981). Inhibition of human platelet thromboxane synthase by 11a-carba-thromboxane A₂ analogs. *Biochem. Biophys. Res. Commun.*, **100**, 184–190

79. Lefer, A.M., Smith, III, E.F., Araka, H., Smith, J.B., Aharony, D., Claremon, D.A., Magolda, R.L. and Nicolaou, K.C. (1980). Dissociation of vasoconstrictor and platelet aggregatory activities of thromboxane by carbocyclic thromboxane A₂, a stable analog of thromboxane A₂. *Proc. Natl. Acad. Sci. USA*, **77**, 1706–1710

80. Halushka, P.V., Mais, D.E., Garvin, M., Kochel, P. and Sightler, H. (1986). Structure activity relationships for 13-azapinane-TxA₂ analogs in platelets and vascular TxA₂/PGH₂ receptors: Evidence for different receptors. In *6th International Conference on Prostaglandins*, Florence, 1986, p. 166. (Fondazione Giovanni Lorenzini)

81. Akbar, H., Mukhopadhyay, A., Anderson, K., Navran, S., Ramstedt, K., Miller, D. and Feller, D. (1985). Antagonism of prostaglandin-mediated responses in platelets and vascular smooth muscle by 13-azaprostanoic acid analogs. *Biochem. Pharmacol.*, **34**, 641–647

82. Ogletree, M., Allen, G., O'Keefe, E., Liv, K. and Hedberg, A. (1986). Activities of various prostanoids at thromboxane receptors revealed by selective receptor antagonists: Studies in human platelets and several rat and guinea-pig smooth muscles. In *6th International Conference on Prostaglandins*, p. 350. (Fondazione Giovanni Lorenzini)

83. LeDuc, L.E., Wyche, A., Sprecher, H., Sankarappe, S.K. and Needleman, P. (1981). Analogues of arachidonic acid used to evaluate structural determinants of prostaglandin receptor and enzyme specificities. *Mol. Pharmacol.*, **19**, 242–247

84. MacIntyre, D.E. and J.L. Gordon (1977). Discrimination between platelet prostaglandin receptors with a specific antagonist to bisenoic prostaglandins. *Thrombosis Res.*, **11**, 705–713

85. Carmo, L.G., Hatmi, M., Rotilio, D. and Vargaftig, B.B. (1985). Platelet desensitization induced by arachidonic acid is not due to cyclo-oxygenase inactivation and involves the endoperoxide receptor. *Br. J. Pharmacol.*, **85**, 849–859

86. Claesson, H.E. and Malmsten, C. (1977). On the interrelationship of prostaglandin endoperoxide G₂ and cyclic nucleotides in platelet function. *Eur. J. Biochem.*, **76**, 277–284

87. Miller, O.V., Johnson, R.A. and Gorman, R.R. (1977). Inhibition of PGE₁-stimulated cAMP accumulation in human platelets by thromboxane A₂. *Prostaglandins*, **13**, 599–609

88. Miller, O.V. and Gorman, R.R. (1976). Modulation of platelet cyclic nucleotide content by PGE₁ and the prostaglandin endoperoxide PGG₂. *J. Cyclic Nucleotide Res.*, **2**, 79–87

89. Gorman, R.R., Wierenga, W. and Miller, O.V. (1979). Independence of the cyclic AMP-lowering activity of thromboxane A₂ from the platelet release reaction. *Biochim. Biophys. Acta*, **572**, 95–104

90. Rybicki, J.P. and LeBreton, G.C. (1983). Prostaglandin H₂ directly lowers human platelet cAMP levels. *Thrombosis Res.*, **30**, 407–414

91. Best, L.C., McGuire, M.B., Martin, T.J., Preston, F.E. and Russell, R.G.G. (1979). Effects of epoxymethano analogues of prostaglandin endoperoxides on aggregation, on release of 5-hydroxytryptamine and on the metabolism of 3',5'-cyclic AMP and cyclic GMP in human platelets. *Biochim. Biophys. Acta*, **583**, 344–351

92. Gerrard, J.M., White, J.G. and Peterson, D.A. (1978). The platelet dense tubular system: Its relationship to prostaglandin synthesis and calcium flux. *Thromb. Haemost.*, **40**, 224–231

93. Owen, N.E. and LeBreton, G.C. (1981). Ca^{2+} mobilization in blood platelets as visualized by chlortetracycline fluorescence. *Am. J. Physiol.*, **241**, H613–H619

94. Rybicki, J.P., Venton, D.L. and LeBreton, G.C. (1983). The thromboxane antagonist, 13-azaprostanoic acid, inhibits arachidonic acid-induced Ca^{2+} release from isolated platelet membrane vesicles. *Biochim. Biophys. Acta*, **751**, 66–73

95. Kawahara, Y., Yamanishi, J., Furuta, Y., Kaibuchi, K., Takai, Y. and Fukuzaki, H. (1983). Elevation of cytoplasmic free calcium concentration by stable thromboxane A_2 analogue in human platelets. *Biochem. Biophys. Res. Commun.*, **117**, 663–669

96. Broekman, M.J. (1984). Phosphatidylinositol 4,5-bisphosphate may represent the site of release of plasma membrane-bound calcium upon stimulation of human platelets. *Biochem. Biophys. Res. Commun.*, **120**, 226–231

97. Berridge, M.J. and Irvine, R.I. (1984). Inositol trisphosphate, a novel second messenger in cellular signal transduction. *Nature (London)*, **312**, 315–321

98. Sekar, M. and Hokin, L. (1986). The role of phosphoinositides in signal transduction. *J. Memb. Biol.*, **89**, 193–210

99. Authi, K., Evenden, B. and Crawford, N. (1986). Metabolic and functional consequences of introducing inositol 1,4,5-triphosphate into saponin-permeabilized human platelets. *Biochem. J.*, **233**, 709–718

100. Rink, T.J. and Hallam, J.T. (1984). What turns platelets on? *Trends Biochem. Sci. Pers. Ed.*, **9**, 215–219

101. Pollock, W.K., Armstrong, R.A., Brydon, L.J., Jones, J.L. and MacIntyre, D.E. (1984). Thromboxane induced phosphatidate formation in human platelets. *Biochem. J.*, **219**, 833–842

102. Watson, S.P. and Lapetina, E.G. (1985). 1,2-Diacylglycerol and phorbol ester inhibit agonist-induced formation of inositol phosphates in human platelets: Possible implications for negative feedback regulation of inositol phospholipid hydrolysis. *Proc. Natl. Acad. Sci. USA*, **82**, 2623–2626

103. Rittenhouse, S.E. (1984). Activation of human platelet phospholipase C by ionophore A23187 is totally dependent upon cyclo-oxygenase products and ADP. *Biochem. J.*, **222**, 103–110

104. Siess, W., Boehlig, B., Weber, P.C. and Lapetina, E.G. (1985). Prostaglandin endoperoxide analogues stimulate phospholipase C and protein phosphorylation during platelet shape change. *Blood*, **65**, 1141–1148

105. Ishii, H., Connolly, T., Bross, T. and Majerus, P. (1986). Inositol cyclic trisphosphate [inositol 1,2-(cyclic-4,5-trisphosphate] is formed upon thrombin stimulation of human platelets. *Proc. Natl. Acad. Sci. USA*, **83**, 6397–6401

106. Gerrard, J.M. and Carroll, R.C. (1981). Stimulation of platelet protein phosphorylation by arachidonic acid and endoperoxide analogs. *Prostaglandins*, **22**, 81–94

107. Siess, W., Siegel, F.L. and Lapetina, E.G. (1983). Arachidonic acid stimulates the formation of 1,2-diacylglycerol and phosphatidic acid in human platelets. *J. Biol. Chem.*, **258**, 11236–11242

108. Daniel, J.L., Holmsen, H. and Adelstein, R.S. (1977). Thrombin-stimulated myosin phosphorylation in intact platelets and its possible involvement secretion. *Thromb. Haemost.*, **38**, 984–989

109. Holmsen, H., Daniel, J.L., Dangelmaier, C.A., Molish, I., Rigmaiden, M. and Smith, J.B. (1984). Differential effects of trifluoperazine on arachidonate liberation, secretion and myosin phosphorylation in intact platelets. *Thrombosis Res.*, **36**, 419–428

110. Connolly, T., Laiving, W. and Majerus, P. (1986). Protein kinase C phosphorylates human platelet inositol trisphosphate 5'-phosphomonesterase increasing the phosphatase activity. *Cell*, **46**, 951–958

111. Litosch, I. and Fain, J. (1986). Regulation of phosphoinositide breakdown by guanine nucleotides. *Life Sci.*, **39**, 187–194

112. Houslay, M., Bojanic, D. and Wilson, A. (1986). Platelet activating factor and U44069 stimulate a GTPase activity in human platelets which is distinct from the qaunine nucleotide regulatory proteins, Ns and Ni. *Biochem. J.*, **234**, 737–740

113. Greenberg, S. (1981). Effect of prostacyclin and 9α,11α-epoxymethanoprostaglandin H$_2$ on calcium and magnesium fluxes and tension development in canine intralobar pulmonary arteries and veins. *J. Pharmacol. Exp. Ther.*, **219**, 326–337

114. Loutzenhiser, R. and van Breemen, C. (1981). Mechanism of activation of isolated rabbit aorta by PGH$_2$ analogue U-44069. *Am. J. Physiol.*, **241**, C243–C249

115. McNamara, D.B., Roulet, M.J., Gruetter, C.A., Hyman, A.L. and Kodowitz, P.J. (1980). Correlation of prostaglandin-induced mitochondrial calcium release with contraction in bovine intrapulmonary vein. *Prostaglandins*, **20**, 311–320

116. Somlyo, A., Bond, M., Somlyo, A. and Scarpa, A. (1985). Inositol trisphosphate-induced calcium release and contraction in vascular smooth muscle. *Proc. Natl. Acad. Sci. USA*, **82**, 5231–5235

117. Mais, D., Knapp, D., Ballard, K., Hamanaka, N. and Halushka, P. (1984). Synthesis of thromboxane receptor antagonists with the potential to radiolabel with ^{125}I. *Tetrahedron Lett.*, **25**, 4207–4208

118. Saussy, D., Mais, D., Burch, R. and Halushka, P. (1985). Identification of a putative TxA$_2$/PGH$_2$ receptor in human platelet membranes. *J. Biol. Chem.*, **261**, 3025–3029

119. Dorn, G., Burch, R.M., Kochel, P., Mais, D.E. and Halushka, P.V. (1985). Alteration of platelet thromboxane A$_2$/prostaglandin H$_2$ receptors by supernatant of platelet homogenates. *Biochem. Pharmacol.*, **36**, 1913–1917

120. Kattelman, E., Venton, D. and LeBreton, G. (1986). Characterization of U46619 binding in unactivated, intact human platelets and determination of binding site affinities of four TxA$_2$/PGH$_2$ receptor antagonists (13-APA, BM 13.177, ONO 3708 and SQ 29,548) *Thrombosis Res.*, **41**, 471–481

121. Burch, R., Mais, D.E., Saussy, D.L. and Halushka, P.V. (1985). Solubilization of a thromboxane A$_2$/prostaglandin H$_2$ antagonists binding site from human platelets. *Proc. Natl. Acad. Sci. USA*, **82**, 7434–7438

122. Burch, R., Mais, D., Pepkowitz, S. and Halushka, P. (1985). Hydrodynamic properties of a thromboxane A$_2$/prostaglandin H$_2$ antagonist binding site solubilized from human platelets. *Biochem. Biophys. Res. Commun.*, **132**, 961–968

123. Mais, D., Burch, R., Oatis, J., Knapp, D. and Halushka, P. (1986). Photoaffinity labelling of a thromboxane A$_2$/prostaglandin H$_2$ antagonist binding site in human platelets. *Biochem. Biophys. Res. Commun.*, **140**, 128–133

10
Mechanisms of action of prostaglandin E_2 and prostaglandin $F_{2\alpha}$: PGE and PGF_α receptors

W. L. Smith, W. K. Sonnenburg, T. Watanabe and K. Umegaki

INTRODUCTION

Prostaglandins are autocoids which normally function near their sites of synthesis to co-ordinate net biological responses among different neighbouring cell types. Responses to PGE_2 and $PGF_{2\alpha}$, the major prostanoids of the E and F_α series of prostaglandins, are mediated by PGE and PGF_α receptors. PGE and PGF_α receptors are membrane-bound proteins which interact specifically with PGE_2 or $PGF_{2\alpha}$, respectively, and, when occupied with ligand, elicit cascades of biochemical events which, in turn, lead to generalized physiological responses, such as luteolysis, contraction or relaxation of smooth muscle, inhibition of water or solute transport and inhibition of lipolysis. In this chapter, we develop the thesis that agonist-occupied prostaglandin receptors interact with specific guanine nucleotide regulatory (N) proteins to cause changes in the concentrations of cAMP, inositol trisphosphate, Ca^{2+} or perhaps other intracellular second messengers. There appear to be at least three different types of PGE receptors interactive with different types of N proteins (N_s, N_i, N_p) and perhaps having different ligand binding properties. In contrast, PGF_α receptors may act only through N_p-like proteins.

The E series and F_α series prostaglandins were the first eicosanoids to be characterized chemically[1] and research in the prostaglandin area focused on these compounds until the mid 1970s. It was then that thromboxane A_2 and prostacyclin (PGI_2) were discovered as relatively labile products of the arachidonate cascade in human platelets[2] and bovine aorta[3,4], respectively.

With the discovery of TxA_2 and PGI_2 and, more recently, the identification of lipoxygenase products[5,6], the earlier general interest in PGE and PGF_α has subsided. Contributing to this shift in emphasis has been a combined confidence in the biological importance of TxA_2 and PGI_2 in haemostasis[7-10] and an uneasiness about the more general significance of PGE and PGF_α. This

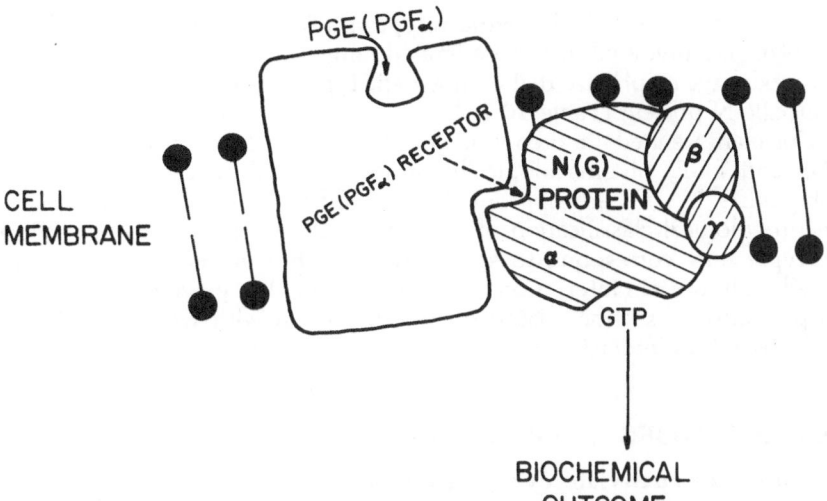

Figure 10.1 Biochemical mechanism of action of PGE and PGF$_\alpha$ receptors. PGE and PGF$_\alpha$ are envisaged as interacting with receptors coupled to guanine nucleotide regulatory (N) proteins. Interactions of an agonist-occupied receptor with a trimeric N protein in the presence of GTP causes dissociation of the N protein into α and $\beta\gamma$ subunits. The results depend on the specific effects of the α and $\beta\gamma$ subunits in the target cell

concern arose from the finding that, unlike PGI$_2$ and TxA$_2$, both PGE and PGF$_\alpha$ can be formed non-enzymically at substantial rates from prostaglandin endoperoxides[11,12]. Moreoever, attempts to demonstrate enzymic synthesis of PGE or PGF$_\alpha$ have not provided simple results[13–16]. Nonetheless, it is clear that there are biological effects for which PGE and PGF$_\alpha$ are uniquely responsible, and there are membrane-bound protein receptors for each of these prostanoids which bind specifically and with high affinity[17,18].

PGE receptors are defined empirically on the basis of binding specificity, the order of potency being PGE$_2$ $\geqslant$ PGE$_1$ > other prostanoids[17,18]. We emphasize the approximate equivalence of PGE$_2$ and PGE$_1$ in this definition because PGE$_1$ can also operate through other receptors[19–21], perhaps PGI$_2$ receptors[20,21], which do not efficiently bind or mediate effects of PGE$_2$. The existence of a PGF$_\alpha$ specific receptor or response requires that the order of potency of prostaglandins for binding the receptor or producing the response is PGF$_{2\alpha}$ > other prostanoids[22].

It should be kept in mind that there is very little information available on any of the prostanoid receptors. To fill in major gaps, we will draw substantially on precedents from the more extensive literature on adrenergic and muscarinic receptors. The theme we wish to develop is that PGE and PGF$_\alpha$ receptors mediate their effects through their abilities to interact with specific guanine nucleotide regulatory (N) proteins to elicit changes in the levels of second messengers such as cAMP, Ca^{2+} and inositol phosphates and perhaps cGMP (Figure 10.1). There appear to be at least three general types of PGE receptors which behave in a manner formally analogous to

α_1-[23,24], α_2-[25-28], and β-adrenergic receptors (Table 10.1); in contrast, PGF$_\alpha$ receptors are involved in a more limited range of events. In accordance with our model, we emphasize that each generic type of receptor functions through a specific N protein (Table 10.1)[29].

Coleman, Kennedy and co-workers have classified the myogenic effects of PGE and PGF$_\alpha$ pharmacologically using a limited series of agonists and antagonists[30-32]. Where appropriate, we address the possibility that their pharmacological classification of PGE and PGF$_\alpha$ receptors into EP$_1$, EP$_2$ and FP types may correspond to some degree with a biochemical classification based on N protein interactions. For purposes of clarity, we have divided the chapter into subsections based on the N protein with which the PGE and PGF$_\alpha$ receptors interact.

PGE RECEPTORS ASSOCIATED WITH N$_i$

Inhibition of adenylate cyclase by PGE

One of the earliest effects found for PGE$_1$ was its ability to inhibit epinephrine-induced lipolysis in adipocytes[33] by preventing the accumulation of cAMP[34]. The ability of PGE$_1$ to blunt isoproterenol-induced increases in cAMP in hamster adipocytes was subsequently shown to be reduced in hamsters that had been treated with a crude source of pertussis toxin[35]. More recently, Murayama and Ui demonstrated that pertussis toxin treatment of adipocytes also diminishes the ability of PGE$_1$ to cause a GTP-dependent inhibition of adenylate cyclase activity in membranes prepared from these cells[36]; associated with this latter effect is a pertussis toxin-dependent, ADP-ribosylation of a protein subunit having the characteristic size ($M_r = 41\,000$) of the α_i subunit of the inhibitory guanine nucleotide regulatory protein N$_i$.

Table 10.1 Classification of PGE and PGF$_\alpha$ receptors based on interactions with guanine nucleotide regulatory (N) proteins

Receptor Type	Function	Examples	Adrenergic Analogy
PGE-N$_s$	Stimulation of adenylate cyclase via increased [α_s]	Thyroid gland[62] Kidney-collecting tubule[54] Hepatocyte[70] Frog erythrocyte[61]	β
PGE-N$_i$	Inhibition of adenylate cyclase via increased [α_i] and [$\beta\gamma$]	Adipocyte[46] Kidney-thick limb[48]	α_2
PGE-N$_p$	Stimulation of Ca^{2+} mobilization, thereby potentiating Ca^{2+}-dependent events	Kidney-collecting tubule[49] Vascular smooth muscle[32]	α_1
PGF$_\alpha$-N$_p$	Stimulation of Ca^{2+} mobilization, thereby potentiating Ca^{2+}-dependent events	Kidney-collecting tubule[102] Vascular smooth muscle[32] Corpus luteum[22]	α_1

Other instances in which inhibitory effects of PGE have been shown to be attenuated by pertussis toxin are in the cases of calcitonin-induced cAMP formation in the T 47 D human breast-cancer cell line[37], PGE$_1$-induced cAMP formation in NG108-15 neuroblastoma × glioma hybrids[38] and insulin release by β-pancreatic cells[17].

The basis for the inhibitory effects of PGE in adipocytes, T 47 D, NG108-15 and islet cells have yet to be explored at the molecular level. However, these effects induced by PGE have characteristics in common with responses mediated by inhibitory receptors known to be coupled functionally to N$_i$. These include adenosine (A$_1$)[35,36,39], somatostatin[40,41], muscarinic cholinergic[38,42,43], dopaminergic (D$_2$)[44], γ-aminobutyric acid (GABA)$_B$[45] and α_2-adrenergic receptors[25-28]. Characteristic responses seen in cell systems in which hormones act via N$_i$ are: (a) that the cAMP elevating effect of forskolin is blocked[26,40]; and (b) that the inhibitory effect is prevented by treatment with pertussis toxin in the presence of NAD[26,28,38,40,44,45]. Inhibition of adenylate cyclase occurs as a result of hormone-induced dissociation of N$_i$ into α_i and $\beta\gamma$ subunits[41]. Increases in the concentration of the $\beta\gamma$ subunit lead to formation of the $\alpha_s\beta\gamma$ (i.e. N$_s$) trimer, thereby decreasing the concentration of free α_s; this, in turn, decreases adenylate cyclase activity. In addition, the α_i formed by dissociation of N$_i$ may exert a direct inhibitory effect on the cyclase catalytic subunit[41].

Association of PGE receptors with N$_i$

PGE binds to hamster adipocyte membranes through a high-affinity site[46] which is probably the receptor mediating inhibition of lipolysis[47]. Grandt et al.[46] were the first to note that GTP and, to a lesser extent, GppNHp and GDP have the unusual effect of enhancing PGE binding in this system; GTP decreases the K_D for PGE binding about 3-fold by increasing the rate constant for association of PGE with the receptor.

Another PGE binding activity which is stimulated by guanine nucleotide derivatives is present in membranes from canine[48] and rabbit renal outer medulla (unpublished observation); PGE binding to adipocyte and outer medullary receptors is also similar with respect both to the stimulatory effects of monovalent cations and to the specificities with which prostaglandins bind. The stimulatory effect of GTP on PGE binding in the canine outer medulla is blocked by pretreating membranes with pertussis toxin plus NAD, but not cholera toxin plus NAD; in addition, pertussis toxin, but not cholera toxin, treatment blocks stimulation by PGE$_2$ of GTPase activity in outer medullary membranes[48]. Thus, the medullary PGE receptor, like the adipocyte receptor, is coupled functionally with a pertussis toxin sensitive-protein, which is most likely N$_i$. The outer medullary PGE binding activity resides in a glycoprotein ($M_r = 65\,000$) which can be solubilized in what appears to be a 1:1 non-covalent complex with N$_i$[48]. It is likely that the outer medullary PGE receptor mediates inhibition of hormone-induced cAMP formation in the thick ascending limb of Henle's loop[49].

There are no synthetic agonists or antagonists known to be specifically reactive with PGE receptors coupled to N$_i$.

PGE RECEPTORS COUPLED TO N_s

Activation of adenylate cyclase by prostaglandins

Prostanoids of the D, E, and I series can stimulate adenylate cyclase in whole cell and membrane preparations from a variety of sources[17,18]. As might be expected, the physiological outcome of cyclase stimulation varies markedly from cell to cell. In some instances, prostaglandins released by one cell type act on different, neighbouring cell types through a cAMP dependent process. In the vasculature, PGI_2 released by endothelial cells causes cAMP formation by both blood platelets[50] and underlying smooth muscle[51] causing inhibition of platelet activation and smooth muscle relaxation[52], respectively. PGE_2, acting via 'EP$_2$' PGE receptors, also causes smooth muscle relaxation[34], again presumably by stimulating cAMP synthesis.

PGE can stimulate or inhibit its own hormone-induced synthesis via an ability to stimulate cAMP production. In the canine renal collecting tubule there appear to be two PGE receptors[53,54]. One of these receptors is an 'inhibitory' receptor which modulates vasopressin-induced H_2O flow[55-58]. The other receptor is coupled to stimulation of adenylate cyclase activity. This latter receptor may be involved in inhibition of arachidonate release and feedback inhibition of hormone-induced PGE production[53]. Similarly, neutrophil activation (and PGE_2 synthesis) induced by f-met-leu-phe is under feedback inhibitory control by a PGE receptor apparently coupled to N_s[59]. The opposite situation occurs in the thyroid. In the thyroid, there are two phases to PGE synthesis. The second phase is cAMP dependent and PGE serves to augment its own synthesis by its ability to stimulate adenylate cyclase activity[60].

Association of PGE receptors with N_s

The concept that there are PGE receptors coupled directly to N_s is based largely on circumstantial evidence, including precedents from work with PGI_2-like receptors and data indicating that GTP affects PGE binding in systems in which PGE is known to simulate adenylate cyclase. Brunton et al.[19] were the first to demonstrate a correlation between PGE_1 binding and increases in cellular cAMP levels in a series of different cell types; however, in the cells examined in this study, PGE_1 bound with more than a one hundred-fold higher affinity than PGE_2, suggesting that binding probably occurred through a PGI_2-like receptor. Later, Lefkowitz and co-workers[61] showed, using frog erythrocyte membranes, that there is a parallel between the abilities of four different prostaglandins to diplace [^{3}H]PGE_1 and to activate adenylate cyclase; importantly, in the frog system, PGE_1 and PGE_2 are approximately equipotent, as expected for a specific PGE receptor. The concept that PGE receptors are coupled directly to N proteins is deduced from the findings that GTP affects PGE binding affinities in frog erythrocyte[61], thyroid[62], adipocyte[46] and kidney membranes[29,48]. That a prostaglandin receptor can be coupled specifically to N_s is deduced from studies on PGE_1-induced GTPase activity in human platelet membranes. Stimulation of GTPase by PGE_1 can be blocked by pretreatment of platelet membranes with cholera toxin plus NAD[63]; cholera toxin functions in most cells to cause the ADP-ribosylation of the α_s subunit of N$_s$[64], thereby causing selective inhibition of the GTPase activity of N$_s$.

While there is reasonable indirect evidence suggesting that PGE receptors function by interacting directly with N$_s$, no 'pharmacologically pure' PGE receptor demonstrably coupled to adenylate cyclase has been solubilized and characterized. Two PGE binding proteins which could well be stimulatory receptors coupled to N$_s$ have been solubilized from liver[65] and brain[66], respectively. The liver receptor was solubilized with Triton X-100 in the presence of PGE. The solubilized receptor is only stable in the presence of ligand. Hayaishi and co-workers have solubilized a PGE binding protein from porcine cerebral cortex with CHAPS[66]. These workers indicate that the solubilized brain receptor is unstable and has a relatively low specific activity, and, thus, may be an unsuitable starting material for purification. PGE binding to the brain receptor is inhibited by GTP[67].

PGE binding activities, probably corresponding to receptors operating via N$_s$ have been characterized in porcine fundic mucosa[68], beef thyroid[62], frog erthyrocytes[61] and rat liver[69–71]. As summarized by Robertson[17], high affinity ($K_D = 1–10\,\mathrm{nmol\,L^{-1}}$) and low affinity ($K_D = 10–100\,\mathrm{nmol\,L^{-1}}$) binding sites for PGE are present in these and several other tissues. In most cases, it is unclear whether the two binding activities correspond to GTP-dependent high- and low-affinity states of the same receptor or, instead, to functionally different receptor populations. Concentrations of the high-affinity receptor[17] are of the order of $0.1–1.0\,\mathrm{pmol\,L^{-1}}$ (mg of membrane protein)$^{-1}$. These specific activities are similar to those typically determined for adrenergic and muscarinic receptors.

Heterologous desensitization induced by PGE

There are adenylate cyclase activation systems involving several different types of hormones (e.g. glucagon, epinephrine, PGE) in which prolonged treatment of a target cell with the hormone leads to a generalized decrease in the ability of the cell to form cAMP, both in response to all stimulatory hormones and to agents such as cholera toxin, NaF and forskolin which act at the postreceptor step[72–77]. In addition, sensitivity to at least some 'inhibitory' agonists, probably functioning via N$_i$, is also reduced[78]. This type of desensitization is termed heterologous or agonist-non-specific desensitiz-ation[72], and is one of the mechanisms through which a cell protects itself from overexposure to stimulatory agonists. Heterologous desensitization requires a longer exposure (several minutes to hours) than homologous or agonist-specific desensitization (seconds to minutes).

Heterologous desensitization of the adenylate cyclase system induced by exposure to PGE$_1$, *presumably* functioning via stimulatory PGE receptors coupled to N$_s$, was first observed in cultured human fibroblasts[74]. N$_s$-like stimulatory activity of fibroblasts was assayed by testing the ability of extracts of fibroblast membranes to reconstitute adenylate cyclase in N$_s$-deficient cyc^- membranes and was found to have been decreased by PGE$_1$ treatment[73]. There was, however, no corresponding change in N$_s$ as measured by the amount of cholera toxin ADP-ribosylation substrate present in membranes from control and PGE-treated fibroblasts. Heterologous desensitization caused by PGE$_1$ did not affect receptor binding or affinity.

PGE-dependent heterologous desensitization has also been shown to occur in rat liver[69]. Treatment of rats with 16,16-dimethyl PGE$_2$ caused a loss in the ability of rat liver membranes to synthesize cAMP when stimulated by glucagon, NaF or forskolin. This general loss of adenylate cyclase activity correlated with decreased levels of N$_s$ as measured both by reconstitution of cyclase stimulatory activity into the cyc^- membrane system and by the amount of cholera toxin substrate. Since 16,16-dimethyl PGE$_2$ appears to act via hepatic stimulatory PGE receptors[70,71], this derivative may act via this receptor to cause a decreased level of N$_s$ and perhaps also cyclase catalytic activity.

It should be noted that the biochemical events responsible for heterologous desensitization are incompletely defined and probably differ among different hormones and even among different cells treated with the same hormone[72,76,77]. One event which is common to heterologous desensitization is an initial increase in the levels of cAMP. In fact, in glioma cells, forskolin and dibutyryl cAMP can mimic the effects of hormones by desensitizing the adenylate cyclase to the stimulatory effects of both hormones and cholera toxin[76]. In contrast, in MDCK cells, heterologous desensitization induced by glucagon can be separated into hormonal and postreceptor (non-hormonal) components[77]; dibutyryl cAMP causes generalized decreases in the responses to stimulatory hormones, but does not affect responses to cholera toxin or forskolin. The fact that increases in cAMP can partially[77] or completely[76] mimic hormone-induced heterologous desensitization suggests that protein phosphorylations are involved. It has not been determined whether N$_s$ and/or the cyclase catalytic subunit are phosphorylated.

Homologous desensitization induced by PGE

Homologous desensitization of the adenylate cyclase system is equivalent to agonist-specific desensitization whereby the response to the stimulating agonist, but not to agonists operating through other receptors, is lost[72]. This type of desensitization has been studied extensively in the β-adrenergic system. Rapid modification of the receptor molecule occurs, rendering the receptor unable to efficiently stimulate adenylate cyclase[72,79,80]. Homologous desensitization of stimulatory receptors such as the β-adrenergic receptor or the PGE receptor apparently involves phosphorylation of occupied receptors by a soluble protein kinase[79,80]. Lefkowitz, Caron and co-workers have suggested that the kinase recognizes cytosolic domains on receptor proteins which are only exposed during agonist binding[80]. Receptor sequestration follows phosphorylation[72,79–81]; however, phosphorylation itself may increase the K_D values for stimulatory ligands and may, thus, be responsible for at least part of the initial desensitization[81]. It is not yet clear whether there is a common mechanism for homologous desensitization of all stimulatory receptors. Curiously, homologous desensitization of stimulatory vasopressin receptors is inhibited by pertussis toxin[82].

The phenomenon of 'down regulation', whereby there is a net loss of receptor sites, is formally equivalent to sequestration (internalization)[72]. There is recent indirect evidence for homologous desensitization of the stimulatory PGE receptor via a cAMP-independent protein phosphorylation step in the kin^- mutant of S49 lymphoma cells[80]. In addition, 'down regulation' of a PGE receptor, where there is a decrease in receptor number but no change in binding affinity, has been shown to occur in liver cells[69,70].

PGE RECEPTORS ASSOCIATED WITH N$_p$-LIKE PROTEINS

Receptors involved in Ca^{2+} mobilization and activation of cAMP phosphodiesterase

Accumulation of cAMP in 1321N1 astrocytoma cells is blocked by carbachol acting via an inhibitory muscarinic receptor[83]. Neither the inhibitory action of carbachol[84] nor the binding of carbachol to astrocytoma membranes[85] are affected by treating the cells with pertussis toxin, but carbachol binding is inhibited by GTP[85]. It is now clear that in 1321N1 cells there is an inhibitory muscarinic receptor coupled to an N protein, dubbed N$_p$[86] (with 'p' being the abbreviation for PIP phosphodiesterase) which differs from N$_i$ and N$_s$. N$_p$ (or N$_p$-like proteins) are thought to be present in most cells and to mediate effects of a variety of hormone receptors[86–88]. N$_p$ functions by activating a phosphodiesterase (phospholipase C) which catalyses the formation of 1,4,5-inositol trisphosphate (IP$_3$) from phosphatidylinositol bisphosphate (PIP$_2$)[87,88]. Inositol trisphosphate causes the mobilization of Ca^{2+} from the endoplasmic reticulum[88]. In 1321N1 astrocytoma cells, Ca^{2+} mobilization leads to activation of a Ca^{2+}-dependent cAMP phosphodiesterase[89], and this is likely to be the mechanism by which carbachol inhibits cAMP accumulation in these cells[89].

There may actually be several N$_p$-like proteins. For example, there is an N protein named N$_c$ (with 'c' being the abbreviation for 'chemotactic') which is involved in the mobilization of Ca^{2+} in neutrophils treated with f-met-leu-phe[90–92]. Unlike N$_p$[86], N$_c$ is readily ADP-ribosylated in reactions catalysed by both pertussis toxin or cholera toxin[92].

In astrocytoma cells, Ca^{2+} mobilization leads to activation of a Ca^{2+}-dependent cAMP phosphodiesterase preventing cAMP accumulation[83,86]. Adrenergic agents acting via α_1 receptors in myocytes appear to elicit an analogous activation of Ca^{2+}-dependent cAMP phosphodiesterase[24]; this latter process is also insensitive to pertussis toxin.

PGE receptors involved in Ca^{2+} mobilization

There are actually no data demonstrating that PGE, acting via a receptor coupled to N$_p$ or a functionally related N protein, can cause the turnover of membrane phosphoinositides and subsequent Ca^{2+} mobilization. However, there is circumstantial evidence which can be interpreted as suggesting that

239

there are PGE receptors coupled to N_p-like proteins in the renal collecting tubule[49] and in some types of smooth muscle containing 'EP$_1$' PGE receptors[30-32], and there are precedents for other prostanoid receptors being coupled to N_p[93,94].

As noted earlier, PGE can inhibit vasopressin-induced water flow in the renal collecting tubule[55-58]. Vasopressin appears to function by binding a stimulatory (V_2) receptor coupled to N_s which causes activation of adenylate cyclase[55,57,95]. PGE inhibits AVP-induced water flow in the collecting tubule apparently by inhibiting cAMP accumulation[55]. The mechanism for this inhibitory effect has been investigated extensively and is still incompletely resolved, but may involve activation of a cAMP phosphodiesterase[49]. By analogy to the muscarinic cholinergic receptor system in astrocytoma cells and the α_1 adrenergic receptor in myocytes, we speculate that the collecting tubule inhibitory PGE receptor is coupled to N_p.

PGE has been shown to elicit both smooth muscle relaxation and contraction acting through 'EP$_2$' and 'EP$_1$' PGE receptors, respectively[30-32]. As discussed above, smooth muscle relaxation caused by PGE is probably a result of PGE acting through a stimulatory ('EP$_1$') receptor coupled to N_s to cause cAMP synthesis[51,52]. In contrast, it seems likely that PGE-induced contractions of smooth muscle[30-32], like those induced by PGF$_\alpha$[93], are elicited by PGE acting via a receptor coupled to N_p to cause Ca^{2+} mobilization. Accordingly, we would anticipate that AH6809, which is reportedly a selective 'EP$_1$' receptor antagonist[32], would block actions mediated by PGE receptors coupled to N_p.

Another example of a prostanoid receptor being coupled to an N_p-like protein occurs with a thromboxane A_2 receptor in platelet cells. Thromboxane A_2 can cause the turnover of inositol phosphates in platelets through a mechanism which is insensitive to pertussis toxin[94]; in addition, thromboxane A_2 functions in platelets to attenuate hormone-dependent cAMP formation by a process inhibited by pertussis toxin and probably involving N_i[96]. Presumably, there are separate platelet TxA$_2$ receptors coupled to N_p and N_i, but only one TxA$_2$-binding activity has been identified in platelets[97].

PGF$_\alpha$ RECEPTORS ASSOCIATED WITH N_p-LIKE PROTEINS

PGF$_{2\alpha}$ is known to act through PGF$_{2\alpha}$-specific processes to cause contraction of iris sphincter muscle in the dog and cat[30-32], involution of the corpus luteum in numerous farm and laboratory animals[98-100] and stimulation of growth in mouse fibroblasts[101]. PGF$_{2\alpha}$ can also cause other effects acting via PGE and thromboxane A_2/PGH receptors[18,30-32]. Importantly, PGF$_{2\alpha}$ rarely stimulates adenylate cyclase activity except in an occasional instance when it is tested at extremely high concentrations[61].

It is likely that PGF$_{2\alpha}$, like muscarinic cholinergic and α_1-adrenergic agonists[102], causes contraction of iris sphincter[30-32] by stimulating IP$_3$ formation and subsequent Ca^{2+} mobilization[93]. In this instance, we speculate that PGF$_{2\alpha}$ functions via a receptor coupled to an N_p-like guanine nucleotide regulatory protein. It is also attractive to speculate that PGF$_{2\alpha}$ operates through a receptor, although perhaps a PGE receptor coupled to N_p, in antagonizing

240

vasopressin-induced water flow in the renal collecting tubule[103]; however, as discussed earlier, the effect of mobilizing Ca^{2+} in the collecting tubule may be to activate a Ca^{2+}-dependent phosphodiesterase, which, in turn, leads to attenuation of cAMP accumulation induced by AVP.

The effect of PGF$_{2\alpha}$ which has been studied most extensively is its luteolytic effect[98–100]. PGF$_{2\alpha}$ acts principally on 'large' luteal cells to inhibit progesterone secretion[104]. The mechanism for this effect probably involves an initial stimulation of phosphatidylinositol bisphosphate hydrolysis and subsequent Ca^{2+} mobilization[105]; that is, an action through a receptor coupled to an N$_p$-like guanine nucleotide regulatory protein. Thus, the luteal PGF$_\alpha$ receptor is likely to be of the same type as that involved in stimulation of smooth muscle contraction. Coleman et al.[32] have actually suggested that the luteal and iris sphincter PGF$_{2\alpha}$ receptors are the same. Their reasoning is that there is a parallel between the potencies of a series of prostanoids to contract dog and cat iris sphincter preparations and their affinities for binding preparations of corpus luteum. There is, however, contradictory evidence summarized by MacIntyre[18], which suggests that there may be pharmacologically distinguishable subtypes of PGF$_{2\alpha}$ receptors in the corpus luteum and in smooth muscle.

The PGF$_\alpha$ receptor of ovine and bovine corpus luteum has been studied by Hammarstrom, Powell, Rao and their co-workers[22,106–110]. There is a clear parallel between the abilities of a large number of prostanoid structural analogues to cause luteolysis and to bind luteal membrane preparations[22,106]. Of the natural prostanoids tested, PGF$_{2\alpha}$ is the most potent in causing luteolysis and is bound most avidly by the luteal receptor. The luteal PGF$_\alpha$ receptor has been solubilized in the presence of ligand using Triton X-100[107]. The solubilized receptor is unstable in the absence of ligand. The molecular weight of the solubilized receptor is estimated to be 107 000. Although most of the receptor is associated with the plasma membrane[107], there may also be PGF$_{2\alpha}$ binding associated with intracellular membranes[108–110].

The nature of the PGF$_{2\alpha}$ receptor involved in stimulating mitogenesis in mouse 3T3 fibroblasts[101] has not been determined. However, it is quite conceivable that, like certain other growth factors[111], PGF$_{2\alpha}$ action in 3T3 cells is mediated via a receptor coupled to an N$_p$-like guanine nucleotide regulatory protein.

ACKNOWLEDGEMENTS

This work was supported in part by National Institutes of Health Grants, AM22042 and AM36485, a Grant-in-Aid from the American Heart Association of Michigan, a National Institutes of Health Predoctoral Traineeship HL07404 (W.K.S.) and an Established Investigatorship from the American Heart Association (W.L.S.).

REFERENCES

1. Bergstrom, S., Ryhage, F., Samuelsson, B. and Sjovall, J. (1963). Prostaglandins and related factors: The structures of prostaglandin E$_1$, F$_{1\alpha}$ and F$_{1\beta}$. *J. Biol. Chem.*, **238**, 3555–3564

2. Hamberg, M., Svensson, J. and Samuelsson, B. (1975). Thromboxanes: A new group of biologically active compounds derived from prostaglandin endoperoxides. *Proc. Natl. Acad. Sci. USA*, **72**, 2994–2998
3. Bunting, S., Gryglewski, R., Moncada, S. and Vane, J.R. (1976). Arterial walls generate from prostaglandin endoperoxides a substance (prostaglandin X) which relaxes strips of mesenteric and coeliac arteries and inhibits platelet aggregation. *Prostaglandins*, **12**, 897–913
4. Johnson, R.A., Morton, D.R., Kinner, J.H., Gorman, R.R., McGuire, J.C., Sun, F.F., Whittaker, N., Bunting, S., Salmon, J., Moncada, S. and Vane, J.R. (1976). The chemical structure of prostaglandin X (prostacyclin). *Prostaglandins*, **12**, 915–927
5. Murphy, R.C., Hammarstrom, S. and Samuelsson, B. (1979). Leukotriene C: A slow reacting substance from murine mastocytoma cells. *Proc. Natl. Acad. Sci. USA*, **76**, 4275–4279
6. Jakschik, B.A., Kuo, C.G. and Wei, Y.F. (1985). Enzymatic formation of leukotrienes. In Lands, W.E.M. (ed.) *Biochemistry of Arachidonic Acid Metabolism*, pp. 51–75. (Boston: Martinus Nijhoff Publishing)
7. Smith, W.L. (1986). Prostaglandin biosynthesis and its compartmentation in vascular smooth muscle and endothelial cells. *Annu. Rev. Physiol.*, **48**, 251–262
8. Fitzgerald, G., Smith, B., Pedersen, A.K. and Brash A. (1984). Increased prostacyclin biosynthesis in patients with severe atherosclerosis and platelet activation. *N. Engl. J. Med.*, **310**, 1065–1068
9. Catella, F., Healy, D., Lawson, J.A. and Fitzgerald, G.A. (1986). 11-Dehydrothromboxane B$_2$: A quantitative index of thromboxane A$_2$ formation in the human circulation. *Proc. Natl. Acad. Sci. USA*, **83**, 5861–5865
10. Weksler, B.B. (1987). Regulation of cyclooxygenase activity in human vascular tissue. In Samuelsson, B., Paoletti, R. and Ramwell, P.W. (eds.) *Advances in Prostaglandin, Thromboxane and Leukotriene Research*, Vol. 17A, pp. 238–43. (New York: Raven Press)
11. Hamberg, M. and Samuelsson, B. (1973). Detection and isolation of an endoperoxide intermediate in prostaglandin biosynthesis. *Proc. Natl. Acad. Sci. USA*, **70**, 899–903
12. Nugteren, D.H. and Hazelhof, E. (1973). Isolation and properties of intermediates in prostaglandin biosynthesis. *Biochim. Biophys. Acta*, **326**, 448–461
13. Pace-Asciak, C. and Smith, W.L. (1983). Enzymes in the biosynthesis and catabolism of the eicosanoids: prostaglandins, thromboxanes, leukotrienes, and hydroxy fatty acids. In Boyer, P.D. (ed.) *The Enzymes*, Vol. 16. pp. 544–604. (New York: Academic Press)
14. Wlodawer, P., Kindahl, H. and Hamberg, M. (1976). Biosynthesis of prostaglandin F$_{2\alpha}$ from arachidonic acid and prostaglandin endoperoxides in the uterus. *Biochim. Biophys. Acta*, **431**, 603–614
15. Watanabe, K., Iguchi, Y., Iguchi, S., Arai, Y., Hayaishi, O. and Roberts, L.J. II. (1987). Stereospecific conversion of prostaglandin D$_2$ to 9α, 11β-prostaglandin F$_2$ and prostaglandin H$_2$ to prostaglandin F$_{2\alpha}$ by PGF synthase. In Samuelsson, B., Paoletti, R. and Ramwell, P. (eds.) *Advances in Prostaglandin, Thromboxane and Leukotriene Research*, Vol. 17A, pp. 44–6. (New York: Raven Press)
16. Tanaka, Y., Ward, S.L. and Smith, W.L. (1987). Immunochemical and kinetic evidence for two different PGH-PGE isomerases in sheep vesicular gland microsomes. *J. Biol. Chem.*, **262**, 1374–81
17. Robertson, R.P. (1986). Characterization and regulation of prostaglandin and leukotriene receptors: An overview. *Prostaglandins*, **31**, 395–411
18. MacIntyre, D.E. (1986). Prostanoid receptors. In Lands, W.E.M. (ed.) *Biochemistry of Arachidonic Acid Metabolism*, pp. 243–267. (Boston: Martinus Nijhoff Publishing)
19. Brunton, L.L., Wiklund, R.A., VanArsdale, P.M. and Gilman, A.G. (1976). Binding of [³H]prostaglandin E$_1$ to putative receptors linked to adenylate cyclase of cultured cell clones. *J. Biol. Chem.*, **251**, 3037–3044
20. Schillinger, E. and Prior, G. (1980). Prostaglandin I$_2$ receptor in a particulate fraction of platelets of various species. *Biochem. Pharmacol.*, **29**, 2297–2299
21. Shafer, A.I., Cooper, B., O'Hara, D. and Handin, R.I. (1979). Identification of platelet receptors for prostaglandin I$_2$ and D$_2$. *J. Biol. Chem.*, **254**, 2914–2917
22. Hammarstrom, S. (1982). A receptor for prostaglandin F$_{2\alpha}$ from corpora lutea. *Meth. Enz.*, **86**, 202–209

23. Lomasney, J.W., Leeb-Lundberg, L.M., Cotecchia, S., Regan, J.W., DeBernardis, J.F., Caron, M.G. and Lefkowitz, R.J. (1986). Mammalian α_1-adrenergic receptor. Purification and characterization of the native receptor ligand binding subunit. *J. Biol. Chem.*, **261**, 7710–7716

24. Buxton, I.L.O. and Brunton, L.L. (1985). Action of the cardiac α_1-adrenergic receptor. Activation of cyclic AMP degradation. *J. Biol. Chem.*, **260**, 6733–6737

25. Regan, J.W., Nakata, H., DeMarinis, R.M., Caron, M.G. and Lefkowitz, R.J. (1986). Purification and characterization of the human platelet α_2-adrenergic receptor. *J. Biol. Chem.*, **261**, 3894–3900

26. Katada, T., Bokoch, G.M., Northup, J.K., Ui, M. and Gilman, A.G. (1984). The inhibitory guanine nucelotide-binding regulatory component of adenylate cyclase: Properties and function of the purified protein. *J. Biol. Chem.*, **259**, 3568–3577

27. Cerione, R.A., Regan, J.W., Nakata, H., Codina, J., Benovic, J.L., Gierschik, P., Somers, R.L., Spiegel, A.M., Birnbaumer, L., Lefkowitz, R.J. and Caron, M.G. (1986). Functional reconstitution of the α_2-adrenergic receptor with guanine nucleotide regulatory proteins in phospholipid vesicles. *J. Biol. Chem.*, **261**, 3901–3909

28. Nomura, Y., Kitamura, Y. and Segawa, T. (1985). Decrease of clonidine binding affinity to α_2-adrenoceptor by ADP-ribosylation of 41,000-dalton proteins in rat cerebral cortical membranes by islet-activating protein. *J. Neurochem.*, **44**, 364–369

29. Smith, W.L., Watanabe, T., Umegaki, K. and Sonnenburg, W.K. (1987). A general biochemical mechanism for prostaglandin actions: direct coupling of prostanoid receptors to guanine nucleotide regulatory proteins. In Samuelsson, B., Paoletti, R. and Ramwell, P. (eds.) *Advances in Prostaglandin, Thromboxane and Leukotriene Research*, Vol. 17A, pp. 463–6. (New York: Raven Press)

30. Kennedy, I., Coleman, R.A., Humphrey, P.P.A. and Lumley, P. (1982). Studies on the characterization of prostanoid receptors: A proposed classification. *Prostaglandins*, **24**, 667–688

31. Coleman, R.A. and Kennedy, I. (1985). Characterization of the prostanoid receptors mediating contraction of guinea pig isolated trachea. *Prostaglandins*, **29**, 363–375

32. Coleman, R.A., Humphrey, P.P.A. and Kennedy, I. (1985). Prostanoid receptors in smooth muscle: further evidence for a proposed classification. In Kalsner, S. (ed.) *Trends in Autonomic Pharmacology*, Vol. 3, pp. 35–49. (London: Taylor and Francis)

33. Steinberg, D., Vaughan, M., Nestel, P.J., Strand, O. and Bergstrom, S. (1963). Effects of prostaglandins on hormone-induced mobilization of free fatty acids. *J. Clin. Invest.*, **43**, 1533–1540

34. Butcher, R.W. and Baird, C.E. (1968). Effects of prostaglandins on adenosine 3′,5′-monophosphate levels in fat and other tissues. *J. Biol. Chem.*, **243**, 1713–1717

35. Garcia-Sainz, J.A. (1981). Decreased sensitivity to α_2 adrenergic amines, adenosine and prostaglandins in white fat cells from hamsters treated with pertussis toxin. *FEBS Lett.*, **126**, 306–308

36. Murayama, T. and Ui, M. (1983). Loss of the inhibitory function of the guanine nucleotide regulatory component of adenylate cyclase due to its ADP ribosylation by islet-activating protein, pertussis toxin, in adipocyte membranes. *J. Biol. Chem.*, **258**, 3319–3326

37. Michelangeli, V.P., Livesey, S.A. and Martin, T.J. (1984). Effects of pertussis toxin on adenylate cyclase responses to prostaglandin E$_2$ and calcitonin in human breast cancer cells. *Biochem. J.*, **224**, 371–377

38. Kurose, H., Katada, T., Amano, T. and Ui, M. (1983). Specific uncoupling by islet-activating protein, pertussis toxin, of negative signal transduction via α-adrenergic, cholinergic, and opiate receptors in neuroblastoma × glioma hybrid cells. *J. Biol. Chem.*, **258**, 4870–4875

39. Stiles, G.L. (1985). The A$_1$ adenosine receptor: solubilization and characterization of a guanine nucleotide-sensitive form of the receptor. *J. Biol. Chem.*, **260**, 6728–6732

40. Reisine, T.D., Zhang, Y.-L. and Sekura, R. (1983). Pertussis toxin blocks somatostatin's inhibition of stimulated cAMP accumulation in anterior pituitary tumor cells. *Biochem. Biophys. Res. Commun.*, **115**, 794–799

41. Katada, T., Bokoch, G.M., Smigel, M.D., Ui, M. and Gilman, A.B. (1984). The inhibitory guanine nucleotide-binding regulatory component of adenylate cyclase: Subunit dissociation and the inhibition of adenylate cyclase in S49 lymphoma cyc^- and wild type membranes. *J. Biol. Chem.*, **259**, 3586–3595

243

42. Florio, V.A. and Sternweis, P.C. (1985). Reconstitution of resolved muscarinic cholinergic receptors with purified GTP-binding proteins. *J. Biol. Chem.*, **260**, 3477–3483
43. Kurose, H., Katada, T., Haga, K., Ichiyama, A. and Ui, M. (1986). Functional interaction of purified muscarinic receptors with purified inhibitory guanine nucleotide regulatory proteins reconstituted in phospholipid vesicles. *J. Biol. Chem.*, **261**, 6423–6428
44. Cote, T.E., Frey, E.A. and Sekura, R.D. (1984). Altered activity of the inhibitory guanyl nucleotide-binding component (N_i) induced by pertussis toxin: Uncoupling of N_i to the catalytic unit. *J. Biol. Chem.*, **259**, 8693–8698
45. Asano, T., Ui, M. and Ogasawara, N. (1985). Prevention of the agonist binding to γ-aminobutyric acid B receptors by guanine nucleotides and islet-activating protein, pertussis, toxin, in bovine cerebral cortex: Possible coupling of the toxin-sensitive GTP-binding proteins to receptors. *J. Biol. Chem.*, **260**, 12653–12658
46. Grandt, R., Aktories, K. and Jakobs, K.H. (1982). Guanine nucleotides and monovalent cations increase agonist affinity of prostaglandin E_2 receptors in hamster adipocytes. *Mol. Pharmacol.*, **22**, 320–326
47. Aktories, K., Schultz, G. and Jacobs, K.H. (1981). The hamster adipocyte adenylate cyclase system. II. Regulation of enzyme stimulation and inhibition by monovalent cations. *Biochim. Biophys. Acta*, **676**, 59–67
48. Watanabe, T., Umegaki, K. and Smith, W.L. (1986). Association of a solubilized prostaglandin E_2 receptor from renal medulla with a pertussis toxin-reactive guanine nucleotide regulatory protein. *J. Biol. Chem.*, **261**, 13430–9
49. Torikai, S. and Kurokawa, K. (1983). Effect of PGE_2 on vasopressin-dependent cell cAMP in isolated single nephron segments. *Am. J. Physiol.*, **245**, F58–F66
50. Gorman, R.R., Fitzpatrick, F.A. and Miller, O.V. (1978). Reciprocal regulation of human platelet cAMP levels by thromboxane A_2 and prostacyclin. In George, W.J. and Ignarro, L.J. (eds.) *Advances in Cyclic Nucleotide Research*, Vol. 9., pp. 597–609. (New York: Raven Press)
51. Miller, O.V., Aiken, J.W., Hemker, D.P., Shebuski, R.J. and Gorman, R.R. (1979). Prostacyclin stimulation of dog arterial cAMP levels. *Prostaglandins*, **18**, 915–925
52. Nakahata, N. and Suzuki, T. (1981). Effects of prostaglandin E_1, I_2 and isoproterenol on the tissue cyclic AMP content in longitudinal muscle of rabbit intestine. *Prostaglandins*, **22**, 159–165
53. Smith, W.L. and Garcia-Perez, A. (1985). A two receptor model for the mechanism of action of prostaglandins in the renal collecting tubule. In Bailey, J.M. (ed.) *Prostaglandins, Leukotrienes and Lipoxins*, pp. 35–45. (New York: Plenum)
54. Garcia-Perez, A. and Smith, W.L. (1984). Apical-basolateral asymmetry in canine cortical collecting tubule cells. Bradykinin, arginine vasopressin, prostaglandin E_2 interrelationships. *J. Clin. Invest.*, **74**, 63–74
55. Grantham, J.J. and Orloff, J. (1968). Effect of prostaglandin E_1 on the permeability response of the isolated collecting tubule to vasopressin, adenosine 3′,5′-monophosphate, and theophylline. *J. Clin. Invest.*, **47**, 1154–1161
56. Schuster, W.L., Kokko, J.P. and Jacobson, H.R. (1984). Interactions of lysyl-bradykinin and antidiuretic hormone in the rabbit collecting tubule. *J. Clin. Invest.*, **73**, 1659–1667
57. Nadler, S.P., Hebert, S.C. and Brenner, B.M. (1985). PGE_2, forskolin, and cholera toxin interactions in rabbit cortical collecting tubule. *Am. J. Physiol.*, **250**, F127–F135
58. Anderson, R.J., Berl, T., McDonald, K.M. and Schrier, R.W. (1975). Evidence for an in vivo antagonism between vasopressin and prostaglandin in the mammalian kidney. *J. Clin. Invest.*, **56**, 420–426
59. Takenawa, T., Ishitoya, J. and Nagai, Y. (1986). Inhibitory effect of prostaglandin E_2, forskolin, and dibutyryl cAMP on arachidonic acid release and inositol phospholipid metabolism in guinea pig neutrophils. *J. Biol. Chem.*, **261**, 1092–1098
60. Levasseur, S., Kostelec, M. and Burke, G. (1984). RHC 80267 inhibits thyrotropin-stimulated prostaglandin release from rat thyroid lobes. *Prostaglandins*, **27**, 673–682
61. Lefkowitz, R.J., Mullikin, D., Wood, C.L., Gore, T.B. and Mukherjee, C. (1977). Regulation of prostaglandin receptors by prostaglandins and guanine nucleotide in frog erythrocytes. *J. Biol. Chem.*, **252**, 5295–5303
62. Moore, W.V. and Wolff, J. (1973). Binding of prostaglandin E_1 to beef thyroid membranes. *J. Biol. Chem.*, **16**, 5705–5711

63. Lester, H.A., Steer, M.L. and Levitzki, A. (1982). Prostaglandin-stimulated GTP hydrolysis associated with activation of adenylate cyclase in human platelet membranes. *Proc. Natl. Acad. Sci. USA*, **79**, 719–723

64. Birnbaumer, L., Codina, J., Mattera, R., Sunyer, T., Rojas, F.J., Hildebrandt, J.D. and Iyengar, R. (1985). Structural basis of nucleotide regulation of receptor binding and transduction of hormone receptor occupancy into positive and negative regulation of cAMP formation: Roles of N proteins. In Cohen, P. and Houslay, M.D. (eds.) *Molecular Aspects of Cellular Regulation*, Vol. 4, pp. 131–182. (Amsterdam: Elsevier Scientific Publishing Company)

65. Smigel, M. and Fleischer, S. (1977). Characterization of Triton X-100-solubilized prostaglandin E binding protein of rat liver plasma membranes. *J. Biol. Chem.*, **252**, 3689–3696

66. Yumoto, N., Watanabe, Y., Watanabe, K. and Hayaishi, O. (1986). Solubilization and characterization of prostaglandin E₂ binding protein from porcine cerebral cortex. *J. Neurochem.*, **46**, 125–132

67. Yumoto, N., Hatanaka, M., Watanabe, Y. and Hayaishi, O. (1986). Involvement of GTP-regulatory protein in brain prostaglandin E₂ receptor and separation of the two components. *Biochem. Biophys. Res. Commun.*, **135**, 282–289

68. Tepperman, B.L. and Soper, B.D. (1981). Prostaglandin E₂-binding sites and cAMP production in porcine fundic mucosa. *Am. J. Physiol.*, **241**, G313–G320

69. Garrity, M.J., Andreasen, T.J., Storm, D.R. and Robertson, R.P. (1983). Prostaglandin E-induced heterologous desensitization of hepatic adenylate cyclase. *J. Biol. Chem.*, **258**, 8692–8697

70. Robertson, R.P., Westcott, K.R., Storm, D.R. and Rice, M.G. (1980). Down-regulation in vivo of PGE receptors and adenylate cyclase stimulation. *Am. J. Physiol.*, **239**, E75–E80

71. Garrity, M.J., Westcott, K.R., Eggerman, T.L., Andersen, N.H., Storm, D.R. and Robertson, R.P. (1983). Interrelationships between PGE₁ and PGI₂ binding and stimulation of adenylate cyclase. *Am. J. Physiol.*, **244**, E367–E372

72. Sibley, D.R. and Lefkowitz, R.J. (1985). Molecular mechanism of receptor desensitization using the β-adrenergic receptor-coupled adenylate cyclase system as a model. *Nature (London)*, **317**, 124–129

73. Clark, R.B. and Butcher, R.W. (1979). Desensitization of adenylate cyclase in cultured fibroblasts with prostaglandin E₁ and epinephrine. *J. Biol. Chem.*, **254**, 9373–9378

74. Kassis, S. and Fishman, P.H. (1982). Different mechanisms of desensitization of adenylate cyclase by isoproterenol and prostaglandin E₁ in human fibroblasts: Role of regulatory components in desensitization. *J. Biol. Chem.*, **257**, 5312–5318

75. Noda, C., Shinjyo, F., Tomomura, A., Kato, S., Nakamura, T. and Ichihara, A. (1984). Mechanism of heterologous desensitization of the adenylate cyclase system by glucagon in primary cultures of adult rat hepatocytes. *J. Biol. Chem.*, **259**, 7747–7754

76. Terasaki, W.l., Brooker, G., deVellis, J., Inglish, D., Hsu, C.Y. and Moylan, R.D. (1978). Involvement of cyclic AMP and protein synthesis in catecholamine refractoriness. *Adv. Cyclic Nucleotide Res.*, **9**, 33–52

77. Rich, K.A., Codina, J., Floyd, G., Sekura, R., Hildebrandt, J.D. and Iyengar, R. (1984). Glucagon induced heterologous desensitization of the MDCK cell adenylyl cyclase: Increases in the apparent levels of the inhibitory regulator. (Nᵢ). *J. Biol. Chem.*, **259**, 7893–7901

78. Hsia, J.A., Hewlett, E.L. and Moss, J. (1985). Heterologous desensitization of adenylate cyclase with prostaglandin E₁ alters sensitivity to inhibitory as well as stimulatory agonists. *J. Biol. Chem.*, **260**, 4922–4926

79. Benovic, J., Strasser, R.H., Caron, M.G. and Lefkowitz, R.J. (1986). β-Adrenergic receptor kinase: Identification of a novel protein kinase that phosphorylates the agonist-occupied form of the receptor. *Proc. Natl. Acad. Sci. USA*, **83**, 2797–2801

80. Strasser, R.H., Benovic, J.L., Caron, M.G. and Lefkowitz, R.J. (1986). β-agonist- and prostaglandin E₁-induced translocation of the β-adrenergic receptor kinase: Evidence that the kinase may act on multiple adenylate cyclase-coupled receptors. *Proc. Natl. Acad. Sci. USA*, **83**, 6362–6366

81. Kassis, S., Olasmaa, M., Sullivan, M. and Fishman, P.H. (1986). Desensitization of the β-adrenergic receptor-coupled adenylate cyclase in cultured mammalian cells: Receptor sequestration versus receptor function. *J. Biol. Chem.*, **261**, 12233–12237

82. Wilson, P.D., Dixon, B.S., Dillingham, M.A., Garcia-Sainz, J.A. and Anderson, R.J. (1986). Pertussis toxin prevents homologous desensitization of adenylate cyclase in cultured renal epithelial cells. *J. Biol. Chem.*, **261**, 1503–1506

83. Meeker, R.B. and Harden, T.K. (1983). Muscarinic cholinergic receptor-mediated control of cyclic AMP metabolism: agonist-induced changes in nucleotide synthesis and degradation. *Mol. Pharmacol.*, **23**, 384–392

84. Hughes, A.R., Martin, M.W. and Harden, T.K. (1984). Pertussis toxin differentiates between two mechanisms of attenuation of cyclic AMP accumulation by muscarinic cholinergic receptors. *Proc. Natl. Acad. Sci. USA*, **81**, 5680–5684

85. Evans, T., Martin, M.W., Hughes, A.R. and Harden, T.K. (1984). Guanine nucleotide-sensitive, high affinity binding of carbachol to muscarinic cholinergic receptors of 1321N1 astrocytoma cells is insensitive to pertussis toxin. *Mol. Pharmacol.*, **27**, 32–37

86. Cockcroft, S. and Gomperts, B.D. (1985). Role of guanine nucleotide binding protein in the activation of polyphosphoinositide phosphodiesterase. *Nature (London)*, **314**, 534–536

87. Nishizuka, Y. (1984). The role of protein kinase C in cell surface signal transduction and tumor promotion. *Nature (London)*, **308**, 693–698

88. Berridge, M.J. and Irvine, R.F. (1984). Inositol trisphosphate, a novel second messenger in cellular signal transduction. *Nature (London)*, **312**, 315–321

89. Meeker, R.B. and Harden, T.K. (1982). Muscarinic cholinergic receptor-mediated activation of phosphodiesterase. *Mol. Pharmacol.*, **22**, 310–319

90. Verghese, M., Uhing, R.J. and Snyderman, R. (1986). A pertussis/choleratoxin-sensitive N protein may mediate chemoattractant receptor signal transduction. *Biochem. Biophys. Res. Commun.*, **138**, 887–894

91. Okajima, F. and Ui, M. (1984). ADP-ribosylation of the specific membrane protein by islet-activating protein, pertussis toxin, associated with inhibition of a chemotactic peptide-induced arachidonate release in neutrophils: A possible role of the toxin substrate in Ca^{2+}-mobilizing biosignalling. *J. Biol. Chem.*, **259**, 13863–13871

92. Okajima, F., Katada, T. and Ui, M. (1985). Coupling of the guanine nucleotide regulatory protein to chemotactic peptide receptors in neutrophil membranes and its uncoupling by islet-activating protein, pertussis toxin: A possible role of the toxin substrate in Ca^{2+}-mobilizing receptor-mediated signal transduction. *J. Biol. Chem.*, **260**, 6761–6768

93. Suba, E. and Roth, B.L. (1986). Prostaglandin $F_{2\alpha}$ activates phosphoinositide hydrolysis in rat aorta. *Fed. Proc.*, **45**, 2985A

94. Houslay, M.D., Bojanic, D. and Wilson, A. (1986). Platelet activating factor and U44069 stimulate a GTPase activity in human platelets which is distinct from the guanine nucleotide regulatory proteins, N_s and N_i. *Biochem J.*, **234**, 737–740

95. Guillon, G., Butlen, D. and Rajerison, R. (1984). Evidence for two molecular forms of solubilized vasopressin receptors in rat kidney membranes: Regulation by guanyl nucleotides. *Mol. Pharmacol.*, **26**, 241–247

96. Avdonin, P.V., Svitina-Ulitina, I.V., Leytin, V.L. and Tkachuk, V.A. (1985). Interaction of stable prostaglandin endoperoxide analogs U46619 and U44069 with human platelet membranes: coupling of receptors with high-affinity GTPase and adenylate cyclase. *Thrombosis Res.*, **40**, 101–112

97. Saussy, D.L., Mais, D.E., Burch, R.M. and Halushka, P.V. (1986). Identification of a putative thromboxane A_2/prostaglandin H_2 receptor in human platelet membranes. *J. Biol. Chem.*, **261**, 3025–3029

98. Goldberg, N.D. and Ramwell, P.W. (1975). The role of prostaglandins in reproduction. *Physiol. Rev.*, **55**, 5325–5331

99. Horton, E.W. and Poyser, N.L. (1976). Uterine luteolytic hormone: A physiological role for prostaglandin $F_{2\alpha}$. *Physiol. Rev.*, **56**, 595–661

100. McCracken, J.A., Carlson, J.C., Glew, M.E., Goding, J.R., Baird, D.T., Green, K. and Samuelsson, B. (1972). Prostaglandin $F_{2\alpha}$ identified as a luteolytic hormone in sheep. *Nature (London) New Biol.*, **238**, 129–134

101. de Asua, L.J., Otto, A.M., Ulrich, M.O., Martin-Perez, J. and Thomas G. (1982). In *Prostaglandins and Cancer: First International Conference*, pp. 309–331 (New York: Alan R. Liss, Inc.)

102. Abdel-Latif, A.A., Smith, J.A. and Akhtar, R.A. (1985). Polyphosphoinositides and muscarinic cholinergic and α_1-adrenergic receptors in the iris smooth muscle. In Bleasdale,

246

J.E., Eichberg, J. and Hauser, G. (eds.) *Inositol and Phosphoinositides*, pp. 275–298. (Clifton, New Jersey: Humana Press)

103. Stokes, J.L. (1985). Modulation of vasopressin-induced water permeability of the cortical collecting tubule by endogenous and exogenous prostaglandins. *Mineral Electrolyte Metab.*, **11**, 240–248

104. Fitz, T.A., Mock, E.J., Mayan, M.H. and Niswender, G.D. (1984). Interactions of prostaglandins with subpopulations of ovine luteal cells. II. Inhibitory effects of PGE$_{2\alpha}$ and protection by PGE$_2$. *Prostaglandins*, **28**, 127–138

105. Raymond, V., Leung, P.C.K. and Labrie, F. (1983). Stimulation of PGE$_{2\alpha}$ of phosphatidic acid-phosphatidylinositol turnover in rat luteal cells. *Biochem. Biophys. Res. Commun.*, **116**, 39–46

106. Powell, W.S., Hammarstrom, S., Samuelsson, B., Miller, W.L., Sun, F.F., Fried, J., Lin, C-H. and Jarabak, J. (1975). Interactions between prostaglandin analogues and a receptor in bovine corpora lutea: Correlation of dissociation constants with luteolytic potencies in hamsters. *Eur. J. Biochem.*, **59**, 271–276

107. Kylden, U. and Hammarstrom, S. (1980). Molecular weight of detergent-solubilized prostaglandin F$_{2x}$ receptor from bovine corpora lutea. *Eur. J. Biochem.*, **109**, 489–494

108. Powell, W.S., Hammarstrom, S. and Samuelsson, B. (1976). Localization of a prostaglandin F$_{2x}$ receptor in bovine corpus luteum plasma membranes. *Eur. J. Biochem.*, **61**, 605–611

109. Rao, Ch. V. (1974). Characterization of prostaglandin receptors in the bovine corpus luteum cell membranes. *J. Biol. Chem.*, **249**, 7203–7209

110. Rao, Ch. V. and Mitra, S.B. (1982). Distribution of PGE and PGF$_{2\alpha}$ receptor proteins in the intracellular organelles of bovine corpora lutea. *Meth. Enz.*, **86**, 192–202

111. Wakelam, M.J.O., Davies, S.A., Houslay, M.D., McKay, I., Marshall, C.J. and Hall, A. (1986). Normal p 21[N-ras] couples bombesin and other growth factor receptors to inositol phosphate production. *Nature (London)*, **323**, 173–176

247

Index